PROGRESS IN CLINICAL PHARMACY: VI

Clinical pharmacy education and patient education

This book reports the proceedings of the twelfth European symposium on clinical pharmacy, which was held in Barcelona in October 1983.

Two of the great challenges facing pharmacy are how better to educate pharmacists to fulfil a clinical or extended role in health-care and how to meet an important part of such a role, that is the better education of patients in the use of medicines. These two complimentary topics were the twin themes of this the largest symposium to be organized to date by the European Society of Clinical Pharmacy.

The plenary lectures were given by leading authorities on the respective themes. William E. Smith, Long Beach Memorial Medical Center, Los Angeles, spoke of the American experience in clinical pharmacy education and Jan-Olof Brånstad, Apoteksbolaget, Stockholm, spoke on patient education. The texts of both these lectures provide a distinguished opening to these proceedings.

As well as papers on the twin themes other papers on relevant contemporary aspects of clinical pharmacy were presented and are published in these proceedings. The subject areas covered include, clinical pharmaco-kinetics, therapeutic techniques, clinical trials, parenteral nutrition, side effects and toxicity of drugs, drug utilization studies and ambulatory clinical pharmacy.

As always this latest book in the series Progress in Clinical Pharmacy provides an authoritative account of current developments in clinical pharmacy in Europe. It will serve as a source of ideas and useful information for any pharmacist contemplating the development of clinical pharmacy services. A particular feature is that it provides examples of clinical services developed and implemented by community pharmacists in collaboration with colleagues in hospital pharmacy. As such it marks an important development in the provision of clinical pharmacy services in the community.

PROGRESS IN CLINICAL PHARMACY: VI

Clinical Pharmacy Education and Patient Education

Proceedings of the 12th European Symposium
on Clinical Pharmacy, Barcelona 1983

Edited by

JOAQUIN BONAL

President, European Society of Clinical Pharmacy
Director of Pharmacy Services
Hospital Sta Creu i Sant Pau, Barcelona

J. W. POSTON

Lecturer, Clinical and Social Pharmacy
Welsh School of Pharmacy,
UWIST, Cardiff

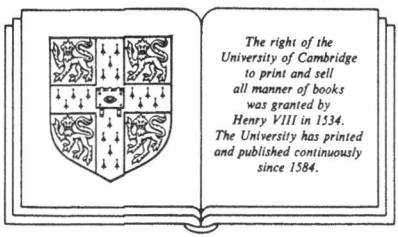

*The right of the
University of Cambridge
to print and sell
all manner of books
was granted by
Henry VIII in 1534.
The University has printed
and published continuously
since 1584.*

CAMBRIDGE UNIVERSITY PRESS

Cambridge

London   New York   New Rochelle

Melbourne   Sydney

CAMBRIDGE UNIVERSITY PRESS
Cambridge, New York, Melbourne, Madrid, Cape Town,
Singapore, São Paulo, Delhi, Tokyo, Mexico City

Cambridge University Press
The Edinburgh Building, Cambridge CB2 8RU, UK

Published in the United States of America by Cambridge University Press, New York

www.cambridge.org
Information on this title: www.cambridge.org/9780521279161

© Cambridge University Press 1984

First published 1984
First paperback edition 2011

A catalogue record for this publication is available from the British Library

ISBN 978-0-521-26610-9 Hardback
ISBN 978-0-521-27916-1 Paperback

CONTENTS

PATIENT EDUCATION AND COMPLIANCE

DRUG EVALUATIONS

CLINICAL PHARMACOKINETICS

Contents   vii

Contents

PREFACE

The European Society of Clinical Pharmacy is convinced that
Clinical Pharmacy is the base for rebuilding Pharmacy Practice. The 12th
European Symposium on Clinical Pharmacy was held in Barcelona (Spain) in
October 1983 and for the first time the meeting was held together with
the XXVIII Congress of the Spanish Society of Hospital Pharmacists. This
provided an excellent opportunity to exchange ideas and experiences
between Spanish hospital pharmacists and colleagues from countries that
participated in the meeting.

Pharmacists from Spain, Holland, Denmark, Sweden, France,
Germany, Switzerland, Norway, Portugal, Italy, United Kingdom, Finland,
Belgium, from Australia, U.S.A., Peru, Argentina and Nigeria, worked
together for three days discussing different aspects of clinical pharmacy.
A total of one hundred and thirty papers were accepted for this meeting
either as platform or poster presentations. Seminars on clinical
pharmacokinetics and a learning resource center were organized simultaneously. More than 600 pharmacists attended the meeting.

A large exhibition was held to show equipment, new drugs and
techniques to be used in clinical pharmacy practice.

The main subjects of the meeting were "Pre and postgraduate
education on clinical pharmacy" and "Patient education and compliance".
Both subjects were discussed in plenary sessions starting with an invited
speaker who gave an introductory lecture followed by a panel discussion.
The invited plenary lecturers were W.E.Smith chief pharmacist of Memorial
Hospital Medical Center from Long-Beach, California, and Jan-Olof
Branstad from Apotёkesbolaget, Stockolm, Sweden.

It is very important to point out that a number of papers
were presented in sessions on "Ambulatory Clinical Pharmacy", most of
them submitted by community pharmacists. This represents a very impor-

step ahead in this field because we are convinced that clinical pharmacy will have a strong influence on health and on society if it is accepted and practised by pharmacists in the community, since it is in the community that most drugs are used.

Only some of the papers presented at the meeting are published in this book because of limited space. The papers are classified according to subjects, and we hope that readers will find many themes of interest and will obtain a representative view of the development of clinical pharmacy in European countries.

Progress on clinical pharmacy VI, contains many new advances in clinical pharmacy compared to previous editions. As the name suggests it provides an up-to-date collection of papers on the progress of clinical pharmacy.

We wish to express thanks to all the members of the Board of the European Society of Clinical Pharmacy to those of the Spanish Society of Hospital Pharmacy, members of the local organizing committee and scientific committee, to the authors of the papers, and to pharmaceutical companies, for their very valuable assistance in the organization of this meeting.

Hospital Sta Creu i S. Pau
Servei de Farmacia
Barcelona - 25. Spain

Dr Joaquin Bonal
President of the European
Society of
Clinical Pharmacy

U.W.I.S.T.
Welsh School of Pharmacy
P.O. Box 13
Cardiff, U.K.

Dr J.W. Poston
U.K. Member
General Committee
European Society of
Clinical Pharmacy

October, 1983

GENERAL COMMITTEE E.S.C.P. (1983)

President:	Joaquín Bonal, Barcelona (Spain)
Vice-President:	Gilles Aulagner, Lyon (France)
Secretary:	Hannu Turakka, Knopio (Finland)
Treasurer:	Dietrich Schaaf, Tübingen (West Germany)
	Paul Amacker, Geneva (Switzerland)
	Rick Clercq, Brussels (Belgium)
	B. Davidson, Stockholm (Sweden)
	Eppo Van der Kleijn, Nijmegen (The Netherlands)
	Nello Martini, Leqnago (Italy)
	Jeff Poston, Cardiff (U.K.)
Bureau-manager:	J.Roy Jonkers, Vithoorm (The Netherlands)
Secretary:	D. van Zanten, Vithoorm (The Netherlands)

GENERAL COMMITTEE A.E.F.H. (1983)

President:	Joaquin Giraldez, Pamplona (Spain)
Vice-President:	Isaac Arias, Vigo (Spain)
National vocal:	Domingo García, Madrid (Spain)
Treasurer:	J.M. Rodriguez, San Sebastián (Spain)
Secretary:	Mª Carmen Martínez, Madrid (Spain)
	Berta Cuña, La Coruña (Spain)
	Mercedes Mendaza, Zaragoza (Spain)
	Antonio Serra, Barcelona (Spain)
	Víctor Jiménez, Valencia (Spain)
	Antonio Benítez, Cuenca (Spain)
	Catalina Buenestado, Sevilla (Spain)
	Sebastián Ibánez, Granada (Spain)
	Miguel Wood, Las Palmas (Spain)

ORGANIZING COMMITTEE

President: Joaquín Giraldez, Pamplona (Spain)
Secretary: Joaquín Bonal, Barcelona (Spain)
Treasurer: Ramón Plá, Tarrasa (Barcelona) (Spain)
                Angel Borrego, Barcelona (Spain)
                Mª Ignacia Ferrer, Hospitalet
                (Barcelona) (Spain)
                Isaías Salagre, Barcelona (Spain)
                Eugenio Sedano, Barcelona (Spain)
                Antonio Serra, Barcelona (Spain)
                Mª Dolores Torres, Barcelona (Spain)
                Luis Triquell, Granollers (Barcelona)
                (Spain)

SCIENTIFIC COMMITTEE

Rik de Clercq, Brussels (Belgium)
Fernando Marcotegui, Pamplona (Spain)
Joaquín Giráldez, Pamplona (Spain)
J. Roy Jonkers, Uithoorn (The Netherlands)
Eppo van der Kleijn, Nijmegen (The Netherlands)
Jeff Poston, Cardiff (United Kingdom)

TRAINING OF PRE/POSTGRADUATES IN CLINICAL PHARMACY IN THE U.S.

W. E. Smith
Memorial Medical Center of Long Beach
2801 Atlantic Avenue
Long Beach, California 90801-1428 U.S.A.

The professional literature of the mid-1960's documented many patient drug-related problems in hospitals. The problems included medication errors (3,14), adverse drug reactions (4,12,16), prolonged hospitalization as a result of adverse drug reactions (4,12,16), drug-drug interactions (9), drug-laboratory test interactions (6), I.V. admixture incompatiblities (8), and drug-induced diseases (11). The providers of clinical pharmacy reasoned that, given an opportunity, pharmacists located in patient-care areas could reduce and prevent many of the drug-related problems. Fortunately, there were some physicians, nurses, and hospital administrators who were interested in improving drug-related services and expanding the role of pharmacists, and they allocated resources to pharmacists to let them demonstrate what they could do.

So, beginning in the mid-1960's, patient drug history interviews, pharmacist participation in patient-care rounds, adverse drug reaction reporting, patient drug-therapy monitoring, answering drug information requests, and patient discharge drug counseling interviews were implemented. Pharmacist clinical activities and, thus, clinical pharmacy in a modern context had started.

What has been accomplished? What can be stated with confidence in 1983? More pharmacists are providing clinical services than ever before in university hospitals and large and small community hospitals. Even so, clinical services are not provided to patients and physicians in even a majority, let along all, of U.S. hospitals.(20) More pharmacy students are provided clinical clerkship learning experiences than ever before. Postgraduate educational programs on clinical subjects are plentiful, and the number of postgraduate clinical residency programs increases each year. Pharmacist paticipation in clinical drug research is increasing. International interest in clinical pharmacy continues at a high level. Clinical services, education, and research by pharmacists are at the highest level ever.

What are the principles, the results, the truths of the past 15 years that will be the basis for expansion in the 1980's? Each of these will be discussed in turn.

Pharmacists can provide effective clinical services if given the time, opportunity, and drug information support. Performance requires knowledge of drugs and their effects on people. It also requires the skill to apply knowledge and the ability to communicate and to work well with others. A desire to perform and a commitment to serve the drug-related needs of patients, physicians, and nurses whenever required are essential. Drug information support gives the clinical staff more time to provide services and also helps expand the scope of clinical practice.

Physicians will support and use the pharmacist's clinical services.(7,10,15,17) Drug knowledge and skill are the basis for a good working relationship with physicians. Knowledge must be specific and accurate; the information must be available and reliable. Physicians must believe that the pharmacist's knowledge and skill will assist them and benefit their patients. Pharmacists and physicians must respect each other's role and responsibilities.

Nurses will support and use the pharmacist's clinical services.(7,17) Knowledge and skill also are the basis for a good working relationship with nurses. They, too, must believe that the pharmacist's services will assist them and benefit their patients. As is the case with physicians, these professionals must respect each other's roles and responsibilities.

Clinical services provided by pharmacists are accepted as appropriate for reimbursement by private and government third-party payers, and various methods have been developed for the payment of clinical services.(2,18)

Patients do benefit from the pharmacist's clinical services. Reduction of drug toxicity, drug incompatibilities, inappropriate use, interactions, and adverse reactions occur daily in clinical programs.(7) Specific examples of pharmacist-regulated therapy that have been documented and evaluated include lower rate of bleeding complications with heparin therapy, lower incidence of nephrotoxicity from the use of aminoglycosides, reduction in serum drug concentrations of no useful clinical value, and reduction in I.V. aminophylline toxicity.

Well-planned and managed clinical pharmacy services are cost effective. Studies that have included the costs for both clinical pharmacy services and drug distribution have resulted in lower patient day costs.(17) Reduction in drug-related problems results in lower patient costs.

In summary, we have demonstrated that a clinical pharmacy program will improve the quality of patient care in hospitals by reducing patient drug-related problems. We have demonstrated that clinical pharmacy services can be provided on a cost-effective basis. We have demonstrated that physicians and nurses will support the clinical pharmacy program and use the pharmacist for drug information. We have learned that the implementation of a successful clinical program needs well-educated and committed pharmacists and competent managers. Together, staff and managers can successfully implement cost-effective services to the benefit of patients, physicians, nurses, and pharmacists. It has been a challenging and exciting period for the profession of pharmacy.

Drug knowledge and the skill to apply knowledge have been the essential components of the successful implementation and growth of clinical pharmacy. In my own situation, it was the desire to utilize the excellent pharmacy education received at the University of California that has continued to be a driving force in my practice and future career plans. The initial five pharmacists for the decentralized pharmacy project in 1966 at the University of California Hospitals joined the project because they wanted a practice which used their drug knowledge. The success of pharmacist clinical practice has led to many changes in the training of pre- and postgraduates in clinical pharmacy in the United States during the decade of the 1970's.

PHARMACY EDUCATION PROGRAMS

To discuss education and training programs, it is necessary to describe briefly the pharmacy education system in the United States.

There are 72 accredited schools of pharmacy. Completion of the educational program will give the graduate either a Bachelor of Science or a Doctor of Pharmacy degree. The schools of pharmacy are members of the American Association of Colleges of Pharmacy. The accreditation of the educational programs of the schools is the responsibility of the American Council on Pharmaceutical Education.

Accreditation may be defined as "the public recognition accorded to an institution or specialized program of study which meets certain established qualifications and educational standards through initial and periodic evaluations." The essential purpose of the accreditation process is to provide a professional judgment of the quality of the educational program offered and to encourage continued improvement thereof.   The American Council on Pharmaceutical Education (ACPE) was established in 1932 and is the national accrediting agency in pharmacy.   The Council is an autonomous agency whose membership is derived through the American Association of Colleges of Pharmacy (AACP), the American Pharmaceutical Association (APhA), the National Association of Boards of Pharmacy (NABP) (three appointments each), and the American Council on Education (one appointment).   The latter appointee serves as a representative of the public in the sense of being a lay person who is not an educator in, nor a member of, the profession for which students are being prepared, nor in any way directly related to the programs being evaluated.   In addition, a panel of public representatives serves in an advisory capacity to the Council.

CLINICAL COMPONENTS FOR THE BACCALAUREATE CURRICULUM

Accreditation standards for the baccalaureate curriculum require clinical sciences and practice as a core component.   While the program may offer elective opportunities for acquisition of differentiated clinical knowledge and skills, the curriculum design is expected to provide clinically-applied courses, as well as clinical clerkships and externships for all students.   Clinical clerkships include intern professional experiences and are primarily acquired in patient care areas.   At the present time, the ACPE considers it reasonable to expect a quantitative experiential component of at least 400 clock hours consisting of a clinical clerkship and externship composite.(1)

CLINICAL COMPONENT OF THE PHARM.D. PROGRAM

The quantity and quality of the clinical experience of the Pharm.D. program are two of the benchmarks of this program.   The training of the doctoral program should assure an experiential emphasis in patient care areas of hospitals and related clinical facilities.   Experience in outpatient areas should include longitudinal experience, as well as studies toward improved ambulatory pharmacy practice.   Clinical services

should be integrated with distribution of drugs so as to relate
adequately to pharmacy practice. Clinical clerkship rotations should be
selected upon predetermined practice foundations, and competencies should
be established accordingly. In addition to a core of experiences,
specialized experiences based on student interest should be developed in
keeping with the standard "that there should be flexibility for students
in choosing programs adapted to their career interests." The clinical
component of the doctoral program should have as a minimal goal one
academic year or 1500 clock hours. Qualitatively, the time should be of
such character so as to be in accord providing a continuity of
professional service and learning experiences. Sufficient experiential
training with ample opportunity for professional decision making and the
acquisition of clinical judgment skills should be provided so as to
assure compliance with the standard that the "program will develop
students professionally more mature than those in the baccalaureate
programs." The professional motivation process is considered to be
closely linked with the quality and quantity of clinical experiences.(1)

A doctor of pharmacy program should prepare pharmacists who
can cope with the complex problems in the delivery of comprehensive
health care; who possess both the knowledge and skill that enable them to
function as specialists in the clinical use of drugs and who can apply
pharmaceutical and biomedical sciences to the practical problems of drug
therapy; who are motivated to participate in the interdisciplinary
delivery of health care; and who can function as easily accessible health
care informants and educators.(1)

TEACHING - CLINICAL CLERKSHIPS

The clinical clerkships are taught by "clinical faculty."
They are active practitioners and possess an adequate understanding of
the basic principles of their respective health sciences to fulfill
capably the instructional tasks to which they have been assigned.

The Department of Pharmacy Services at Memorial Medical Center
of Long Beach has clinical faculty. Doctor of Pharmacy students from the
University of California, San Francisco, and the University of Southern
California Schools of Pharmacy obtain 50% to 100% of their clinical
clerkship education at Memorial Medical Center.

Memorial Medical Center of Long Beach is a 998-bed, nonprofit
community teaching medical center. The medical staff consists of 1000

private practicing physicians. The medical education program consists of
113 residents in medicine, ob-gyn, pediatrics, pathology, radiology,
family practice, and surgery.

The Medical Center consists of three hospitals: Children's,
Women's, and Memorial. A full range of inpatient care is provided, newborn to geriatric, emergent, acute and critical care, medical, surgical,
psychiatric, chemical dependency, and rehabilitation. It is a medical
center committed to excellence, quality of care, and equipped with the
latest technology.

The innovations of the pharmacy department are identified as
follows:

Decentralized Pharmacy Service
Pharmacists' Clinical Practice
Pharmacy Technicians
Unit-dose Drug Distribution
Drug Information Service - regional
Pharmacokinetics Service
Reimbursement System
Group Drug Purchasing Program

The pharmacist clinical practice is focused on the following
functions:

Clarify incomplete prescription
Question incorrect prescription
Answer physician drug information requests
Answer nurse drug information requests
Provide drug use education (physician, nurse, patient)
Monitor patient's drug therapy
Provide medication dosing guidelines
Perform drug research
Drug utilization review
Safe and efficient drug distribution

These functions are based on the triad of service-teaching- research.
Clinical pharmacists should practice in such a triad. Quality patient
care service requires competent clinical practitioners who can teach and
increase their knowledge from research activities.

The pharmacy staff currently totals 111: 47 pharmacists of
which 33 practice full time clinically; 1 management and 8 clinical
residents; 43 technicians; secretarial and support staffs.

The clinical pharmacy program at Memorial Medical Center has gained the support of the medical and nursing staffs. Clinical drug information and pharmacokinetic services are an integral and essential part of patient care. Hospital administration believes pharmacist clinical services affect the quality and costs of patient care in a positive manner. The pharmacist's daily practice provides an academic challenge and requires the pharmacist to increase drug knowledge continuously. During the past ten years, more pharmacist time is being spent on the implementation and monitoring of selected and approved drug dosing guidelines. Dosing guidelines exist for the following types of therapy: anticoagulation (heparin and warfarin); aminoglycosides; aminophylline; I.V. insulin for high-risk pregnancy; pain control; and hyperalimentation (peripheral and central). Physicians will prescribe a dosing guideline, and the pharmacist will implement the request by ordering the drug, appropriate lab tests and necessary adjustments during the course of therapy. The pharmacist must successfully complete experience and an examination to become qualified to implement a dosing guideline without additional staff assistance. The utilization of the dosing guidelines by the medical staff has doubled in the past year. Re-audits of the pharmacists' performance is now in process to be completed by March 1984. These audits are to measure the impact of these pharmacist clinical services on the patients' hospitalization. I believe students learn best in an environment in which they see and can participate in clinical practice services that they will provide after graduation from pharmacy school. Clerkship experiences, such as those described in the following paragraphs, are being provided to students for each of the accredited schools of pharmacy.

The student and resident will spend four or six weeks in the Drug Information Service (DIS). They receive extensive instruction in the best reference sources for different question types; prepare written answers for actual questions; and work with the drug reference files.

The student and resident spend four to six weeks in the Pharmacokinetics Service. They will assist with the scheduling of drug levels; perform computer simulations using digital and analog computers; prepare consultation reports; learn the working relationships with the laboratory department; and learn the kinetic literature.

The student and resident will spend four to six weeks per clerkship. At least five clerkships will be completed in a year. The

Inpatient clinical clerkships are completed in the satellite pharmacy services. The student will perform patient drug interviews, monitor drug therapy, answer drug information questions, participate in medication dosing guideline activities, become familiar with I.V. therapy and equipment, participate in drug distribution activities, participate in patient care rounds, and provide seminars to nursing staffs.

Conferences are held to discuss clinical subjects. Small group conferences are held with the director of pharmacy services to discuss the management of a clinical pharmacy program.

Some clerkships are offered in ambulatory care settings. The student will practice for four to six weeks with the clinical faculty member as both clinical and dispensing services are provided.

POSTGRADUATE TRAINING

Postgraduate education and training for pharmacists are available as residencies, fellowships, and continuing education seminars. The American Society of Hospital Pharmacists (ASHP) has provided leadership in postgraduate education and training since 1962. The ASHP established accreditation standards for general hospital pharmacy residencies in 1962. The statistics for 1984 ASHP residencies are: 151 residencies classified as special clinical, clinical, or general hospital pharmacy. There are 335 residents in training in 1983-1984.

Special clinical residencies are now accredited for: psychopharmacy, nutritional support, oncology, geriatrics, ambulatory care, drug information, pediatrics, and nuclear pharmacy.

Residencies near accreditation status are: advanced residency in management, and a residency in pharmacokinetics.

The accreditation standards include requirements for: qualifications of the preceptor; qualifications of the training site; scope of pharmacy services provided at the training site; goals and learning objectives for resident program; documentation and evaluation of resident performance; areas of emphasis; extramural experiences; and research projects.

Each program requests accreditation status. A site visit is made, and the ASHP Commission on Credentialing recommends accreditation status to the ASHP Board of Directors. Re-accreditation with site surveys is performed on a six-year cycle.

The residency experience provides the student with greater clinical experience and knowledge. It assists the student in career selection and preparation for a clinical career. Many of the changes in hospital and clinical pharmacy services have resulted from resident projects.

A fellowship differs from a residency. The major objective of the clinical fellowship is to develop a pharmacist's competencies in the scientific research process, including writing research proposals, conducting research, evaluating results, and reporting the research. The research training and experience involves clinical studies relating to the use of drugs in the care and management of patients in the respective differentiated clinical areas represented by the fellowships.

A minor objective of the fellowships is to refine pharmacists' competencies in providing clinical services in the respective practice areas represented by the fellowships.

The ASHP now administers fellowships for: cardiovascular pharmacotherapy, clinical pharmacokinetics, critical care pharmacy, geriatric pharmacotherapy, infectious disease pharmacotherapy, oncology pharmacotherapy, pediatric pharmacotherapy, pharmacy nutritional support, and psychiatric pharmacotherapy. The annual stipend for the fellow is provided by grant funds from several pharmaceutical manufacturers.

Continuing education is provided by seminars and correspondence courses. Many states require a specified number of continuing education hours for relicensure. Subject matter covers a wide spectrum of pharmacy topics.

STUDY COMMISSION - PHARMACY

In 1974, the National Study Commission on Pharmacy was appointed under the sponsorship of the American Association of Colleges of Pharmacy. I had the privilege of being a member of the Commission. Its membership totalled 12;eight members were not pharmacists or pharmacy educators. Membership included: university presidents, deans, physicians, a nurse, and representatives from the pharmaceutical industry. Pharmacy was represented by two practitioners, a dean and a faculty member. The charge to the Commission was to recommend what pharmacy education should be to prepare students for practice for the year 2000 and beyond. The final report of the Commission, entitled "Pharmacists for the Future," was published in 1975.(13)

Consultants were invited to meet with the Commission and to comment on the following questions: What do pharmacists now do? What could pharmacists do? What should pharmacists do? We heard comments from the 89 consultants that ranged from, "We do not need pharmacists," to, "We need pharmacists to provide clinical services beyond that which is in existence at this time."

It is important to realize that the Commission could have recommended the discontinuation of pharmacy education; pharmacists as professionals are no longer needed. The members, the majority of whom were not pharmacists, would have made such a recommendation if they had reached that conclusion. The Commission's conclusion after two years of study was that pharmacists are needed, but they need to be educated to practice with a focus on drugs and how they affect people.

Some of the key concepts in the final report are:

1. Pharmacy is a knowledge system as it generates, tests, applies, transmits, and utilizes knowledge.

2. Drug regulations will continue to increase. Governmental control and regulation are probably the strongest external force shaping and determining the evolution of pharmacy, and thereby the practice of pharmacists. There is no reason to expect that the future will bring any appreciable decrease in such control; in fact, the reverse is more likely. As new and more powerful drugs are developed, even greater regulation may be deemed necessary.

3. Pharmacy has many differentiated roles, i.e., community, hospital, industry, education. Pharmacists are differentiated by what they know, what they can do, and how and where they practice.

4. Pharmacy education should be designed as a competency-based curriculum. The faculty is responsible for the curriculum. Students should be educated at schools which have the resources available in a university health sciences center, i.e., medical, nursing, dental schools; teaching hospital, library, etc. There should be a core curriculum for every pharmacy student plus courses and experiences for the pharmacist differentiated roles; i.e., hospital and community practice, management, etc.

Many other important recommendations were made. The Commission expected it would take 8 to 10 years before the impact of the report could be measured. The report has had an impact, and a greater impact is expected in the near future. I recommend this report be added to your reading list.

FUTURE DRUGS AND TECHNOLOGY

Pre- and postgraduate training of pharmacists for clinical practice need to emphasize future drugs and technology.

Two recent quotes from pharmaceutical executives emphasize the potential impact of new drugs on practice in this decade:

"The 1980's offer the possibility and promise of advances in society's battle against disease, disability, and suffering that will equal or surpass those of the 1940's when much of the modern age of medicine was forged." J. J. Horan, Merck & Co., 1979.

"The 1980's would far outstrip the 1960's and 1970's in new product innovation and development on the threshold of significant new advances in many areas." Joseph Williams, Warner-Lambert.

There have been 56 new drugs approved for use in the United States in the past two years. There are 160 drugs pending approval, plus 46 oncology drugs under study. Many drug companies are developing cooperative relationships with companies in Japan and Europe. As drugs are developed and researched in other countries, they could appear in the United States. New drugs have become a worldwide arena. Pharmacy students and pharmacists need to recognize this arena and adjust their educational efforts accordingly.

At a conference in September 1983, Dr. Donald C. Brodie, Adjunct Professor of Pharmacy and Medicine, University of Southern California, discussed "Planning for Technological Change."(5) His study of high technology will result in a paper entitled, "Impact of High Technology on Pharmaceutical Education." He conceptualized the high technology era as "The Moving Frontier."

The Moving Frontier consists of technology, demographics, social, economic, and societal attitudes.

Technology consists of: Automated Systems, Bioelectronics, Biologicals, Diagnostic Techniques, Targeted Disease Drugs, Drug Delivery Systems, Drug Development in Space, Genetic Engineering, Organ Transplantation, Patient Care, Reproduction Science, and Therapies.

Drug categories include: Antiarthritics, Antibiotics, Antineoplastics, Antiobesity, Antiviral, Cardiovascular, Immune Substances, Neuropeptides (Endorphins), and Specific Drugs.

Drug delivery systems include: drug polymer complex systems, hydrogels, osmotic technology, pumps, transdermal technology, and transmucosal technology. The education of pharmacists for clinical

practice must begin to include high technology. The drug component of
new technology will be significant. Pharmacy will be affected. How to
educate, how to keep up-to-date are important questions that need
answers.

CONCLUSION

Each of us practices and studies at a time of rapid change
regardless of the country in which we live. Drugs and drug therapy are
international. A greater number of American pharmaceutical manufacturers
perform clinical research in Europe and Japan, then market these drugs in
the United States. Patients, drugs, physicians, pharmacists, nurses, and
hospitals exist in every country. What is different is traditional roles
of the professionals, social and political factors in health and hospital
care.

I believe it is critical for pharmacists to assess their
current and past practice environment and, at the same time, assess their
future. What will the future become if current trends continue? What
should the future become if the profession can make needed changes in
practice and education? It is a requirement of a health profession to
conduct such analyses and to make necessary changes. Otherwise,
pharmacists cannot meet the changing needs of those we serve--patients,
physicians, and nurses.

The 1980's is a decade of opportunity. The expansion of
clinical pharmacy services to all hospital patients who need them in this
era of cost control, coupled with new drugs and technology, presents
unique challenges and opportunities to pharmacists and pharmacy
educators. How well hospital pharmacy practitioners and educators
recognize the opportunities and develop specific methods and strategies
to prepare, perform, and defend cost-effective clinical services will
determine how many patients in hospitals will receive the benefits in
this decade. To help ensure success, I offer the following comments for
your consideration and appropriate action.

Strategic planning

Hospital pharmacy societies exist to promote the interests of
their members. I suggest a more important reason for their existence is
the development and expansion of clinical pharmacy services for patients
in hospitals. Every organized hospital pharmacy society should develop a
strategic plan committed to the implementation of clinical services for

patients in all hospitals within their specific geographical area. This
strategic plan would include: (1) identification of patients who need
clinical services; (2) the best method to provide and document the
services; (3) recognition of the political, legal, and economic hurdles
to overcome; (4) identification of educational programs needed for both
staff and managers; and (5) active solicitation of physician, nurse, and
hospital management involvement and support to achieve the objectives.

Pharmacy management

Without competent and effective management, clinical services
will not be successfully developed, implemented, and maintained. To
ensure that adequate resources are allocated for clinical services is a
pharmacy management task. Schools of pharmacy are not preparing
graduates for management positions. At the minimum, schools need to
identify students with the aptitude and potential for leadership and
provide them with principles of management in their educational program.
Six specific areas of clinical pharmacy management need study and review;
these areas are the following:

1. The hospital management's decision-making process,
including how decisions are made and by whom, and what data and justification are required for a program proposal;

2. The working relationship between the director of pharmacy
and immediate supervisor, including the requirements for a good working
relationship;

3. The proper location of the pharmacy department in the
hospital's organizational structure, specifically determining if pharmacy
is a clinical or material department, and to what level of management the
pharmacy director reports;

4. Management methods to produce both financial and clinical
results, including a good work-measurement system;

5. Methods to increase productivity of the staff, including
how computer technology and other techniques can be used most effectively
for clinical services and drug distribution systems; and

6. Developing essential skills to function effectively in
interdisciplinary situations.

Hospital pharmacy societies must play an important role in
developing and fostering greater management expertise within hospital
pharmacy. In my judgment, this demands a high priority of attention by
society leadership.

Clinical services

The first step for successful implementation of a clinical
pharmacy program is a definition of the services to be provided. This
definition must be made by the pharmacy staff. If the pharmacy staff
does not know what it wants to do and why, how can hospital management,
medical, and nursing staffs be expected to support the proposed changes?
The definition will include each clinical activity to be provided by
pharmacists, as well as the expected benefits for patients, physicians,
and nurses. With these definitions and a personal commitment to succeed,
pharmacy managers and staff can be successful.

"How to study your own hospital" and "what patients need
clinical services" are two questions that need better answers before
clinical services will expand in hospitals. It is important to realize
that hospital specificity determines what and how services are provided.
People in key management positions (administration, nursing, pharmacy,
and medical staff leadership) and hospital goals, objectives, and
facilities are all important factors to be considered in the design of
cost-effective services for a hospital. As a result, pharmacy management
must develop methods for studying any hospital that will produce the best
program design for that hospital. Data to be collected and analyzed will
include, (1) patient types and number of patients per service; (2) number
of hospital service areas; (3) systems for the delivery of drugs and
number of doses administered per patient day by dosage form and by time
of day; (4) medical staff visit patterns to the hospital; and (5) pharmacy department workload and facilities. These data will translate into
decisions of centralized versus decentralized systems, scope of unit-dose
drug packaging programs, personnel requirements, and impact on nursing
time and that of other hospital personnel. This is an excellent topic
for seminars, resident projects, and graduate student research.

Inherent in the question of which patients need clinical
services is the suggestion that not all patients need pharmacists'
clinical services. Those who do need clinical services need to be
identified; knowing the number and type of patients will determine a
reasonable staffing requirement and, therefore, costs for services. This
is a selective approach that fits well with the era of cost limits, and
it is an approach that I believe hospital management will support. A
study of a hospital patient population should focus on selected drugs:
drugs in which dosage is affected by quick changes in patient status,

drugs that require serum concentrations, drugs that interact with other drugs, and drugs that could have a toxic effect on blood, kidneys, or liver.

Pharmacy education

Pharmacy education is entitled to accept some of the credit for the successful implementation of clinical services. Without a pharmacy education that gave sufficient confidence to the pioneers of clinical services, the accomplishments of the past 15 years would not have been realized.

The challenges before pharmacy education are even greater if clinical pharmacy services are going to be fully effective. These challenges include three elements: knowledge-in-depth, research, and service.

Clinical pharmacists require the broad knowledge and skills of a generalist in the use of drugs. Specific knowledge, or knowledge-in-depth, is also required. Clinical teaching must include assignments that require the student to learn at least one subject in great depth. The student must experience the time required, the amount of literature to be reviewed, how to make judgments on the subject matter, and the self-confidence that results from knowledge-in-depth. The skills developed from this experience will be used throughout the graduate's career as drug information changes.

Greater participation by schools of pharmacy in research to help implement changes in professional practice is needed. It would be helpful if schools of pharmacy would take more of a lead role in the needed research.

Each school of pharmacy that uses hospitals as sites for student teaching should assist in the development of comprehensive clinical services. Students need to learn in environments where the clinical faculty members perform the services the students are being educated to provide after graduation. Credibility is lost when the services at the teaching sites are less than complete.

Teaching, research, and service are the responsibilities of a school of pharmacy. Faculty members need to recognize the importance of clinical services to their own personal growth and support. Without continual growth and success in the profession, how long will pharmacy education and, therefore, faculties continue to be supported? When faculty members finally realize the importance of the success of clinical pharmacy, many conflicts within pharmacy education can be resolved, and educational programs will advance.

Pharmacy is a service profession, and the pharmacist's mission is to serve the drug-related needs of patients, physicians, and nurses. Drug therapy in the modern hospital is a primary modality of patient care. Most hospital patients receive drugs, and the number of drug orders and doses prepared and administered is staggering. The pharmacy leadership in each hospital should ask the following questions: What are the drug-related problems in my hospital? What are the alternatives for solving these problems? What are the roles for the pharmacists in my hospital? I am confident that clinical pharmacy services is the answer to these questions.

The 1980's is a decade of rapid change in the financing of hospital care. It is a decade of opportunity for pharmacists. Clinical pharmacy services can reduce costs, increase hospital efficiency, and improve the level of patient care in a cost-effective manner.

A clinical pharmacy practice brings its own rewards to the pharmacist. To be an expert in the clinical use of drugs presents a lifelong challenge of learning and self-study. It brings professional respect from physicians and nurses and places the pharmacist in the mainstream of caring and healing. A career in clinical pharmacy is an open-ended opportunity for those who seek its rewards.(19)

REFERENCES

1 American Council on Pharmaceutical Education. Second printing of the
    Seventh Edition of The Accreditation Manual. (1979)
2 American Society of Hospital Pharmacists. (1979). Final report of the
    task force on payment of pharmacy services. Bethesda, MD.
3 Barker, K.N. & McConnell, W.E. (1962). How to detect medication
    errors. Mod Hosp., 99:95-103.
4 Barr, D.P. (1955). Hazards of modern diagnosis and therapy: the price
    we pay. JAMA, 159:1452-6.
5 Brodie, D.C. (1983). "Planning for Technological Change." Presented to
    Second Annual Symposium, Pharmacy and Therapeutics Committees,
    Memorial Medical Center of Long Beach, California.
6 Cripps, G.W., et al. (1973). Significance of drug-altered laboratory
    test values. Am J Hosp Pharm, 30:603-6.
7 Fink, A., et al. (1982). Assessing whether a clinical pharmacy program
    is meeting its goals. Am J Hosp Pharm, 39:806-10.
8 Fowler, T.J. (1967). Some incompatibilities of intravenous admixtures.
    Am J Hosp Pharm, 24:450-7.
9 Hansten, P.D. (1971). Drug Interactions. First Edition. Philadelphia,
    PA.: Lea & Febiger.
10 Moody, P.M., et al. (1970). Attitudes of hospital personnel toward
    unit dose at the University of Kentucky Hospital. Am J Hosp
    Pharm, 27:473-9.
11 Moser, R.H. (1969). Diseases of Medical Progress: A Study of
    Iatrogenic Disease. Third Edition. Charles C. Thomas.
12 Ogilvie, R.I. & Ruedy, J. (1967). Adverse drug reactions during
    hospitalizations. Can Med Assoc J, 97:1450-7.
13 Pharmacists for the Future, The Report of the Study Commission on
    Pharmacy. (1975). Ann Arbor, MI: Health Administration Press.
14 Schimmel, E.M. (1964). The hazards of hospitalization. Ann Intern Med,
    60:100-10.
15 Simon, J.R., et al. (1968). Attitudes of nurses, physicians and
    pharmacists toward a unit dose drug distribution system. Am J
    Hosp Pharm, 25:239-47.
16 Smith, J.W., et al. (1966). Studies on the epidemiology of adverse
    drug reactions. Ann Intern Med, 65:629-40.
17 Smith, W.E. (1973). The economic feasibility of clinical pharmacy in
    the hospital setting: personnel costs. Pharmacy and
    Development HSMA, Dept. HEW, Contract HSM-110-71-208 Document
    PB-220-616 U.S. Department of Commerce, National Technical
    Information Service.
18 Smith, W.E. & Weiblen, J.W. (1979). Charging for hospital
    pharmaceutical services: product cost, per diem fees and fees
    for special clinical services. Am J Hosp Pharm, 36:355-9.
19 Smith, W.E. (1983). Clinical pharmacy in the 1980's. Am J Hosp Pharm,
    40:223-9.
20 Stolar, M.H. (1979). National survey of hospital pharmaceutical
    services, 1978. Am J Hosp Pharm, 36:316-25.

PATIENT EDUCATION AND COMPLIANCE WITH TREATMENT - SWEDISH
EXPERIENCES

Jan-Olof Brånstad
Apoteksbolaget AB, S-105 14 Stockholm

First of all I would like to express my gratitude for the in-
vitation to this congress and for the honour of having the privilege to
present Swedish experiences of patient education to this audience.

We all see the need for good and thoroughly prepared patient
education, but at the same time it feels urgent to point at the fact that
within the field of drugs this is still not the most important problem.
For many countries the overshadowing problem is to make good and cheap
basic drugs available in order to prevent and cure perilous diseases. It
is important to keep this in mind. But at the same time I think that we
who live in countries with a well-organized drug supply are in the position
- by reporting our experiences - to enable those countries that today
struggle with great problems in the field of drug supply to avoid making
the mistakes we made when it comes to patient education. Not so many years
ago we who work within pharmacy and the doctors were completely satisfied
just with having the right drug prescribed in the right dose and handed out
to the right person. Today we know that it is also a question of getting a
correct use of the drug and this is achieved through education and information.

A large number of inquiries have shown that the patients'
compliance is bad. Between one fourth and half of the patients in outpatient care do not follow the prescriptions. Too many patients are forced
to seek medical care because they have used their drugs incorrectly.

We who occupy a professional part within the field of drugs are
well aware of the important role played by drugs in medical care. For a
large number of diseases drugs have meant a gradual improvement of the
treatment. It has resulted in a reduction of personal suffering and at the
same time a decrease in costs both for the individual and society. In our
fairly well-organized European countries many people, however, have a
distrust towards drugs. This distrust is partly due to ignorance and partly

to some tragedies with drugs where they have caused servere damage because of insufficient control. Mass media have shown very great interest
in the negative sides of drug therapy. At least in Sweden, this has meant
that side effects of drugs is a popular topic in magazines and newspapers.
This has created a distrust towards drugs. From this follows that patient
education is not only a question of how to convey knowledge but also how
to influence attitudes.

In for instance many pharmaceutical magazines and journals and
at pharmaceutical congresses many ideas and plans have been presented of
how to improve patient education and patient information. Even if these in
many cases are reports of practical activities, at least I personally have
the impression that many plans and ideas are never carried out in reality.
The patient education that I will outline here today is neither original
nor unique, but I think it may be of some interest because it is an endea-
vour to introduce some information systems in all pharmacies in a country
with the aim to improve patient education. It is also a part of the efforts
to show that pharmacy in the first place aims at getting the best possible
drug therapy at the treatment of diseases, independently of whether the
drug is sold on prescription or not.

Pharmacy in a country has developed gradually in cooperation
with the medical care of that country, that is with doctors and nurses in
outpatient and inpatient care.

Health care today in Sweden is regarded as being clearly a task
for the public sector. Responsibility for individual-oriented health
services and for medical care, both outpatient and inpatient, rests with
26 County Councils.

A new law on health and medical care is effective since the
first of January this year. The overall goal for health and medical care is
good health and treatment on equal conditions for the whole population in
the country. The new law among other things describes the position of the
single patient and marks a new attitude in daily work, a positive belief
in the individual's own ability, also when it comes to assuming the responsibility for his own health. Medical-care treatment shall, as far as possible,
be planned and persued after consultations with the patients. This means
that patients need increased knowledge of their body and soul, about diseases and treatment alternatives and about the organization of the health-
and medical-care system.

Increased demands are placed on information to the patients.

The new law also underlines the importance of comprehensible information.

The first legal regulations in Sweden about pharmaceuticals were given in 1675. Ever since then, the pharmaceutical field has been subject to a firm governmental control.

Until 1971 the Swedish pharmacies were private enterprises. They were owned by pharmacists with so-called personal privileges and these owners had been appointed by the Government with proposals from the National Board of Health and Welfare.

Since January 1, 1971, the National Corporation of Swedish Pharmacies (Apoteksbolaget) has held the exclusive right to the public distribution of drugs in our country. The County Councils have the right to operate their own hospital pharmacies, but in 25 of the County Councils the directors have given Apoteksbolaget the responsibility for coordinating the drug supply for the inpatient care also. The guidelines for the activities of the Company were laid down in an agreement made between the Government and the Company.

The Company was required, among other things to
- provide information and statistics, independent of producer influence, about drugs,
- make sure that the personnel engaged in drug distribution meet all safety requirements.

Today there are about 750 pharmacies for outpatient service, about 70 of which also have inpatient service, i.e. they are hospital pharmacies. The total number of hospital pharmacies in Sweden is 130, of which about 100 are owned by Apoteksbolaget. The number of small hospital pharmacies without outpatient service is today 40 and more of the hospital pharmacies will also get outpatient service.

All the pharmacies are organized in about 60 pharmacy groups. A pharmacy group corresponds geographically mainly to the medical-care district. This means that in almost all groups at least one hospital pharmacy is included.

An example of the development of the cooperation with medical care during recent years is the location of pharmacies. In 1970 only 3% of the pharmacies were located close to medical-care institutions. Now we are approaching the state where every third pharmacy is situated either in a hospital or in a health center.

As patient education must influence both knowledge and attitudes in order to achieve good compliance, it is often impossible to reach

this goal simply by giving information at the drug treatment in connection
with illness. When used correctly, the drug is the most important tool when
treating a disease - this understanding must be conveyed already at an
early age. Therefore it is important to reach schoolchildren with information and education on drugs and the role of drugs in the treatment of
diseases. The pharmacies in Sweden have during the last few years taken a
very active part in the instruction of schoolchildren in the last grades
of the upper section of comprehensive school. During the school year 1982/
83 pharmacists gave lessons in about 40% of all classes in grade 9. This
means education of approximately 50,000 teenagers. During two hours they
are given a description of
- the role of drugs in the treatment of illness
- how the drug acts in the body
- practical advice for the use of drugs.

     This education has been evaluated both as to attitudes and
knowledge. A few examples: In one attitude inquiry 175 schoolchildren were
included. About 70% thought that drug education at school is important and
that the educational material was easy to understand. When asked how much
they felt they has learned during this education period, 6% answered many
new things, 78% some new things and 16% nothing new. In an inquiry on the
influence on knowledge, 150 pupils participated. One question was the following: "You have received a drug on prescription. On the label it says: 1
tablet 3 times daily. You take the first tablet at eight o˜clock in the
morning. When shall you take the second and the third tablet and when shall
you take the first one next day?" The replies were considered correct only
if all three part questions had been correctly answered. Before training,
18% answered correctly but after training 75%. To summarize it can be said
that the participation of pharmacists in the instruction on drugs at school
has been appreciated by the schoolchildren and the training has given them
important basic knowledge. A majority of the teachers find the cooperation
of a pharmacist necessary which is very important, as it is the teachers
who decide if the specialist is to participate or not.

     During summer we have compiled educational material for the
youngest schoolchildren. Soon this material will be sent to all teachers in
grades 1 to 3. The material comprises a number of pictures that can easily
be transformed into overheads, with a brief text. It describes how to prevent, alleviate and cure infectious diseases. This is an area well-known to
all children. The idea is that the teacher shall use this material when the

children in his class have been vaccinated against some infectious disease,
when one of the children has been affected with pneumonia or a similar
disease or in connection with epidemic flu.

The public can be reached in several different ways: through
patient organizations, pensioners´ associations, etc. However, there is a
period in life which, surprisingly, has not been used very much so far and
that is when a person is hospitalized. This is especially relevant for
patients in medical clinics who are there for examination, and the examination in many cases is followed by life-long drug treatment. An important
goal is to make the patient so well-informed that he dares to ask the doctor about the medication which he shall later handle by himself. We have
made a video-film intended to be shown in medical wards called "Ask about
your medication". In this film, three people - two elderly persons and one
young man - put questions to the nurse and to the doctor. The questions
raises are such as everyone should ask before starting a medication. In the
film is also shown different preparation forms and how to use them as well
as simple aids to remember when to take the medicine. At present this film
is lent to a large number of hospitals through the hospital pharmacies.
Both patients and medical-care personnel have been very enthusiastic about
this way to activate the patients in medical-care wards about questions
concerning their future medication.

In one inquiry we asked about 50 inpatients about this film.
75% found that it raises a subject which is important; 45% said the film
had given them something to think about and 95% thought that one should
continue to show the film on the ward.

Even if there are several different ways to reach the public
outside the pharmacies with patient education, our most important opportunities to give information come when the drugs are delivered at the
pharmacy. It is obvious that it is in these connections we can best motivate our activities. Having access to the drug package that the patient
shall later use and to the supplementary written information, if any, provide us with a unique opportunity for rational and individually adapted
information.

In Sweden the pharmacies are visited each year by 60 million
customers, that is a Swede visits a pharmacy 7-8 times yearly on an average.
Naturally there are great variations.

75% of the customers are women and the older a person gets,
the greater is the number of pharmacy visits. Of these 60 million customers

visits, 35 million take place because of mild disorders, so-called self-care. Through investigations we can show that about 90% of all illness conditions do not result in contacts with a doctor. We know that for a large number of the mild disorders different tricks and so-called household remedies are used. These have often been learnt from parents or from magazines. We also know that about 9 out of 10 customers come to the pharmacy knowing more or less exactly what drug to buy.

By analysing the sales of certain articles in the food shops and the sales in pharmacies, one rapidly reached the conclusion that there is not always a clear connection between what is best sold to alleviate temporary illness and the knowledge we have of what is best documented. In this field I believe that pharmacy in more countries than in Sweden has shown lack of interest and purposefulness in its activities. We have in a very unsatisfactory manner informed about what is the best therapy for temporary disorder, for example irritating cough, sore throat, aching muscles, etc. Perhaps the fact is that our insufficient information and lack of education of the public has favoured the sales of a number of humbug preparations. We decided to change this state of affairs a few years ago. As our pharmacies are organized in about 60 pharmacy groups, geographically spread to follow the corresponding organization of medical care, this was the level at which the information was coordinated. Within each such geographical area the best therapy was discussed for the about 30 most common temporary disorders. It was also discussed at what symptoms of illness self-care should be abandoned and a doctor consulted instead. If this concept is to be accepted both by pharmacies and medical-care personnel, it is tremendously important that everybody feels that they share the responsibility for the recommendations. We must realize clearly that when seeking this unity based on scientific grounds, many persons with advisory and recommendary functions must revise their views and recommendations. If this is done in a proper manner, it is actually a question of further education, that is to make pharmacy and medical-care personnel accept that what was the opinion of science 10-15 years ago, for instance, has changed since then. Mostly these recommendations have been compiled in a booklet describing in a simple way the characteristics of each illness and giving instructions for self-care in the best way and when it is adviseable to seek a doctor. These written recommendations can then be read at home and if a person turns to medical care or to a pharmacy, he will meet the same advice. Even if many persons may ignore these problems, it must be

essential that professionally working pharmacy clearly states for instance
which is a good or bad cough preparation, remedy for hemorrhoids or constipation, etc. The evaluation made has also shown that this information
has given very good results.

Some examples: With the exception of colds, people had in 30%
of the cases changed from the earlier treatment of mild disorders to the
recommended treatment. Furthermore another 30% stated that they already
applied the recommended therapy but considered it an advantage to know
that this treatment in fact agreed with the one recommended by medical care
If the sales statistics are studied, it is clear that there has been a
considerable shift towards recommended drugs. Before the information activi
ties started, the number of persons at a health center were counted who
contacted medical care to get advice on self-treatment. Here the result
was that the share of people seeking advice for self-treatment of their
illness was 20%. A corresponding study after the information activities
showed that the share was then 11%. Thus the strain on medical care had
been almost halved for states of illness where the pharmacies can give the
best service, that is give advice and at the same time efficient drug
treatment.

In comparison with most other European countries Sweden has had
relatively few nonprescription drugs. It is obvious that the medical expert:
with the decisive influence if a drug should be available only on prescription have not previously estimated the pharmacies´ possibilities to
give advice on self-care especially highly. This has changed dramatically
in recent years. Effective anti-cough drugs, nasal drops for decongestion
of the nasal mucosa, hydrocortisone for the treatment of eczema, preparations for treatment of cutaneous mycotic infections - these are examples
of medicines that were earlier on prescription but that during the last few
years have been changed into non-prescription drugs. The pharmacists abilit)
to judge when the symptoms of a customer indicate a more serious disease
that should lead to treatment by a physician, to recommend suitable treatment at mild states of sickness and to influence those who are clearly
treating themselves incorrectly, all this has highly contributed to this
development. Concerning patients who treat themselves incorrectly, it is
often hard to prove effects of active information. At least in Sweden there
is a large group of above all elderly people who make excessive use of
stimulant laxatives. We know today that these people will sooner or later
risk after-effects that lead to hospital care. Active information from the

pharmacies may have a good influence, which the following study proves.

All customers who during a certain period visited the pharmacy asking for a large package of peristaltic stimulant laxatives, that is 100 tablets or more, were informed about the risks. The information from the pharmacy influenced 30% of the customers so that they chose a more lenient preparation and 12% to buy a smaller package. On the other hand nobody refrained from buying a laxative. As to the reaction of the customers to the information from the pharmacy, a little more than 10% were very positive and almost 40% were positive whereas 13% were negative or even very negative. It would have been desirable also to have been able to follow up this inquiry to study the long-term effects. However, we did not have that possibility.

Without exception, the most important role of the pharmacies when it comes to education and information appears in connection with the sale of prescription drugs. That is the last chance of influencing the patient towards a correct drug treatment in order to regain health and to avoid side effects.

In the guidelines for the Swedish pharmacies' information, it is clearly stated that "the pharmacies shall when required give practical instructions on application and the personnel shall in each transaction, as far as possible, try to make sure that the customer knows how to handle the drug correctly. The pharmacistsshall with sound judgement provide information on drug effects when requested or when the pharmacy believes it necessary for the correct use of a particular drug." This means that the pharmacy shall repeat part of the information that the prescribing doctor should have given and also supplement this by such information as only the pharmacy can give, for instance technical instructions.

In a systematic study of all Swedish drugs, were selected in the first place drugs that at each transaction should be accompanied by oral and written information. With this as a basis an information system has been built up. The Swedish pharmacies are at present going through a stage of technical development, computerization, which will be completed in 1988. The computer among other things takes care of pricing and writes out labels. Through numerical codes the computer can also signal that written and oral information should be given. For example, a number of informational messages repeating the information of the doctor about the effects of the drug are included:
- Reactions may be temporarily slowed (for instance in driving).

Drugs concerned are for example antihistamines, tranquilizers, certain psycho-pharmacological preparations.
- May cause dryness of the mouth. Pay particular attention to dental hygiene. Drugs concerned are for example anticholinergics and some psycho-pharmacological preparations.

Totally about 20 such informational messages are at present included in the system.

Furthermore approximately 30 informational messages on practical use and for instance how to store drugs are included. These are for example "must be swallowed whole", "to be inserted into the rectum", "to be kept in a refrigerator", "to be applied thinly", etc.

At present a total of about 40% of all prescription drugs are covered but the system will certainly be enlarged.

The computer produces a small side label that is not put into the package but acts as a message to the pharmacy personnel. If the numerical code is preceded by the letter F or B, this means that the message concerned is already included in the marking from the producer. If no such marking exists, the drug is provided with a small label with the text in question. Then when the drug is handed out to the patient, the computer-produced label serves as a check note and the patient gets the oral information adapted especially to him. This means that it is sometimes enough just to print at the label or the marking, but on other occasions the message must be more clearly explained. For some informational messages there are also supplementary pamphlets, for example for drugs influencing reactivity or drugs causing dryness of the mouth. In pharmacies where pricing and labelwriting is done manually, the numerical code in question is transferred from the price-list to the prescription form and then serves as a basis for any supplementary marking and oral information.

The introduction of this system has been followed by evaluations of patient attitudes and influence on patient knowledge. Some examples:

"How would you prefer to be informed about drugs at the pharmacy?"	
- Oral information	32 %
- Written information	42
- Oral and written information	24
- I do not know	2

The combination of oral and written information was not included in the interview form but was listed spontaneously by the interviewed persons.

```
"How do you like it that the pharmacy gives information in this way?"
- Good                96 %
- Fairly good          2
- Neither good or bad  2
- Less good            0
- Not good             0
```

       95% found the information "Very easy to understand" or "Easy to understand.

       On the question "Do you miss anything you want to know?" 51% said "Yes" and 49% "No".

       Almost all those who wanted to know more wanted more information on possible side effects.

       An example of the influence on knowledge:

"Which drugs should not be taken together with tetracyclines?":	Control group	Test group
- Iron and headache powders with caffeine	2 %	0 %
- Iron and preparations for constipation	4	4
- Iron and antacids	10	76
- Iron and large doses of vitamin C	2	1
- Iron and certain cardiac remedies	2	2
- I do not know	80	17

       The control group got no information at the pharmacy and thus they indicate how much the patients remember of the information given by the doctor. The test group, on the other hand, was given information at the pharmacy, among other things that one should not take iron preparations and tetracyclines or antacids simultaneously. The interviews were made by telephone a few days after the day the drugs had been handed out at the pharmacy.

       The pharmaceutical patient education and patient information are put to a test at the seemingly simple customer contacts. Every patient being attended to at the pharmacy must be given optimum education. There has been and there still is a clear tendency to be selective and make

efforts only when it is "heroic", for example to prevent fatal interactions. But daily patient education, that is education aiming at every
patient and this means at an equilibrium about 10 million occasions
yearly in Sweden, it does not feel and is not especially heroic. Naturally
it is also directed to sick people who cannot or are incapable of showing
spontaneous gratitude or happiness which of course is important to stimulate further educational activities. It is a demanding task to try to
enter into the needs and wishes of the patient concerned when it comes
to drug information. It is not enough for pharmacists who only have good
knowledge - social responsibility and great enthusiasm are also needed.
We do not know yet how 10,000 employees in the Swedish pharmacies will be
capable of fulfilling the present intentions and the signals given by the
information system. But we are so optimistic that we are already preparing
next step! Among the Swedish public there is a large group of people who
want more information on their drug treatment. In Sweden like in many
other countries a discussion concerning the introduction of informational
package inserts has been going on for many years. The Swedish drug industry,
that accounts for about half of the drugs sold in Sweden, does not possess
production lines enabling the insertion of written information unless vast
investments are made. Special written information for each drug also
entails certain disadvantages, for instance it will be hard to survey for
the person carrying the primary information responsibility, that is the
physician. Information on drugs with similar application areas, however,
shows a number of features in common. This we bear in mind. Very soon we
will have produced about 60 information sheets covering most prescription
drugs in Sweden. This work has been carried out in the following way: Our
Information Department has compiled a preliminary text following a certain
pattern. This text has then been checked by medical experts and the drug
industries concerned. The written material has the headings in common.
The pharmacy writes the name of the drug in question. From the introductory text can be seen that the written information repeat and supplements
the doctor's information. If anything in this information is not clear,
ask at the pharmacy, but if the patient has other questions concerning
the treatment, these questions should be put to the doctor.

Under the heading "How does the medicine work?" an explanation
is given in simple language how the drug should influence the disease in
question.

Under the heading "How shall I take the medicine?" the brief

dosage instructions transferred from the prescription on to the pharmacy's
label are elucidated. Here is also stated if the drug should be taken in
special relation to meals and if the preparation form requires special
attention or use, that is a repetition of some of the special information
from the pharmacy.

Under the heading "Can I get side effects?" such side effects
are listed that the patient can notice himself. For mild side effects it
is described how and if they can be avoided or alleviated. For more serious
side effects there is a division between those when a doctor should be
contacted immediately and those when a doctor should be consulted as soon
as possible.

Under the heading "Who should avoid to take this medicine?"
above all those medicines are listed that should not be used during
pregnancy or breast-feeding.

Under the heading "How shall I keep the medicine?" the patient
receives in writing the same information that is also given orally when
the drug is delivered at the pharmacy.

The trial activities with this written information have now
been going on for a little more than a year in about twenty pharmacies.
Parallel to these trial activities the attitudes and knowledge of the
public have been investigated, practical handling at the pharmacies has
been studied and we have kept a very sensitive ear to the reactions by the
doctors, especially after the second visit by the patient. Before the trial
activities started, all doctors had been informed and had had the opportunity of reading and reflecting on the written information. In the first
round, 15 information sheets were included, corresponding to about 25% of
the prescription drugs in Sweden delivered in outpatient care. During this
autumn another ten will be issued and they will be supplemented by another
ten at year-end. During 1984 we estimate that all the about 60 information
sheets will be ready.

In practice, the delivery is organized in the following way: The
patient hands in his prescription. We strive to achieve a calm and secluded
area for the information but all pharmacies do not yet have this modern
standard. By means of an alphabetical list the prescriptionist receiving
the prescription can rapidly check if and in that case which information
sheet or sheets should be given to the patient. When this trial activity
is put into effect in all pharmacies, the computer will signal which information sheets to hand out. The patient can then in peace and quiet

during 2-4 minutes study this written information. In the meantime the prescriptionist transfers data from the doctor's prescription to the computer. The computer prices the drug and writes out a label while the prescriptionist collects the prescribed drug. After checking, signing the label and labelling the drug package, the prescriptionist returns to the patient at the counter. The prescriptionist tells him about the information included in the system I described a little while ago, and the patient then has the opportunity of asking questions if there is anything that is not quite clear in the written or oral information.

A study of patient attitudes to this written information comprised about 200 patients who were interviewed twice: once at the pharmacy counter and once by telephone, 3 to 7 days after the visit to the pharmacy. The aim of the interview at the pharmacy was partly to get their telephone number, partly to ask certain questions that were then repeated at the telephone interview. As 15 written sheets were included in the trial activity, we planned to get ten interviews per sheet with the exception of one information sheet for which 50 interviews were conducted. The rate of reply was very high, 96%. The patients find the information on the information sheets very important or important. No significant change takes place between the interview at the pharmacy and the one by telephone.

Only very few patients regard any of the types of information as unessential or very unessential. The most common reason for this is that they think that the information should be given by the doctor.

92% of the patients think that the information is easy or very easy to understand. One person only finds the information hard to understand.

The percentage of patients finding that they missed something in the information has been reduced to 14%. Most of them state that they wish more information on side effects. Among other remarks it has been noted that about one third of the patients spontaneously give positive opinions about the information. There were also spontaneous opinions of the following kinds:
- One is too nervous during the visit to the doctor to comprehend the information.
- One wants to study the information in peace and quiet, several times if necessary.
- After the visit to the doctor one is too tired for oral information.

Some patients have furthermore spontaneously stated that the

information has helped to reduce their worries for the medication and
that it has increased their motivation to take the drug.

The aim of the knowledge study was to investigate the influence
of the information sheets on the patient´s knowledge of his drugs. Patients
who had been prescribed some kind of tetracycline were included in the
study. It covered a little more than 200 patients, divided into two groups:
one control group who was not given any information by the pharmacy, and
one test group receiving information sheets in the way I just described.
By using a control group it is possible to measure how much the patients
know about tetracyclines when they come to the pharmacy.

No greater difference in knowledge between the control and the
test groups could be noted concerning the most correct way to take a drug
in two doses per day.

Of the patients in the control group and the test group 76%
and 89% respectively gave the right answer. The dominating part of the
public thus has good knowledge about how to take one tablet twice daily.

On the other hand there were great differences in knowledge
between the control and test groups as to the effects of tetracyclines.

"Do you know in which of the following ways the ... (name of drug) works?"	Control group	Test group
- It prevents virus from multiplying	2 %	4 %
- It prevents tetracyclines from multiplying	3	2
- It prevents bacteria from multiplying	9	63
- It kills virus	8	2
- It kills bacteria	24	17
- I do not know	54	12

Here it is important to note that 54% of the patients in the
control group, that is patients who only have the doctor´s information,
give the answer "I do not know". Only 9% give a correct answer. In the
test group the corresponding figure for "I do not know" is 12% and 63%
give a correct answer to the question "How do tetracyclines work?".

The ambition at all drug treatment must be that the patient
knows why he shall take his drug and how it works.

There were also great differences in knowledge between the
control and test groups when it came to knowing the interaction of tetracyclines with ordinary nonprescription drugs.

In the test group 54% gave the correct answer when asked which drugs cause interactions with tetracyclines. 30% gave the reply "I do not know". In the control group 9% knew the right answer whereas 86% gave the alternative "I do not know".

Finally an example of what is remembered from the written material informing which patient group should avoid tetracyclines.

"Do you know which of the following groups should avoid taking ... (name of drug)?"	Control group	Test group
- Women with hypertension	4 %	6 %
- Persons driving	3	4
- Persons with bad teeth	1	1
- Pregnant women	10	62
- Persons drinking alcohol often	14	9
- I do not know	68	18

Of the patients in the control group 10% knew that pregnant women should avoid tetracyclines. 68% gave the alternative "I do not know". In the test group the situation was more or less the reverse: 62% could give the right answer whereas 18% gave the "I do not know"-replay.

In a similar study we tested the knowledge of patients right after they had read the information at the pharmacy. We were interested in finding out if there were any differences between short-term memory and long-term memory. We did not find any such difference, that is the inquiry gave approximately the same results as the one I have just accounted for.

To summarize I can say that concerning the written information we feel fairly convinced that we have found the right extent regarding volume and contents. When the system is introduced all over Sweden and we have reached a state of equilibrium, that is when we have reached all those who are on continuous medication or long-term medication, we believe that about 10 million information sheets will be needed annually.

The attentive listener has of course noted that none of these studies had tried to measure compliance. So far we have not got any good such studies. Naturally we are trying to fill this gap as soon as possible. But everyone who has thought about and read compliance studies knows that this is very complicated indeed. What we will try to analyse is the cases

when the patient used his drug incorrectly due to ignorance or misunderstanding. To us, compliance has been too much of just one-way communication. The medical-care law in force in Sweden as of this year gives the
individual the unrestricted right to decide himself if he should for
instance start or continue his medication. I am optimistic and I believe
that within a few years we will be able to report some kind of measure of
how the influence on attitudes and knowledge in its turn influences
compliance, that is how the patients take their medicines.

I said at the beginning that mass media and above all weekly
magazines and journals have influenced attitudes towards drugs in such a
direction that many people have misunderstood the role of drugs in the
treatment of diseases. The most important thing, of course, is to concentrate on those occasions when medication shall actually take place. But
we have found that it is also a question of meeting the weekly press
through similar information channels. Four years ago we started publishing
a customer journal called "Apoteket" (The Pharmacy). This journal is
published four times a year and is given free of charge to pharmacy
customers. Each issue consists of 400,000 copies and in general it is out
of stock at the pharmacies within two months. The aim of this journal is
also to follow up our informational and sales activities concerning para-
pharmaceuticals. - Incidentally, I can also mention that the pharmacies in
Sweden sell more than half the amount of all tooth-brushes sold in Sweden.
High quality in combination with low prices has been an efficient means of
competition. - The journal shall also spread general knowledge about
common diseases and their treatment as well as information and advice in
the field of self-care.

The publication of "Apoteket" has been followed by a number of
studies on the views of the readers on the journal, but I will not bore you
with yet another lot of figures. One exception, however: In a large inquiry, about 60% of the persons interviewed said the information they got
from the journal "Apoteket", they did not get anywhere else. Just this
reply, taken in combination with the fact that the readers greatly appreciate the journal, is motivation enough for us to continue publication.

In recent years Sweden has become a popular tourist country.
Our islands, lakes, rivers and deep forests attract tourists. Sweden has
what we call the "common right access" allowing both Swedes and tourists
access to most parts of the Swedish nature. Also, Sweden has a large number
of immigrants from for instance Finland, Greece, Yugoslavia and Turkey.

Tourists and immigrants often speak a language which is not understood by
the pharmacy personnel. Therefore we have compiled the oral and written
information which the pharmacy shall give in ten different languages.
Here you put a mark in front of the relevant information. A complicating
fact is that the pharmacy personnel cannot know from where the person not
speaking Swedish comes. To cope with this, we have turned it all around:
on the counter in Sweden pharmacies there is a board with ten flags. On
this we ask the customer not speaking Swedish to point out the flag of
his country so that he can get the dosage instructions in the right
language.

Patient education is partly a question of organization. But
most important of all is to have enthusiasts working, who pave new ways
and who serve as models. Sometimes it is enough with spreading the experiences of the enthusiasts. Two Swedes who serve as models when it comes to
patient education are Gunnar Karlsson and Jan-Erik Ögren. They have both
achieved much in spreading Swedish pharmacy through close cooperation
with the doctors and nurses in local medical care. In a poster they
present further details in addition to what I have described here.

Patient education is la Sagrada Familia of pharmacy. It is all
the time being extended further. Active pharmacy both towards patients and
towards medical care demands continuous further education. To keep the
pharmacists´ drug knowledge at a high level, to increase understanding for
the patients´ behaviour and the possibilities of grasping patient education - this is a large and interesting complex of problems ant it would
demand another hour to report Swedish experiences in this field. But perhaps there will be time to revert to this on another occasion.

Teaching Therapeutic Problem-Solving to Clinical Pharmacy
Students

R.J. Cipolle
College of Pharmacy, University of Minnesota,
Minneapolis, Minnesota 55455, USA

L.M. Strand
University of Utah, Salt Lake City, Utah

A.S. Pancorbo,
Wayne State University, Detroit, Michigan

The trend in pharmacy practice toward patient-oriented services
has emphasized the need for pharmacy students to acquire fundamental
problem-solving skills in addition to establishing a strong knowledge
base in pathophysiology and therapeutics. It is the pharmacist's
ability to problem solve and provide recommendations based on the best
professional judgment and current scientific knowledge that separates
the professional from the technician.

Some Pharmacy educators have recognized the need for didactic
training in problem solving techniques, and a few formal courses have
been designed. These courses are important, but their success is
limited by the lack of a common, structured approach to the problems
addressed on a daily basis in clinical pharmacy practice, namely the
assessment of a patient's drug therapy. Assessing drug therapy is a
common function in all pharmacy practice settings. Therefore a common
problem solving approach will help students resolve problems related
to drug therapy regardless of the clinical situation.

We have developed and implemented a structured approach for
pharmacy students to assist them to acquire important problem-solving
skills which can be directly applied in clinical practice. Central to
this structured approach is the Pharmacist's Workup of Drug Therapy.
The Pharmacist's Workup of Drug Therapy represents a thought process
which is designed to be consciously learned and practiced by all
pharmacy students. It is analogous to the physician's workup of the
patient but differs in its purpose, knowledge-base, interpretation of
information and therefore differs in outcome. The primary purpose of
the physician's workup is to arrive at an appropriate diagnosis to
solve a medical problem. The Pharmacist's Workup is used to assess a

patient's drug therapy needs and resolve problems related to drug
therapy. Much of the same patient information is processed in both
the Pharmacist's Workup and the physician's workup, but due to
different purposes and knowledge-bases, the information is interpreted
differently by pharmacists than by physicians. Therefore, the
information provided by the pharmacist is unique and necessary for the
comprehensive care of the patient.

There are seven major categories of the Pharmacist's Workup of
Drug Therapy. The first section deals with patient data collection,
which includes description of the patient, medical problem list
(or diagnoses), present medications, history of medication use, and
history of compliance. The second section guides the student through
a Pharmacologic Review of Systems. The function of each organ system
is reviewed as it pertains to the use of medications. Each of these
categories is addressed from the "how will the DRUG affect this
patient?" and "How will this PATIENT'S condition affect the drug
therapy?" points of view. Throughout the Pharmacist's Workup of
Drug Therapy, the student is prompted with a list of focus questions
which guide the student to collect all of the most appropriate
information. As an example, in the Pharmacologic Review of the renal
system, the student is prompted to determine whether the patient's
renal function would alter the elimination of any medications as well
as whether any of the medications used by this patient can alter renal
function or tests used to estimate renal function.

After these two data collection sections are completed, the
student is required to integrate all of the information about the
patient and the drug therapy and formulate an ASSESSMENT OF DRUG
THERAPY or a "PHARMACIST'S PROBLEM LIST". The format for the
Pharmacist's Problem List is a list of the patient's medical
problems and the relationship of each to drug therapy. This section
is where the student must create a list of patient problems that are
the responsibility of the pharmacist to resolve. Each entry of the
PHARMACIST PROBLEM LIST is numbered and dealt with sequentially
through the final four steps of the workup.

The next section is the DESIRED THERAPEUTIC OUTCOMES. Here the
student sequentially lists the goals of drug therapy for each of the

numbered problems identified in the PHARMACIST'S PROBLEM LIST
section. The format of desired therapeutic outcomes include:
elimination of disease and/or symptoms, normalization of laboratory
values, production of desired drug concentrations, and enabling the
patient to be compliant with required drug regimens.

The next section requires the student to list all of the possible
THERAPEUTIC ALTERNATIVES which might accomplish the goals listed in
the previous section. In this section, the format includes routes
and modes of drug administration as well as various pharmacologic
agents which could possibly result in the desired therapeutic
outcomes. This section draws on the student's pharmacology and
therapeutics data base.

The next section guides the student to formulate a PHARMACIST'S
RECOMMENDATION FOR DRUG THERAPY. Here the student must select the
best choice from the previously listed THERAPEUTIC ALTERNATIVES. This
section allows the student to experience the decision-making portion
of drug therapy. The student's recommendation must be in a complete
format including drug, a dosage regimen individualized for each
patient, a route and method of administration, and the most
appropriate duration of therapy.

The final section in the PHARMACIST'S WORKUP OF DRUG THERAPY
guides the student to create a PLAN FOR MONITORING DRUG THERAPY.
Here the student learns to create a plan to ensure that his/her
recommendations will produce the desired effects and minimize the
undesired or toxic effects. The student lists the tests or information
required and how often each of these parameters must be evaluated to
ensure that the desired outcomes are occurring. The format also
requires the student to list the information or tests required and
how often each much be evaluated to ensure the undesired and toxic
effects of each recommended drug regimen are minimized.

A significant and unique aspect of the Pharmacist's Workup of Drug
Therapy, is its ability to assist the student to think systematically
and analytically when assessing drug therapy. A series of questions
follow each major section of the Pharmacist's Workup. These questions
represent the context in which the patient information should be
interpreted by the pharmacy student. Each section guides the student

to logically evaluate all drug-related problems and all relevant solutions. When used appropriately, the Pharmacist's Workup functions as a framework in which the student can integrate drug-specific knowledge with the patient-specific information for each clinical situation.

This orderly problem-solving approach and the rationale for each section is formally presented in the classroom. In this setting the student is taught to integrate drug-related information and patient-related information to continuously assess each patient's drug therapy needs and determine the appropriate amount of drug in every situation.

After the Pharmacist's Workup is formally presented in the didactic setting, the student must apply the approach throughout the clerkship experience. In the clerkship setting, preceptors focus on the student as an assessor of drug therapy. Students follow the Pharmacist's Workup thought process for each patient situation encountered. This problem-solving approach guides the student to act only when adequate information has been collected and after the student's drug recommendations have been documented. With practice, each student becomes very proficient using this approach.

In summary, a structured problem-solving approach to clinical pharmacy education and practice has been described. This approach guides the student in developing a systematic and analytic method of thinking about patient's drug therapy problems. Our experience with this teaching method has been most positive. Students find their abilities to identify drug related problems and determine the best solution is enhanced considerably. Faculty and preceptors find that this structured approach is very useful to determine and document each student's ability to function in the clinical setting.

PHARMACIST'S WORKUP OF DRUG THERAPY

DESCRIPTION OF THE PATIENT

Patient Age, Sex and Race:
1. Is the patient at risk to experience side effects from certain drugs because of his/her age, sex or race?
2. Is the patient's metabolism and elimination of certain drugs affected because of his/her age, sex or race?

Height:
Lean body weight calculations are dependent on height.

Weight:
How does this patient's weight affect dosage calculations?

Lean Body Weight
Kinetic parameters are calculated by lean body weight.
[Male   = 50 + 2.3 (no. of inches greater than 5'0")
 Female = 45 + 2.3 (no. of inches greater than 5'0")]

PROBLEM LIST - DIAGNOSIS
1. What are the patient's medical problems or complaints?
2. Is the problem defining a specific indication for drug therapy?
3. Are these problems which can be caused by inappropriate drug therapy?
4. Does the disease affect the way the drug is handled in the body?

PRESENT MEDICATIONS
1. Considering the patient's problems and symptoms mentioned in the previous section, what medications, routes of administration, dosages, and durations, has the patient been taking to improve the situation? (prescribed and/or not prescribed)
2. Have the medications produced the desired therapeutic outcome?
3. Are these medications contributing to some or all of the problems experienced by the patients?
4. What organ systems can be affected by the medications?

MEDICAL HISTORY (Past, Surgical, Hospital)
1. Have the present medical problems been treated previously?
2. Is a past problem defining a contraindication for a specific drug therapy?
3. Is there anything in the patient's previous medical history which could affect the action or effectiveness of drugs?

MEDICATION HISTORY
1. Is there a history of success or failure of past drug therapy for similar medical problems?
2. Has some medication in the past altered a body system that will affect the disposition of current drug therapy?

ALLERGIES
1. Do potential allergies exist (drug, food, etc.)?
2. Have any allergic reactions occurred in the past?
3. What is the nature and significance of any allergic reactions?

SMOKING/ALCOHOL HISTORY
1. Is the smoking/alcohol history significant to affect drug disposition?
2. Is the smoking/alcohol history significant to contribute to the patient's problems?

COMPLIANCE

Patient:
1. Are there therapeutic failures in the past that would suggest a lack of adherence to prescribed drug therapy?
2. What is the social history and living conditions of the patient that may affect adherence to prescribed medication regimens?
3. How reliable is my source of information?

Drug Delivery System:
1. How reliable is my source of information?
2. What is the evidence that the patient has received the medication as prescribed?
3. Is there any evidence to suggest problems with pharmaceutical formulations presently employed?

PHARMACOLOGIC SYSTEMS REVIEW
1. Is the condition of an organ system defining an indication for drug therapy?
2. Are present drugs affecting the patient by producing a pharmacologic effect?
3. Are present drugs affecting the patient by producing a toxic effect?
4. Is the condition of the patient's organ systems affecting the disposition of a drug? (absorption, metabolism, distribution, elimination)

Vital Signs: Temp, Heart Rate, Blood Pressure, Respiration:
1. Are there deviations from normal which could be due to drug therapy?
2. Are there deviations from normal which could affect drug therapy monitoring?

Renal:
Is the patient receiving a drug that can alter renal function?
Function Tests: BUN, serum creatinine, creatinine clearance

Liver:
Is the patient's liver function affecting the elimination of certain drugs? Are certain drugs producing toxic effects in the liver?
Function Tests: SGOT, liver enzymes, proteins, coags

Cardiovascular:
Is the patient experiencing side effects from certain drugs manifested in the cardiovascular system? (arrhythmias, tachycardia)
Function Tests: pulse, blood pressure, EKG reading

Pulmonary:
Does the patient have COPD which may contraindicate the use of certain drugs?
Function Tests: chest x-ray, arterial blood gases, pulmonary function tests

Blood:
Are coagulation studies needed to determine liver function or therapeutic end-points for anticoagulation?

Function Tests: CBC, differential

Fluid Status:
Is the patient's fluid status sufficiently abnormal to affect laboratory values used to monitor drug therapy?
Function Tests: Electrolytes, acid-base determinations

GI:
Is the condition of the patient's GI tract affecting the absorption of orally administered drugs?

GU:
Is the condition of the patient's GU system defining an indication for drug therapy?

Musculoskeletal:
How is the patient's musculoskeletal system defining an indication for drug therapy?

Neuro/Mental:
Determine patient's baseline status so potential side effects may be identified?

Skin:
Determine patient's baseline status so potential side effects may be identified?

EENT:
Determine patient's baseline status so potential side effects may be identified?

PERTINENT LABS
1. What tests are needed to determine efficacy of present drug therapy?
2. What tests are needed to determine if present drug therapy is cause of toxicity?
3. What baseline laboratory values are needed in anticipation of therapeutic effectiveness and toxicity monitoring of drugs?

PHARMACIST'S ASSESSMENT OF DRUG THERAPY/PHARMACIST'S PROBLEM LIST:
1. Are each of the present drugs producing the desired effect?
2. Are any of the present drugs contributing to the patient's problems (toxicity, ineffective)?
3. Does any portion of the present drug therapy require changing? (dose, drug, route, duration, addition, deletion)
4. What new therapeutic indications are present in this patient?

DESIRED THERAPEUTIC OUTCOMES
1. What are the optimal therapeutic outcomes for each of the problems identified in the pharmacist's problem list?

THERAPEUTIC ALTERNATIVES:
1. What other drug regimens might produce the desired response?
2. What are the risks and benefits of each of the potential alternative drug regimens?

PHARMACIST'S DRUG RECOMMENDATION AND DOSAGE INDIVIDUALIZATION:
1. Considering the therapeutic alternatives in this patient, what drug regimen should be instituted?
2. What changes need to be made in existing drug therapy (add, delete drugs?)
3. What specific dose, route of administration, dosage formulation, regimen and duration of therapy has been selected for each drug?

PLAN AND RATIONALE FOR CONTINUED DRUG MONITORING:
1. What information do I need to ensure that the recommended drug therapy is producing the desired effect?
2. What information do I need to ensure that the recommended drug therapy is not causing problems?
3. With what frequency and for what duration do I need to collect the relevant information?

CLINICAL PHARMACY IN THE PHARMACEUTICAL EDUCATION IN DENMARK

M. Rasmussen
Dept. of Pharmaceutics, Royal Danish School of Pharmacy
2 Universitetsparken, DK-2100 Copenhagen, Denmark

Abstract. In Denmark a new syllabus for the pharmaceutical education was instituted in 1980. The 5-year-study includes the following subjects: chemistry (37%), biology (25%), pharmacy and social pharmacy (20%) and apprenticeship (18%). During the first 6 months of the study, the students deal with subjects as chemistry, statistics, pharmacy and social pharmacy, pharmacognosy, microbiology and pharmacology (pharmacokinetics) in the School of Pharmacy. The following 11 months they serve an apprenticeship in a retail pharmacy. For the last 5 months of this first part of the study, the students return to the School of Pharmacy and read subjects such as pharmacy, social pharmacy, pharmacognosy, botany, mathematics and physics. In the third year the subjects are inorganic, organic and physical chemistry and physics. The fourth year consist mainly of biological subjects such as biology, biochemistry, microbiology, pharmacology, biopharmaceutics, chemistry of natural products and analytical chemistry. The fifth and final year comprehend control and evaluation of drug products, medical chemistry and pharmacognosy. These subjects are mandatory and occupy one third of the fifth year. During the last two thirds of the year the students are occupied within one of the areas: formulation and production, analysis and control or distribution and information. The students may select a number of courses within or amongst the three areas. One of the courses is clinical pharmacy.

INTRODUCTION

In Denmark there is only one School of Pharmacy. Therefore a new syllabus, which was started in 1980, affects all pharmacy students in the country. The School of Pharmacy matriculates 160 students and graduates about 70 pharmacists a year. The study is prescribed to five years but in average the students take 6-7 years to graduate, only 3-7 students per year have graduated within the fixed time over the last three years.

PART ONE OF THE STUDY

The first part of the study is prescribed to two years and having passed this examination the students are licensed to work as registered pharmacy technicians.

Table 1. Part one of the study

Months	Subject	Lectures & Seminars (h)	Laboratory practice (h)
	Chemistry	61	80
	Statistics	39	
	Pharmacy	58	
6	Social pharmacy	98	
	Pharmacognosy	4	18
	Pharmacology	49	
	Microbiology	14	
11	Apprenticeship		
	Mathematics	39	
	Physics	47	
5	Pharmacy	40	
	Social pharmacy	36	36
	Pharmacognosy	42	44

Table 2. Subjects in social pharmacy

1st year	Organization and function of pharmacies
	Prescription rules
	Taxation
	Basic social medicine
	Concepts of illness and drug therapy
	Drug legislation
	Drug distribution
	Drug utilization
	Production and marketing of drugs
	Drug control system
	Sociological methodology
Apprenticeship:	Projects on drug distribution or drug utilization in the local community
2nd year	Research methodology
	Scientific theory
	Sociology of the welfare state
	Sociology of the social and health care sectors
	Projects about subjects important to the health of the population, e.g. clinical iatrogenesis, nutrition, work environment

Within the first six months the students attend courses of a
variety of subjects (table 1) with the purpose to give them some insight
in the broad sprectrum of pharmacy and to prepare them for the 11-month-
apprenticeship in a retail pharmacy. During the apprenticeship the students are distributed all over Denmark practicing pharmacy and working on
two minor projects: one in traditional pharmacy and one in social pharmacy.
The project in social pharmacy is restricted to be within drug distribution
or drug utilization in the local community. When the students return to
the School of Pharmacy, they are examined in routines, rules and laws of
pharmacy practice with respect to individual drug preparation, proficiency
in raw materials of drugs, and handling of medical articles and drugs.

For the next five months the students attend courses in the
subjects that are included in the part I examination i.e. mathematics/
physics, pharmacy, social pharmacy and pharmacognosy (table 1) for which
written examinations are held.

The course in social pharmacy is not familiar to pharmacists
in all European countries, and the content of the subject differs from
country to country. The subjects are shown in table 2 (Hansen et al.).

PART TWO OF THE STUDY

The third year of the study is devoted to chemical and physical
sciences whereas the fourth year is mostly devoted to the biological and
biological adjoining sciences (table 3). In the beginning of the fifth
year all students have to pass courses in control and evaluation of drug
products, pharmacognosy, medical chemistry and work environment (table 3).
Thereafter the student can choose among different courses within the three
areas:

1. formulation and production
2. distribution and information
3. analysis and control

The students may select a number of courses according to their special
interests. They have to make a minor research project for about 3 months
so it is essential that there is a mutual connexion between courses and
topic of the project.

One of the optional courses offered is clinical pharmacy.

Table 3. Part two of the study

Year	Subject	Lectures & Seminars (h)	Laboratory practice (h)
3rd	Inorganic chemistry	54	88
	Physical chemistry	81	56
	Organic chemistry	120	176
	Physics	71	28
4th	Analytical chemistry	18	88
	Chemistry of natural products	50	
	Biopharmacy	44	48
	Pharmacology	78	
	Microbiology	36	44
	Biology	75	28
	Biochemistry	57	
5th	Control & evaluation of drug products		70
	Pharmacognosy	37	44
	Medical chemistry	48	
	Work environment	33	

Several optional courses min. 4.5 modules[*]

Research project 3.0 modules

[*]1 module ~ 110 working hours for the students.

CLINICAL PHARMACY

The course in clinical pharmacy is based upon the traditional pharmaceutic sciences. The objective of the course is to give the students insight in cases of hospitalized patients - the somatic, psychiatric and social aspects - to such an extent that they will be able to evaluate the medical treatment and on this basis cooperate with physicians, nurses, patients and any one else involved in the pharmacotherapy to achieve the optimal treatment.

The teaching methods involve lectures, seminars, colloquial lessons, a trainee period in a hospital, minor projects and a presentation of projects from the hospital trainee period.

After a few introductory lectures on clinical pharmacy practice and clinical pharmacy education - development and present status in different countries - the students are grouped within the following subjects: drug handling, clinical trials, drug monitoring, drug distribution and

large volume parenterals. Each group has 2-3 students. Each year a new
topic within each group will be chosen and there will be given one theoretical and one clinical lecture on each of these 5 topics. All students have
to attend all lectures irrespective of group and topic. Table 4 shows some
of the subjects in each main group.

All subjects are more or less cross-linked, consequently a
careful choice of the special topics within each group should give the
students a general knowledge of the scope of clinical pharmacy.

During the trainee period each student spends 20 hours in a
ward to work with clinical tasks concerning a special topic. The student
draws up a report on the practical task and presents it to the other
students of the course. The students work together on the task in each
group, which means that it will sum up to 5 presentations of 5 reports.

The students are also trained to solve theoretical and clinical
problems by use of scientific papers given to them - one task on each main
subject, i.e. 5 tasks for all students.

In the end of the course the students have to pass a 4-hour
written examination. The marks passed or failed are given.

Table 4. Examples of topics within the main subjects of
          clinical pharmacy

    I. Drug handling

      1. handling of cytostatics
      2. biopharmaceutical problems
      3. training programmes for patients before
         discharging

   II. Clinical trials

      1. ethical and legal aspects
      2. design
      3. adverse drug reactions

  III. Drug monitoring

      1. clinical pharmacokinetics
      2. clinical microbiology

   IV. Drug distribution

      1. distribution systems
      2. medical auditing
      3. use of EDP-systems

    V. Large volume parenterals

      1. parenteral nutrition
      2. dialysis

REFERENCES

Hansen, E.H., Henriksen, H.H., Kruse, P.R. & Sørensen, E.W. (1982)
Social pharmacy, Royal Danish School of Pharmacy. A poster
presented at the F.I.P. Congress, Copenhagen.

EDUCATION IN CLINICAL PHARMACY FOR COMMUNITY PHARMACISTS

Fernandez,P., Bonal,J., Bonet,R., Eritja,R., Escuin,M.,
Gonzalez,B. Society of Pharmacists of Barcelona. Continuing
Education Commitee

Nowadays, Postgraduate Continual Education (C.E.), is a
necessity for all Professionals, and specially for Health Professionals.

To plan C.E. one has to bear in mind certain factors:

- The C.E. is directed to practising professionals, specially
to those who have a busy working day and so have very little time free.

- There is no guarantee that practising professionals can take part in the sequential courses as their business commitments frequently prevents this, even though they have the best will.

- It is essential to give priority in programming C.E. so
that what they learn should have maximum scientific and social accomplish
ment.

- The C.E. must be guided in such a way that knowledge so obtained could be immediately applicable in daily routine, this is the best
way to stimulate the participation and to observe practical results.

- The fundamental aim of the C.E. is to achieve enough motivation so that every professional feels the need for self-learning in the
field that suits him so that at the time of programming the C.E. it is
essential to bear in mind these points quoted, in short they are as follows:

- Programs that adapt to professional working hours.
- The activities will not be sequentials but completely independent in themselves.
- The priority of these programs should result in the formation of pharmacists as a specialist in drugs.
- And parallel to the C.E. it has to program practical activities which are going to motivate a professional of community pharmacy.

In 1978 as a result of opinions a Continuing Education Commitee, was set up which was made up of hospital and community pharmacists.
After various changes and under standing it clearly, a program for C.E.
was organized in 1981.

The experience and the results so obtained during its 3 years
working are shown here.

The objective of the present program is to put in to practice
clinical pharmacy in Community Pharmacy.

The course gives instructions in Physiopathology and Pharmacological applications mainly related to chronic type of pathology.

The knowledge of Anatomy and Physiopathology (Fig.1) is given
by a Doctor specialist in the mentioned subjects, with deep enough knowled
ge so that Therapeutical effect of the drug could be understood. The lectures on pharmacology are given by Hospital Pharmacists. The bibliography
is attached to the papers which are handed out at the beginning of the
course.

FIGURE 1.- CLINICAL ORIENTATION OF THE COURSES.

PLANING SCHEME OF EACH COURSE:

- Theory of Anatomy.
- Physiopathology.
- Pharmacology: choice of treatment.
  Technique.
  Toxicity and interactions.
  Pharmacokinetic.
  Dosage rules.
- Bibliography.
- Function (work) of Community Pharmacists in the Prevention
  and Treatment.
- Assessment.

Once the theory part is over, a "Round table conference" is
held in which all the professors of the course take part and work as Mo-
derators, Coordinators of C.E.C., they talk about the work of a Community
Pharmacists as regards to prevention and treatment of pathology under
discussion.

Assessment consists in presenting real or imaginary clinical case.

Questions are asked on pharmacological treatment about the said case and reasoned answers are given by the pharmacists, after studying the available documents.

C.E.C. which were held between the period of Feb.1981 and June 1983 as well as their duration in hours and the number of attendants are included in figure 2.

FIGURE 2.- C.E.C. FOR COMMUNITY PHARMACISTS (FEB.81 - JUNE 83).

COURSE SUBJECTS	Hours Duration	Course Realized	Attend
Physiopath. & Treat. of Cardiac Diseases	10	8	98
" " Respir. Diseases	10	3	93
" " Renal Diseases	10	2	86
Live saving and First Aid	40	2	82
Clin.Pharm. on Community Pharm. seminar	5	3	119
Drug interactions seminar	5	3	277
Biochem. bases, diet.& Phychol. of Nutr.	10	1	40
Formulas	31	1	100

The Clinical Pharmacy on Community Pharmacy seminar is considered as a preamble necessary for the development of the C.E.C. course. This is what really makes the pharmacist see the need to change the image to obtain a new concept of following our profession.

The clinical pharmacy will not be really important if we cannot succeed in extending this concept to Community Pharmacists, we must not forget that 90% of the drugs are consumed through National Health Service.

C.E.C. are decentralized, they have been held at different towns of Barcelona Area, with the object of assisting the spread of the courses in the Provincial, Regional or National atmosphere. A Part of Physiopathology has been recorded on Video tapes. At present we have the following recordings. (Fig.3).

FIGURE 3.-   RECORDED VIDEOS

- Physiopathology and treatment for cardiopathy.
- Lung: Its structure and function.
- Renal Physiology.

                         VIDEOS UNDER PREPARATION

- Physiopathology of the Hypertension.

The statistical information of the development of the course is shown in figure 4.

FIGURE 4.-
                                                  33 PHARMACISTS
          PROFESSORS WHO PARTICIPATED: 48   15 PHYSICIANS

          TEACHING HOURS: 271
          NUMBER OF PROFESSIONAL ASSOCIATED IN BARCELONA IN 1983:3664
          NUMBER OF PROFESSIONAL ASSOCIATED WHO HAVE ATTENDED
          AT LEAST ONE COURSE: 565 (15.4%)

In figure 5 one can see courses under preparation.

FIGURE 5.-   COURSES UNDER PREPARATION

- Physiopathology, Treatment and Prevention of Rheumatic
  illnesses.
- Physiopathology, Treatment and Prevention of Hypertension
- Program for Home Study Course.

As the courses were successful, Coordinator, Dr. J. Bonal, has been invited to present this programme at the following centers. Figure 6.

Since the aim of the C.E. is to put into practice Clinical Pharmacy into Community Pharmacy, it has stimulated certain group of workers, who start activities of Clinical Pharmacy in their own Community

```
┌─────────────────────────────────────────────────────────────────────┐
│ FIGURE 6.-                                                            │
│            CENTERS AT WHICH THE PROGRAMME HAS BEEN INVITED            │
│                                                                       │
│ ├ Society of Pharmacists of Oviedo. 1981                             │
│ ├ Society of Pharmacists of Gerona. 1982                             │
│ ├ Society of Pharmacists of Jaen. 1982                               │
│ ├ Pharmacists Journey of Andalucia. Sevilla 1982                     │
│ ├ National Congress of Pharmaceutical Science of Portugal. Lisbon 1982│
│ ├ Delegation of Pharmacists school of Tarragona. Tortosa 1983        │
│ ├ National Pharmacists Journey of Las Palmas of Gran Canaria 1983    │
│                                                                       │
└─────────────────────────────────────────────────────────────────────┘
```

Pharmacy. Actually 4 of these groups exist, with an active participation of a considerable number of Pharmacists. Three of these groups prepared information about groups of Pharmacologists, guiding as much to Community Pharmacy as to the patients. Other group has done work on Epidemiology about the treatment for the patients under National Health Service, who have chronic obstructive pulmonary disease (C.O.P.D.) in one defined area of Barcelona.

CONCLUSIONS

It can be seen from the pharmacists number who attended the course has been satisfactory and well accepted.

The teaching method has shown its efficency by completing its objective. Motivating Community Pharmacist to put into practice Clinical Pharmacy.

Results of this motivation are 2 communications which they present in this Congress, in which a very important number of Community Pharmacists have Collaborated.

In the end we offer to all those schools that are interested material and the course method.

INTRODUCTORY COURSE TO CLINICAL PHARMACY: EVALUATION AFTER 1O YEARS

Bonal,J., Castro,I., Altimiras,J.

Pharmacy Service

Hospital de la Santa Creu i Sant Pau. Barcelona

INTRODUCTION

In 1974 we started in our pharmacy service of the hospital "de la Sta. Creu i S. Pau" a two week course called " Introductory course to Clinical Pharmacy ". The main objective of this course was to stimulate and spread the philosophy and concepts of clinical pharmacy and to orient people on their way to study and practice.

Because of the lack of experience in these types of teaching activities and because there were no other courses with similar orientation in our country, we first established the program by intuition and in the following years, we modified it progressively looking for an orientation according to the hospital pharmacy needs, and paying attention to the specific opinions and suggestions of the course participants.

After ten years of experience, we think that it would be interesting to analyze the evolution of the course on the one hand and on the other to ask for the opinion of the people that have taken the course about the quality of it and in what way the course has influenced their daily practice.

EVOLUTION OF THE COURSE

It is interesting to see how the course program has been changing from year to year since the first course in 1974. At the begining most teachers were physicians. In the first year only 38'2 % of the teachers were pharmacists and only 17'6 % were pharmacists from our service. In 1983, in the tenth course, 70'8 % of the teachers were pharmacists and 54'1 % were pharmacists from our service. The annual evolution of the teachers is shown in figure 1. We can see how the pharmacists have increased in relation to physicians and also that the proportion of pharmacists from our service has increased significantly. There is no doubt that, besides the personal usefulness of this course for the

participants in addition the participants have been an important instrument
of education and stimulation within their our own pharmacy service.

Courses have been scheduled for 55 - 60 contact hours of
theoretical and practical activities. The proportion between both
activities has been changing, increasing the practical activities and
decreasing lectures, specially in the last few years, as can be seen in
figure 2.

On the other hand, the kind of practical activities has also
been modified. During the first five years, the practical part consisted
mainly in taking rounds with a medical team in some selected wards of the
hospital. The intention of this was to familiarize pupils in the taking
of such rounds with the care team.

Nevertheless, after these first years, we found that such
activities were not very useful, probably because of the number of pupils
and the number of physicians usually taking such rounds. For this reason,
after the 6th course (1979) we modified the practical program and organized
seminars of clinical application in groups of 5 students coordinated by
one pharmacist from our service with experience in the theme of the
seminar.

The change was successful and was well accepted and consequently
the number of seminars was increased. We scheduled 5 in the 6th course,
10 in the 7th, 8th and 9th and 13 in the 10th.

Also as a form of practical teaching selected clinical cases
are studied and discussed by small groups from the first course on. These
cases are presented by the students in a final session, with all the rest
of the students and professors of the course.

The number of participants in these ten years has been about
300, twelve from foreign countries like Portugal, Italy and France. The
rest have been Spanish hospital pharmacists wich means about 50 % of the
total number of Hospital Pharmacists in Spain.

EVALUATION OF THE COURSE

In order to evaluate the effectiveness of the course and the
degree of satisfaction of the participants of these ten years, we mailed
a simple questionaire that is shown in figure 3.

```
FIGURE 3.-   Questionaire to evaluate the course of introduction to
             clinical pharmacy.
             1.  Do you think that the course of introduction to clinical
                 pharmacy is useful and/or necessary?.
             2.  Have you been able to improve your daily work as
                 pharmacist in some aspect because of the course?.
             3.  If yes, What has improved?.
             4.  If not, Why not?.
             5.  What would you suggest to improve the course?.
```

We mailed 250 questionaires because some addresses were unknown and we got 87 answers which is about 35 %.

The answers to question 1 were positive 100 % of the answers considered the course useful and 72 % also necessary.

92 % recognize that they have improved some aspect of their daily work through the things that they learned during the course. The activities improved are shown in figure 4.

```
FIGURE 4.-   Activities improved because of the course.
             Drugs distribution system . . . . . . . .        33 %
             Drug information service. . . . . . . . .        61 %
             IV admixtures and/or TPN programs . . . .        27'5 %
             Approach to  team care . . . . . . . . .        54 %
             Drug compounding and control. . . . . . .        10 %
             Others. . . . . . . . . . . . . . . . . .        31 %
```

Those that did not feel that their daily work has improved at all or as far as they consider necessary, gave the reasons shown on figure 5.

```
FIGURE 5.-   Reasons of insufficient improvements.
             Problems with the hospital administration . . . . 4 cases
             Problems with the structure of the pharmacy
                                     service. . . . . . . . 6 cases
             Lack of time because they took the last course. . 5 cases
```

The last question asked for suggestions to improve the course. 10 of the answers suggested repeating the course after some years, 9 suggested increasing the practical part of the course, (they probably took one of the first courses). 4 suggested organizing monographic courses at a later date and finally 3 said that the course ought to be longer.

CONCLUSIONS

1. The percentage of unanswered questionaires is relatively high. That was predictable in this type of mailed questionaire.

2. The low level of response, oblige us to evaluate the results. Behind the unanswered questionaires there may be some degree of unsatisfaction or lack of interest.

3. Nevertheless, in the answers received clearly the usefulness of the course is absolutely recognized. In addition, a lot of them considered the course also necessary for the education of clinical pharmacists.

4. There is quite a large recognition that the course has been useful to change and improve some aspects of the daily practice.

5. Unfortunately there is a group that can not improve their practice at least not enough because they have difficulties with the hospital administration or with their own pharmacy service. That can be symptomatic of a lack of understanding from the people responsible for the hospital or a lack of initiative from some heads of pharmacy services.

INFORMATION PHARMACIST - A NEW POSTGRADUATE EDUCATION IN
SWEDEN

S.G.Lindgren
Hospital pharmacy, University Hospital, S-581 85 Linköping,
Sweden

Structure of pharmaceutical education in Sweden

The swedish society is very organized and the pharmaceutical
sphere is no exception. Because of a small population the number of pharmacies is only about 700 which with few exceptions belong to "Apoteksbolaget"
The National Corporation of Swedish Pharmacies.

The number of pharmacists is about 5000 of which 4000 are
working in pharmacies. The education and structure of pharmacy personnel
is seen from fig 1. Note that Sweden has three categories of employees in
the pharmacies of which the pharmacist and the prescriptionist have acade-
mical training of different depth but both leading to authorization by the
state to dispense and to be head of a pharmacy as well. Note that no more
pharmacy technicians are educated and those who are working today have the

Fig 1. Education and structure of pharmacy personnel in Sweden. Figures in
the boxes are the approximative number of each category. The number
in brackets under "pharmacist" are those working in pharmacies.

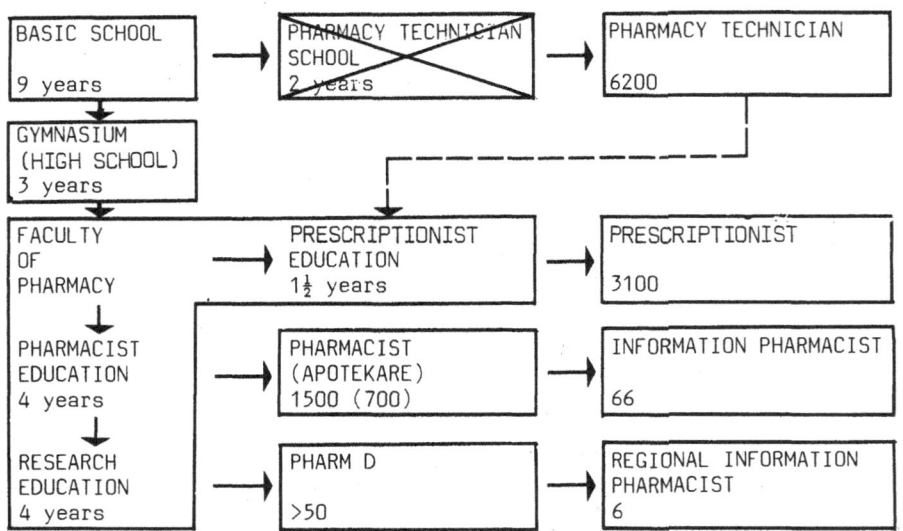

possibility to convert themselves to prescriptionists.

The reasons for such a change is twofold. The main reason is a need for good and homogenous competence among the personnel in all contacts with patient and the prescriber. Another reason is the technical development and automatization which diminishes the need for typing, calculating registration and billing and other parts of pharmacy technicians work.

Health-care and pharmacy service

Swedish health care is run by the 25 county councils and is organized in four levels. The base is the primary care where most of the doctors are employed by the county council. When there is a need for hospital care, increasing specialization in three levels is available (fig 2).

To suit the health-care organization the pharmacies are organized in groups covering the same area as the local health-care district. Above this level there are six region offices and a head office for Apoteksbolaget in Stockholm (fig 2).

Regional information pharmacists

There has always been a great need for information from the pharmacist and most countries have developed systems to meet the need for drug information in the hospital. In the beginning of the seventies Apoteksbolaget created six new positions as regional information pharmacists at the university hospitals. Their main tasks are:

* Organize and give drug information to the hospital
* Work in the Drug & Therapeutics Committé

Fig 2. Correspondence in organisation between pharmacy service and health care in Sweden.

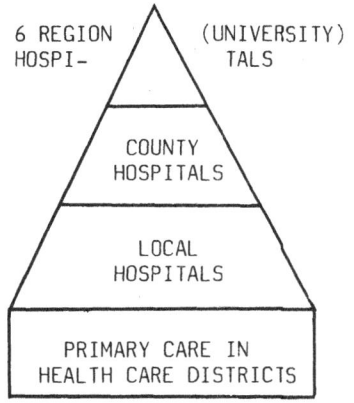
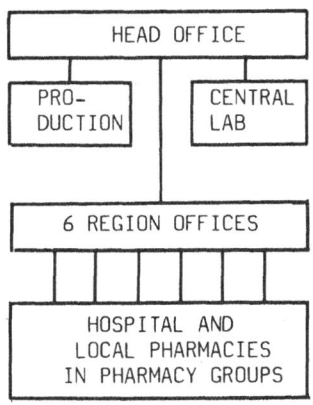

* Give impulses and knowledge and cooperate in drug related research work
* Improve information and education standard among the pharmacy personnel
* Participate in educational work directed to other health-care personnel

Information pharmacist education

During the seventies the structure of the relation between medical care and pharmacy has changed in Sweden. A lot of pharmacies have been
established in health care centers and a new type of cooperation between
primary care and pharmacy has been born. One of the resulting effects is
an increased need for improved information capability at the pharmacies.
To give support to pharmacies in a local pharmacy group and to try to improve and increase information to the patient 66 new positions as information pharmacists were founded. They were given basic pedegogic training
and could in seminars discuss their potential role. The main body in their
training was a 14-month course in "Applied pharmacology" which was held on
a regional level where the local regional information pharmacist was responsible for the detailed program.
The participating pharmacist had to do selfstudies in anatomy and physiology according to detailed reading instuctions and a lot of training questions. Lists of suggested reading and training questions were also distributed when the main subjects were attacked. After self-study periods of
about one month when they could use 25 % of their contracted time for studies, that particular part of the course was concluded by two days of joint
lectures, seminars and discussions. The disposition was:
Day 1 Pharmacological lectures and discussions; clinical lectures and
seminars; comprehensive discussions on choice of therapy.
Day 2 Seminars and discussions about:
* Problems requiring a comprehensive knowledge in the subject of interest
* The local drug formulary, why these drugs are recommended and if the
  recommendation is obeyed
* The practical use of the knowledge of that particular therapeutic group
  what concerns both pharmacy personnel and prescribing physicians.
The first three months were devoted to general pharmacology,biopharmacy
pharmacokinetics and general subjects using a booklet called "Basic principles of pharmacology" written by the regional information pharmacists and
teachers at the faculty of pharmacy. Different areas of therapy were then
covered during the rest of the 14 month course. The following topics were
treated during the introductory part on biopharmacy and related subjects:

Absorption	Pharmacokinetics	Drugs in the childhood
Distribution	Pharmacodynamics	Drugs and the elderly
Drug metabolism	Therapy control	Drug interactions
Excretion	Clinical evaluation	Side effects of drugs
Dosage forms	Compliance	Drug information and advertizing
Ways of administration		

Continous training. After this start a number of positions have changed
bearer but there is still a need for this education of information pharmacists and this training is organized on a nationwide scale where the regional information pharmacist is responsible for a certain therapeutic
area. This continous basic course for the new information pharmacists has
a circulation time of about two years. The regional information pharmacist
is also responsible for the further training of the information pharmacist by arranging regional meetings twice a year with lectures and seminars in drug fields of interest.

Duties for the information pharmacist. What is the purpose with this position and why has Apoteksbolaget put all these efforts in the education of
information pharmacists? The intention is a contribution to a more efficient use of drugs by implementing improvements in drug information to the
public. Their tasks as described by their employers are:
* Work for application of the policy of Apoteksbolaget in the local pharmacy group
* Assist in planning, arranging and realizing information activities
  in the local pharmacy group concerning the formulary
* Give feedback to the management about the need for information and
  education activities
* Participate in and coordinate the work with the formulary in the
  pharmacy group based on local drug recommendations from the Drug & Therapeutics Committee or other agreements with the local health care.
They can spend half their working time on these activities.

All of the information pharmacists have also worked with booklets on self-
care in cooperation with local physicians and nurses. The text is directed
to the public and gives advices how to cure or treat minor illnesses.
The booklet is spread by pharmacies and health-care centers with the aim
that they may contribute to a more efficient use of health-care resources.

DESIGNING AN IN-SERVICE TRAINING PROGRAMME TO FACILITATE
THE DEVELOPMENT OF CLINICAL SERVICES IN A REGION

P. R. Noyce
Pharmacy Dept , The Royal Free Hospital, London, NW3 2QG, U.K.
B. Davies
Pharmacy Dept , Guy's Hospital, London. SE1 9RT, U.K.

Background

The training of clinical pharmacists in U.K. has been
approached in various ways: in London a one-year full-time Masters course
has been established (Noyce & Hibberd 1980) and in Birmingham a two-year
day-release programme (Ashcroft et al. 1982). The London course produces
a maximum of eight graduates a year and these are shared amongst four
Health Regions. In South East Thames Region, which covers the south east
section of London and the counties of Kent and East Sussex, the Regional
Pharmaceutical Officer was enthusiastic to establish a more widespread
development of clinical pharmacy across the Region than could be achieved
quickly by the small number of graduates. The Regional Pharmaceutical
Education Working Group, in responding to this demand, recognised that
widespread development of clinical pharmacy was only likely to be
stimulated if facilitators were established in local hospital pharmacies
and proposed a scheme to be organised to train them. The authors' task
then became to design a scheme for training middle-managers (i.e. Staff
Pharmacists) to become self-motivating foci for the development of
clinical pharmacy in their base departments.

TABLE 1 - KEY COMPONENTS OF TRAINING PROGRAMME

1 Roles and Working Situations of Course Members.

2 Aims and Perspectives in Developing Ward/Clinical Services.

3 Learning Methods.

4 Staff Development and the Facilitator Role.

5 Problems of Pioneering Developments and Self-Help.

6 Major exercise on Devising an In-service Development
Programme at the Base Hospital Pharmacy.

7 Implementation Process/Management of Change.

Approach and Constraints

At the preliminary stages in design, it was recognised that
the programme needed to combine education in topics relevant to clinical
pharmacy development alongside training in skills to facilitate the
development process. Learning methods in clinical pharmacy and
management of change were topics that readily came to mind - in other
words a blend of professional and managerial skills were necessary in
performing a facilitator role. A complete list of the topics identified
as key components are given in Table 1. A major practical exercise at
the base department was considered an essential feature of the programme
and dictated that it be run as two modules.

The design team had to accept that there would be no pre-
selection of course members, the time available for training was minimal
and on return to work no extra resources would be available to fund
developments. Since course members would also have to cope with the
problem of "transfer" of course material to work (Noyce 1980) and be
self-motivating, underlying themes of the programme were engendering a
self-reliant approach and sharing experience.

Course Design

The overall format adopted was a two-day residential module,
followed by eight months work experience and concluding with a single
review day, with an emphasis on demonstrating techniques and practical
exercises. The detailed programme is given in Table 2. A four-hour
session was devoted to learning scenarios which could be readily adapted
in base departments in handling clinical pharmacy topics.

Since time was short, a pre-course questionnaire was used to
orientate members to the course: a device previously successfully
employed (Noyce et al. 1978). Through a tutor-guided discussion in small
groups it was possible to ascertain details of individual working
situations and provide an opportunity to share perceptions and expectations of the training event. Two presentations followed to provide a
perspective on clinical pharmacy development; the first an analysis of
activity in an adjacent Health Region and the second, the wider
implications as seen by a senior pharmacy manager.

The concept of learning and available methods were then
introduced as a prelude to practical sessions. The applicability of
procedural manuals as a means of guidance and reference was explored and
some practice given in their preparation. Various formats for in-service

TABLE 2 — PROGRAMME FORMAT

	Components	Format
1	Establishing individual course member's roles, working situations, aspirations, level of development.	Pre-course questionnaire and and small group discussion.
2a)	Analysis of ward pharmacy practice in adjacent Region.	Lecture.
b)	Resource, organisational and training implications of clinical pharmacy development.	Lecture.
3a)	Teaching and learning techniques.	Lecture and film.
b)	Procedural manuals as vehicles for guidance and reference.	Small group exercise with demonstration examples.
c)	Learning formats for clinical pharmacy.	Demonstrations and exercises.
d)	Performance review — criteria for assessing performance, including peer review.	Lecture and small group discussion.
4	Coaching, Staff Appraisal and counselling.	Films, small group discussions and personnel simulation exercise.
5a)	Practical problems in implementing training in Ward/ Clinical pharmacy.	Tutorial
b)	General approach to pioneering developments and self help.	Tutorial
6	Preliminary work in designing and in-service development scheme.	Guided individual work. Design strategy had to be completed in 1 month.
7a)	Implementation of development scheme.	Written progress reports at 3 and 6 months.
b)	Review of implementation of scheme (with particular emphasis on rate of progress, realism of expectations, obstacles encountered, tactics adopted).	Second module Individual presentations in small small groups.
c)	Summary of experience in implementing individual schemes.	Tutorial.
d)	Management of change.	Lecture.
e)	Training and development of clinical pharmacy in another Region.	Tutorial.

clinical pharmacy training were then comprehensively demonstrated. The section on learning methods was concluded with a presentation on performance review.

The components of staff development — coaching, counselling and appraisal, are difficult to inculcate quickly and so training films were used with a personnel simulation for practice.

Course members were then prepared for their projects in clinical pharmacy developments which were to cover the first six months of two year strategic plans. Contributions were made on a general approach to operational developments and the problems encountered in providing clinical pharmacy training. A strategic plan in development and an action time-table for the first six months had to be registered by each course member within one month of the end of the first module and subsequently three to six monthly written progress reports prepared.

Review

At the end of the two-day module, and again just prior to the second module, course evaluation questionnaires, covering all sessions, were circulated. These showed that the two-day module was immediately assessed overall to have a relevance of 80%, which was generally sustained with a rating of 68% after eight months of practical experience.

On the review day each course member gave a thirty minute presentation in small groups on his experience of implementing his action plan. The emphasis in this session was on process rather than outcome, to provide course members with the opportunity to learn from their own experience key points in the management of change, which generally can only be considered hypothetically. In particular attention was directed towards whether the planned time-table was maintained and the reasons for deviation, the obstacles encountered and appropriate coping mechanisms, and the opportunities presented and whether these were fully exploited. Alternative approaches were explored where helpful. Several common issues were identified from the collective experience of the course membership which were germane to the management of change:

      unexpected changes in demands and resources;

      necessity of tactical plan in order to exploit opportunities;

      need for means of measuring progress;

      importance of gaining commitment of managers and staff to plans;

scope for reorganising work;

unrealistic aims.

The review day, apart from providing an opportunity to consider the attitudinal and organisational barriers to change, also acted as a motivation to sustain planned developments. If the intended widespread development of clinical pharmacy, as originally envisaged by the Regional Pharmaceutical Officer, was to be achieved beyond the training programme then a continuing mechanism in motivation was necessary. Thus at the end of the course a Regional Clinical Pharmacy Working Group was established.

ACKNOWLEDGEMENTS

We acknowledge the opportunity provided by Mr. J. C. Barfield, Regional Pharmaceutical Officer and Mrs. N. Coker, Chairman of the Regional Pharmaceutical Education Working Group to design and monitor this training programme and for support in its execution.

REFERENCES

Ashcroft, C.E., Harris, D. and Panton, R. (1982). Training pharmacists in clinical pharmacy. Pharm. J., 229, 496-7

Noyce, P.R. (1980). Education and Training. In Textbook of Hospital Pharmacy, eds. Allwood, M.C. and Fell, J.T., pp 47-67. Oxford: Blackwell Scientific.

Noyce, P.R., Fullerton, S.E. and Ware, J.R. (1978). Development scheme for senior pharmacy managers in National Health Service. Fédération Internationale Pharmaceutique, Cannes.

Noyce, P.R. and Hibberd, A.R. (1980). Launch of the London M.Sc. in Clinical Pharmacy. Pharm. J., 225, 473-474.

A STRATEGY FOR POSTGRADUATE TRAINING IN CLINICAL PHARMACY
IN NORTH WEST THAMES REGION

J.A.CROMARTY
Northwick Park Hospital, Harrow, Middlesex, U.K.

North West Thames Regional Pharmaceutical Service has accorded priority to the development of patient services in its overall strategy for pharmacy services in the next decade. A combination of formal postgraduate education and in-service training schemes in clinical pharmacy is regarded as a key factor in this development.

M.Sc. CLINICAL PHARMACY, UNIVERSITY OF LONDON

In response to a considerable demand for postgraduate education in clinical pharmacy in South East England, a Master of Science (M.Sc.) degree course in Clinical Pharmacy commenced in October 1980 (Noyce & Hibberd 1980). The course is jointly organised by North West Thames Regional Pharmaceutical Service and The School of Pharmacy, University of London. Health Authorities in London release pharmacists possessing several years experience of hospital pharmacy for the one year duration of the course. This M.Sc. course is designed to advance pharmacists' knowledge and experience of drug selection and the clinical use of drugs. It also provides pharmacists with an appreciation of clinical research methodology and its application to therapeutic problem solving. The M.Sc. students spend approximately half their time at The School of Pharmacy and the other half attached to clinical firms at Northwick Park Hospital for the first six months of the course. During this period they receive 175 hours of formal lectures and tutorials and 125 hours of practical laboratory work. For the remainder of the course each student undertakes a practical research project which often takes the form of a clinical pharmacokinetic study. On completion of the M.Sc. course, these pharmacists return to their base hospitals to participate in the development of local clinical services and training schemes.

REGIONAL CLINICAL PHARMACY TRAINING SCHEME

This training scheme has been devised on a regional basis in order to minimise duplication of effort among M.Sc. graduates and to

maximise the utilisation of available expertise throughout the Region.
Each M.Sc. graduate in Clinical Pharmacy within the Region has been
involved in the development of the scheme and acts as a tutor for 2
trainees. The scheme comprises two 3 month periods during which
pharmacists attend two 3 day residential courses and spend two 1 week
attachments at their tutor's base hospital. Both during these attachments
and whilst working at their own hospital, the pharmacists complete a
number of set exercises including prescription monitoring, medication
history taking, patient counselling, case presentations, comparative
drug evaluations, pharmacokinetic problems and case studies.

The two 3 day residential courses involve lectures, seminars
and workshops on prescription monitoring, biopharmaceutics,
pharmacokinetics, therapeutic drug monitoring, interpretation of
laboratory data, drug information, ward pharmacy and interview
techniques.

A maximum of 20 trainees will be selected to undergo this
training scheme during any one 6 month period. These trainees will be
monitored both prior to and following completion of their period of
training in order to assess the influence of the scheme on clinical
pharmacy practice.

Much of the training material available on the scheme may be
used by trainees when they return to their base hospitals. In this way
it is hoped to extend the opportunities for clinical pharmacy training
to all pharmacists within the Region.

Noyce, P.R. & Hibberd, A.R. (1980). Launch of the London M.Sc. in
    Clinical Pharmacy. Pharm. J. 225, 473-474.

BACKGROUND TO THE IMPLEMENTATION, AT A REGIONAL LEVEL, OF A
PAIN TREATMENT UNIT

F. SEIJO
Neurosurgery Service. Ciudad Sanitaria. Oviedo (Spain)
R.M.SIMO
Pharmacy Service. Ciudad Sanitaria. Oviedo (Spain)

INTRODUCTION

Approximately a third of the population of the developed countries is affected by acute or chronic pain, while in Spain expediture on
pain amounts to some two per cent of the Gross National Product, that is,
some five hundred and fifty thousand million pesetas in the year 1982.(In
Simposio Mecanismos Básicos del dolor, Madrid, Oct. 1982).

According to figures taken from the Catalogue of Pharmaceutical Specialities 1983, in December 1982 there were 429 registered medicines
with analgesic properties available on the Spanish market, in a total of
791 presentations. In the group "non-narcotic antipyretic analgesics", consisting of 160 specialities in 311 different presentations, only 30% of
these former had only a single active agent in their make-up, the rest –
being combinations more or less debatable, but in any case of doubtful therapeutic benefit and with greater risks entailed in their use.

Despite such great expenditure and the exorbitant number of preparations available, pain remains a serious problem which is still a long
way from a solution, leading to a general recognition that the use of these
drugs needs to be modified, as indeed do certain attitudes towards them.

In the Ciudad Sanitaria of Oviedo (CSO), a teaching hospital
with 1200 beds, a number of steps have been taken since 1981 with the aim
of acheiving an improved and more rational analgesic therapy, while ensuring that the activity, effectiveness, safety and cost of the treatments
are the most appropiate to each kind of pain and to each patient suffering
pain.

Consumption has been studied over this two year period, while
at the same time informative sessions have been organized for specific Clinical Services, and seminars for hospital staff. The use of morphine has
been introduced, administered both orally and intrathecally, for cases of
terminal neoplasic pain, and the surgical techniques have been perfected.

CONSUMPTION OF ANALGESICS

As is the case with any other kind of drug, the consumption of analgesics deduced from the quantities dispensed by the Pharmacy Service may give an approximate idea of a hospital's prescription practice, but is not qualitatively valid as on occasions not all those units dispensed are actually administered to patients. Despite this drawback, however, its usefulness as an approximation is widely recognized.

The Defined Daily Dose is considered as the average maintenance dose for the main indication (or one of the main indications) of a drug, per day. (W.H.O., 1979). The DDD is therefore a technical unit of measurement and comparison. When appropriately defined and interpreted, the total number of DDD prescribed or sold per 1000 inhabitants and per unit of time may yield an approximate estimate of the number of people or patients in a given population who happen to be treated with a particular drug. (W.H.O. 1979).

For population statistics DDD is expressed per 1000 persons per day, while the concept of DDD per 100 bed-days is used to evaluate or compare the consumption of drugs in or between hospitals. The term bed-day is also a technical expression of measurement and is defined as the average number of patients in the hospital or each ward per day.

The Nordic Council on Medicines has been establishing, since 1975, the DDD for the majority of drugs used in the Nordic countries. It is from this source that the DDD values for acetylsalicylic acid, acetaminophen, d-propoxyphene, morphine, methadone, meperidine and pentazocine have been drawn. For the DDD of dipyrone the values of TRIQUELL et al. have been accepted. The DDD used are set out in Table 1.

In Table 2 the DDD per 100 bed-days consumed in the CSO are compared for the years 1981 and 1982, giving a total of 14,47 and 14,02.

Table 1. Defined daily doses (DDD)

Opioids

Morphine	0,030 g
Meperidine	0,24 g
Methadone	0,025 g
Pentazocine	0,2 g
D-propoxyphene	0,3 g
Codeine	0,24 g
Tilidine oral	0,12 g
Acetylsalicylic Acid	3 g
Acetaminophen	2,5 g
Dipyrone inj.	6 g
Dipyrone oral,rectal	3 g

Table 2. Analgesic use in the CSO.

DDD per 100 bed-days

Analgesic	1981	1982
Morphine	0,01	0,08
Meperidine	1,08	1
Pentazocine	0,17	0,15
D-propoxyphene	0,036	0,031
Codeine	0,076	0,18
Tilidine	0,044	0,037
Salicylates	4,2	3,8
Acetaminophen	0,02	0,28
Dipyrone	6,93	6,92
Assoc.Analgesics	2,07	1,69

The modifications which have taken place may be readily observed from
the aforementioned Table, with an appreciable increase in the consumption
of codeine, morphine and acetaminophen, and a decrease in that of the
salicylates, while that of dipyrone has remained stable.

In order to compare the values obtained and be able to draw some
conclusion, the only data available are those of HARTVIG   et al., who
carried out a five year consumption study at the University Hospital of -
Uppsala (HUU), and those of TRIQUELL   et al . who did a similar study, o-
ver a four year period at the Hospital General of Granollers (HGG). The   -
comparative data are set out in Table 3, in which differences of significance appear, permiting certain conclusions
to be drawn:

a) As regards the narcotics, if the orally
administered DDD were to be added, the HGG
would reach a figure of 4,8 DDD per 100 -
bed-days, while the HUU would increase to
11,5 DDD per 100 bed-days.

b) Acetaminophen shows completely diffe -
rent consumption for the three hospitals. It

Table 3. Comparison of certain values of
DDD per 100 bed-days in three hospitals.

Analgesics	CSO 1981	HGG 1981	HUU 1980
Parent. narcotics	1,26	1,79	7,2
Salicylates	4,2	5,9	2,8
Acetaminophen	0,02	2,35	5,9
Dipyrone	6,93	3,5	–

should be pointed out that, until a few months ago, there was only one o-
rally-administered form for adults on the Spanish market.
c) Dipyrone has not been used for several years in many countries and yet
in Spanish hospitals it is widely employed.
d) More work along these lines will be need to be able to form reliable conclusions and so define the average number of analgesic DDD per 100 bed-days.

MORPHINE RESERVOIRS

So as to demonstate the need for a pain treatment unit to be
opened, a survey was made of all those patients who were referred to the
Neurosurgery Service, due to pain, over a twelve-month period. Table 4 shows
the type and number of surgical operations carried out in this time, 42 of
which correspond to percutaneous rhizotomy for trigeminal neuralgie, and 18
to implantation of morphine reservoirs for intrathecal administration, a
technique that is worth more detailed commentary.

This new method of analgesia by morphine has been made possible
by the discovery of opiate receptors at the medular level. It was first employed experimentally in animals, and subsequently WANG   et al . confirmed
intense, segmentary and long-lasting analgesia in man. Data contributed by
YAKSH, among others, demonstrated that morphine acted not only indirectly,

Table 4. Surgical operations carried out over a twelve-month period for
states of pain.

Percutaneous rhizotomy for trigeminal neuralgie	42
Percutaneous radiofrequency lumbar rhizotomy	6
Implantation of morphine intrathecal reservoirs	18
Implantation of epidural neural stimulators	2
Subtotal resection of sensory root for major trigeminal neuralgie .	5
Trigeminal tractotomy	1
Dorsal root rhizotomy	2
Temporal arteria ligature (Horton's Cefalea)	1
Total	**77**

but also had a direct effect at the medular level.

The first two patients in this present experiment were injected with the dosage of morphine dissolved to 2 ml in physiological saline
solution. For the rest of the patients the formulation indicated by LAZOR-
THES   et al. was used: hyperbaric morphine solution containing 333 mg of
morphine Hydrochloride and 6,66 g of glucose per 100 ml, prepared in ampoules each containing 2 ml.

Administration was by an intradurally derived deposit whose
reservoir was installed in the gluteous region.

Morphine reser-
voirs are used in the treatment of patients with chronic pain secondary to neoplasia in an advanced stage, the characteristics of
which are as set out in
Table 5.

Table 5. Criteria for the placement of a morphine reservoir

- Malignant pain
- Pain developing over more than a month
- Unbearable pain (3 - 4/4)
- Pain in the lower half of the body
- Pain resistent to conventional treatment
- Survival of more than a week and less than six months
- Intrathecal morphine test: greater than twelve hours

The commencement and duration of analgesia are variable, with
the effect beginning to be noted 5 to 10 minutes after intrathecal administration and reaching its maximum analgesic level after 15-20 minutes,
with an approximate duration of from 24 to 36 hours.

The side-effects of the intrathecal morphine are few and in a
very small number of cases make it necessary to withdraw the reservoir. -
Perhaps the most frequent of these is an itching sensation not confined to
the medular segments, but often noticeable in the palate, neck and trunk.
Steroids do not improve this itching, though it may be controlled with
mild antihistamines.

Nausea and vomiting, another of the most frequent side-effects,
is normally controlled with oral metoclopramide.

THE ANALGESIC COMMITTEE

Initially, a neurosurgeon and a clinical pharmacist were responsible for the steps taken and for following up the patients results. Later, a psychiatrist, an anaesthetist and a specialist in internal medicine joined the team, which was recognized by the Hospital Management as the Analgesic Committee, whose functions are those habitually carried out in those Centres where pain units exist (BONICA & BUTLER), and which may be summarised as follows:

- Diagnosis of the cause of pain, if not known.
- Treatment.
- Assistance to Services with patients presenting chronic pain.
- Out-patient treatment.
- Teaching and informing health workers inside and outside the hospital.
- Epidemiological, pharmacological and technical research.

To discharge these functions within the hospital, all the consultations requested by the Clinical Services, and the subsequent follow-up of patients, are carried out; information sheets are published; there are on-going studies of the utilization and consumption of analgesics,and the progress of patients undergoing treatment is evaluated fortnightly.

Outside the hospital, one day a week is devoted to out-patient consultations; written information on methods and precautions to be observed during treatment is sent to the physicians who will attend the patient once at home and informational sessions with out-patient medical personnel are envisaged.

REFERENCES

BONICA J J, BUTLER S H (1978). The management and function of pain centres. In Swerdlow M (ed.), Relief of Intractable Pain. Chapter 3.
HARTVIG P et al. (1982). The influence of a Hospital Drug Committee's recommendations on the use of analgesics as evaluated by drug-use data. J. Clin. Hosp. Pharm. 7: 161-167.
LAZORTHES Y et al. (1980). Analgésie par injection intrathécale de morphine. Neurochirurgie 26: 159-164.
NORDIC COUNCIL ON MEDICINES (1975). Drug dose statistics. List of Defined Doses for Drugs Registered in Norway. Oslo.
TRIQUELL LL et al. (1983). Changes in analgesics patterns. Progress in Clinical Pharmacy V. Cambridge University Press.
WANG J K et al. (1979). Pain Relief by Intrathecally Applied Morphine in Man. Anesthesiology 50: 149-151.
WHO (1979). Studies in Drug Utilization, Methods and Application. Regional Publications. European Series, 8. Copenhague.
YAKSH T L (1981). Spinal Opiate Analgesia: Characteristics and Principles of Action. PAIN 11: 293-346.

MONITORING OF PRESCRIPTION PATTERNS IN DISTRICT MEDI_CINE BY A·DRUG INFORMATION SYSTEM (SIF-USL)

N. Martini, L. Castellani, G. Scroccaro, and L. Bozzini
Hospital Pharmacy Service - Borgo Roma - Verona, Italy

INTRODUCTION

In 1980 the Italian Parliament approved the law which institu_tes the NHS, whose main feature is the decentralization of the health ca-re organization, via the institution in the 20 italian regions of local health councils, named Unità Sanitarie Locali (USL).

With respect to the pharmaceutical sector, almost all USL have instituted a specific service to coordinate and control drug related activities and assistance.

In order to control drug expenditure and to provide educatio-nal programs, a drug information system specifically for local health co_uncils has been implemented; this system, called SIF-USL (Sistema Informa_tivo Farmaci per le Unità Sanitarie Locali), is substantially based on the intensive computerized monitoring of drug prescriptions in a clearly defined area and with respect to a known population, for administrative and epidemiological use (Andreani, Fiorica et al., 1983).

Three major reasons stress the relevance of a tool like the SIF-USL:
- the continuous and impressive increase in total drug expenditure in the last few years in Italy;
- the existence of important differences in drug use and drug expenditure across similar situations;
- the necessity to bridge the administrative and medical aspects of drug use by combining educational programs and expenditure surveillance.

This paper presents some preliminary results obtained by pre-scriptions monitoring in the USL n° 25 of the Regione Veneto, whose popu-lation is approximately 300.000 and is served by 76 community pharmacies and by 340 doctors (891 inhabitants/doctor).

DESCRIPTION OF THE SYSTEM AND PRELIMINARY RESULTS

Input procedures: the SIF-USL system includes the standard in_put of the following drug prescription data: pharmacy code - patient's identification - prescribing doctor and drug trade name. The prescrip-tions monitoring can be made monthly on total drug prescriptions or on samples for selected periods of time.

The data presented here are derived from the input of all drug prescriptions (993.518) in the period January-March 1983.

Output programs: the key-feature of the SIF-USL system is the linkage of the file of pharmaceutical products (with their administrative -oriented coding) with two files which have been created and are updated to provide the translation of the products and prescription codes into the names of the active principles, therapeutic class(es) and defined dai ily doses (DDD) of each active principle (or their combinations).

The various types of output programs run by SIF-USL system are:
- Program 1: identification of general prescription parameters and control of administrative data;
- Program 2: analysis of drug prescriptions by therapeutic class (es) and group(s);
- Program 3: analysis of drug prescriptions by active principles;
- Program 4: analysis of drug prescriptions by therapeutic group and acti ve principle;
- Program 5: identification of prescription parameters and drugs prescribed by each doctor.

TABLE I: Incidence of various therapeutic classes on total drug expenditu re and prescriptions (January - March 1983)

THERAPEUTIC CLASSES	% ON TOTAL EXPENDITURE	% ON TOTAL PRESCRIPTIONS
Antibiotics	15.4	12.9
Antiulcer agents	7.6	1.5
"Vasodilators"	6.6	4.8
NSAID	5.5	5.9
Topical preparations	5.3	8.3
Mucolytic agents	4.5	5.8
Hypotensive agents	4.4	3.5
Hormones	4.1	3.0
"Tonics"	3.6	3.8
Antiplatelets drugs	2.7	1.4
Liver cell "protectors"	2.7	2.6
"Central neutrophics"	2.4	0.7
Vitamins	2.4	4.5
"Peripheral neutrophics"	1.8	0.8
Antilipemic drugs	1.6	0.7
Diuretics	1.5	2.5
Antianginal agents	1.4	1.6
Analgesics-Antipyretics	1.4	2.8
"Thymus extracts"	1.4	0.1
Antidepressants	1.3	1.4
Spasmolytics	1.2	2.1
Antiemetics	1.1	1.2
Others	20.1	28.1
	100.0	100.0

TABLE II: The 20 drugs mostly incident on total drug expenditure (January
         - March 1983)

	% ON TOTAL EXPENDITURE	% ON TOTAL PRESCRIPTIONS
1. Ranitidine	5.8	0.8
2. Citicoline	2.4	0.7
3. Flunarizine	2.2	0.5
4. Calcitonin	2.1	0.3
5. Cefuroxime	2.0	1.1
6. Ticlopidine	1.5	0.2
7. Tymostimoline	1.3	0.1
8. Naproxen	1.3	0.8
9. Gangliosides	1.3	0.3
10. Ambroxol	1.2	0.9
11. Amoxicillin	1.2	1.1
12. Diclofenac	1.0	0.8
13. Ursodeoxycholic ac.	0.9	0.2
14. Cimetidine	0.9	0.2
15. Dipyridamole	0.9	1.0
16. Co-trimoxazole	0.9	1.2
17. Fosfomycin	0.9	0.2
18. Vitamins	0.9	1.6
19. Dihydroergotoxine	0.8	1.1
20. Atenolol	0.7	0.3
	30.2	13.4

TABLE III: Incidence of expenditure (%) and exposure (DDD/1000 inhabi-
          tants/day) (January - March 1983) for antibiotics

	% ON TOTAL EXPENDITURE	DDD/1000 INHABITANTS/DAY
Cephalosporins	34.3	2.15
Penicillins	11.8	5.11
Aminoglycosides	11.3	0.23
Sulfonamides + Trimethoprim	5.8	3.60
Urinary antiseptics	5.6	2.06
Others	31.2	- -
	100.0	13.15

TABLE IV: Incidence of expenditure (%) and prescription (%) (January – March 1983) for some questionable and/or useless drugs

VASODILATOR AGENTS	% ON TOTAL EXPENDITURE	% ON TOTAL PRESCRIPTIONS
Flunarizine	34.4	10.2
Dihydroergotoxine	13.0	25.2
Suloctidil	10.2	4.4
Nicergoline	8.1	6.6
Pentoxifylline	6.0	4.0
Vincamine	5.5	4.4
Buflomedil	4.0	2.7
Others	17.9	42.5
	100.0	100.0

"ORGAN – EXTRACTS"	% ON TOTAL EXPENDITURE	% ON TOTAL PRESCRIPTIONS
Thymus extract	38.3	4.6
Cortex extract ± other sustances	15.7	21.8
Liver extract ± other sustances	12.7	36.9
Liver and cortex extract ± other sustances	24.6	22.4
Others	8.4	14.3
	100.0	100.0

"TONICS"	% ON TOTAL EXPENDITURE	% ON TOTAL PRESCRIPTIONS
Carnitine + Vit. B12	13.8	6.1
Asparginine	9.6	11.0
Phosphoserine + Phosphotreonine + other sustances	8.1	6.7
Pyrisuccideanol	6.7	2.1
Piracetam	5.4	3.9
Protein hydrolysates + other sustances (os)	6.7	8.2
Others	49.7	62.0
	100.0	100.0

DISCUSSION AND CONCLUSIONS

The importance of outputs which tabulate consumption, cost and prescription patterns by active principles and therapeutic classes, should be underlined as a very simple idea, but rarely used.

DDDs file is a further step in evaluating some drugs as tracers of problems in the community and to identify the fraction of the population exposed to a specific treatment (Andrew, 1982).

By examining the incidence of various therapeutic classes on total drug expenditure and prescriptions (Table I) and by the analysis of active principles prescribed (TABLE II), it can be recognized that: the 56.5% of total drug expenditure accounts for drugs with well-established therapeutic value; the 16.1% accounts for drugs with controversial therapeutic efficacy and 27.4% concerns drugs for which no adequate controlled clinical trials exist, supporting their clinical value.

On the italian market, as in the majority of western european countries (Spain, France and West Germany), a very large number of trade names and fixed combinations is present; besides some completely useless or obsolete products are still being prescribed (TABLE IV), although these drugs have long been withdrawn from the market in many countries. Very similar patterns of drug prescriptions are recently reported from Spain (Laporte, Porta et al. 1983).

Combining drug code with prescribing doctor's code of drug prescriptions, is possible to identify the "therapeutic profile" for each doctor, in terms of general prescription indexes, active principles prescribed and corresponding therapeutic classes. These "therapeutic profiles" are monthly issued to each doctor by a specific therapeutic Committee of the USL n° 25, which controls the data obtained and plans educatio nal programs.

REFERENCES

Andreani A, Colombo F, Fiorica E, Mandelli M, Mosconi P, Tognoni G, Bozzi ni L, Martini N. A drug information system (SIF-USL) for admi nistrative and epidemiological use. 1983; in press.

Laporte J-R, Porta M, Capella D. Drug utilization studies: a tool for determining the effectiveness of drug use. Br J Clin Pharmacol 1983; 16: 301-4.

Andrew M. Drug utilization statistics: a review. In: Progress in clinical pharmacy IV, eds. Ostino G, Martini N, Van der Kleijn E. Else vier Biomedical Press. 1982; 95-106.

USE OF AEROSOLS IN THE GRANOLLERS GENERAL HOSPITAL
IMPORTANCE OF THE PATIENT'S TRAINING

PARDO,C., MAS,M.P., AGUSTI,C., SAGALES,M.
Granollers General Hospital. Pharmacy Service. Granollers.
Barcelona. Spain

INTRODUCTION

The drugs administered by means of inhalers make up one of the main basis in the patient's treatment with such a type of pathology as asthma or chronic obstructive pulmonary disease. Some of reasons why they are so widely prescribed are the comfort in administering it, and a lower incidence of adverse effects when using this type of administration(DUKES M.N.G. 1980), getting therapeutic effects similar to other routes.

We can find studies in which the therapeutic efficiency of the bronchodilator drugs administered by inhalation is very much related to the usage technique (OREHEK,J. 1976) (SHIM,C. 1980). The correct usage of inhalers implies the knowledge of a relatively simple technique. But curiosly it has been demostrated (GOADY,T.J. 1976)(EARIS,J.E. 1978)(AGUSTI A.G.N. et al 1983) that there is a high number of patients who use the spray incorrectly. Due to the importance of the administration technique a variety of programmes have been studied, so as to find the most comfortable and efficient method, having tested the efficacy in all of them (DARR,M.S. 1981) (ROBERTS,R.J. 1982) (O'BEY,K. 1982).

MATERIAL AND METHODS

A group of patients admitted to Granollers General Hospital was studied. All of them were inhalers users. The period studied lasted from the 1st of April to the 15th August 1983.

Two pharmacists were in charge of the study. They interviewed the patients,studying whether they had been taught how to use the spray while being in Hospital, or in an out patient's clinic, and who had been the person in charge of teaching them the technique of administration. The technique of inhaler administration was studied too.

To value the technique of administration the patients had to take the drug as they usually did, without giving them any kind of information. Four points were analyzed according to the instructions written in the patient package insert of the drug (Ventolin® patient package inserts. Lab. Glaxo). Table I.

---

1. POSITION OF THE MOUTHPIECE IN THE MOUTH

2. DEEP EXPIRATION BEFORE INHALATION

3. INHALATION

4. MAINTENANCE OF THE APNEA FOR 15-30 SECONDS

Table I.- Aspects to be considered in the correct use of inhalers

In the cases where the technique had been incorrectly done after the first administration, the patients had to be taught orally, putting emphasis on the mistakes they had made. The technique was revalued the next day using the technique previously described, for a maximum of 3 days.

RESULTS AND DISCUSSION

Forty-six patients have been studied, 28 of them (60.8%) were men and 18 (39.2%) women. Two groups were made according to the use of the inhalers technique. 30 patients (65%) used the inhaler incorrectly, and 16 (35%) correctly. These figures are similar to the ones found by Agusti et ál (AGUSTI, A.G.N. et al 1983) in a research performed in a hospital geographically very close to ours, having found in this case that 61% of patients did it incorrectly and 39% correctly. The average age of the patients in the groups previously described was sixty years in both cases. The patients were asked about who had prescribed the inhalers and who had taught them how to use them. In Table II are presented the results of the patients who were seen in outpatient clinics and in Table III those of hospitalized patients.

It should be pointed out that in the community environment, the physician is the person who usually assumes the patient's formative function. It should be said as well, that in two patients with a wrong technique, no-one had trained them before. In another four patients with a wrong technique, two patients had followed the patient package insert alone, in the other two they had followed it with the support of a physician.

From studying the hospital environment we find that the nurse and the physician usually train the patient.

The period during which patients had been taking inhaled drugs was studied. In the group of patients with incorrect technique was a prevalence of patients who had been taking it for less than a year (34%) and 47% had been taking it for 3,4,5 or more years (Figure 1).

	CORRECT TECHNIQUE	%	WRONG TECHNIQUE	%	TOTAL
PHYSICIAN	5	(28)	13	(72)	18
NURSE	0	(0)	2	(100)	2
PATIENT PACKAGE INSERT	1	(20)	4	(80)	5
OTHERS	0	(0)	1	(100)	1
NOBODY	0	(0)	2	(100)	2
	6	(21)	22	(79)	28

Table II. Method used to train the out patients in the use of inhalers.

	CORRECT TECHNIQUE	%	WRONG TECHNIQUE	%	TOTAL
PHYSICIAN	6	(75)	2	(25)	8
NURSE	4	(36)	7	(64)	11
PATIENT PACKAGE INSERT	0	(0)	1	(100)	1
OTHERS	0	(0)	1	(100)	1
NOBODY	0	(0)	0	(0)	0
	10	(48)	11	(52)	21

Table III. Method used to train the hospitalized patient in the use of inhalers.

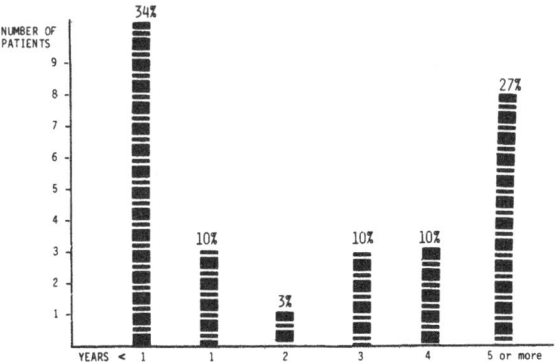

Figure 1. The period during which patients with incorrect technique had been taking inhaled drugs.

Analyzing the group of patients who used the inhaler incorrect
ly (Figure 2) we can see that the most repetitive mistakes were the lack
of synchronization between inhalation and pressing the canister [(20 patients (30%)] and the lack of previous expiration before inhalation more
over, not keeping the apnea the adequate time after inhaling happened in
14 cases (22% of patients).

These data will suggest the necessity to put more emphasis on
the greatest problematic stages. 70% of patients made more than one mista
ke simultaneously and only 30% made a single mistake.

After the educational process developped by the pharmacists,
(Figure 3), it was noticed that 47% of patients acquired a correct techni
que in the first day, 33% after the second day an 7% in the third day.

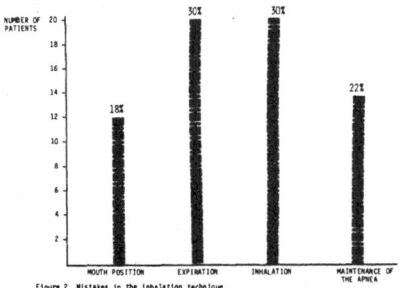

Figure 2. Mistakes in the inhalation technique.

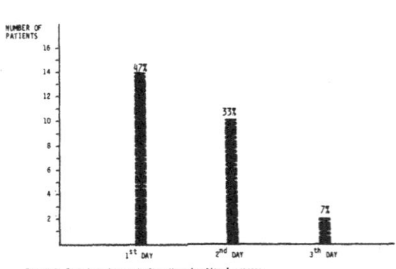

Figure 3. Technique improved after the educational process.

Only one case (3%) patients was unable to improve the technique after 3 days of training. It is important to point out that a greater
number of sessions are necessary in order to achieve an acceptable techni
que thought there's a wide group which improves highly after the first vi
sit.

CONCLUSIONS

Inhaled drugs are widely used in our environment, though usually in a wrong way.

It is necessary to put emphasis on the training practice in or
der to avoid this problem, buy using more sophisticated methods in the ca
se of patients who are difficult to be trained.

In order to get the maximum therapeutic yield of inhaled drugs,
both, the community and the Hospital Pharmacists have the opportunity to

collaborate with physicians and nurses due to their optimal situation to carry out this function because they keep strongly in touch with the patients.

REFERENCES

AGUSTI,A.G.N. et al (1983). Asma bronquial y broncodilatadores en aerosol: empleo incorrecto en nuestro medio. Servei de Pneumologia i Al-lergia Respiratoria, Hospital Clínic i Provincial. Facultat de Medicina. Universitat de Barcelona (in press).

DARR,M.S. et al (1981). Content and retention evaluation of and audiovisual patient-education program on bronchodilators. American Journal of Hospital Pharmacy. $\underline{38}$: 672-675.

DUKES,M.N.G. (1980). Meyler's side effects of drugs. Editor: Dukes,M.N.G., Griffin,J.P. Excerpta Medica. 9 th ed. pp. 222-225. Amsterdam.

EARIS,J.E., BERNSTEIN,A. (1978). Misuse of pressurised nebulisers. British Medical Journal, $\underline{1}$: 1554.

GOADY,T.J., STEWART,C.J. (1976). Use of pressurised aerosols by asthmatic patients. British Medical Journal, $\underline{1}$: 833.

O'BEY, K. et al (1982). An education program that improves the psychomotor skills needed for metaproterenol inhaler use. Drug Intelligence and Clinical Pharmacy. $\underline{16}$: 945-948.

OREHEK, J. et al (1976). Patient error in use of bronchodilator by asthmatic patients. British Medical Journal. $\underline{1}$: 833.

ROBERTS, R.J. et al (1982). A comparison of various types of patient instruction in the proper administration of metered inhalers. Drugs Intelligence and Clinical Pharmacy. $\underline{16}$: 53-59.

SHIM,C., WILLIAMS,H. (1980). The adequacy of inhalation of aerosol from Canister Nebulizers. The American Journal of Medicine. $\underline{69}$: 891-894.

Ventolin® patient package inserts. Lab. Glaxo.

EXPERIENCE OF CLINICAL PHARMACY IN COMMUNITY PHARMACY

Coordinator: Serra,J. Medical Adviser: Sanchis,J.
Authors: Blanchart,M. Alvareda,A. Balcells,R. Barabad,L. Blanca,J. Creus,J
Esteban,M. Figueras,X. Fontanet,J. Fuentemilla,E. Fuentemilla,M. Garcia,A.
Garrabou,M. Grau,G. Jordana,J. Manet,D. Martí,M. Martinez,M. Masdeu,M. Mo-
ya,A. Pardell,P. Pau,T. Pereita,M. Suades,J. Troiano,R. Torres,L. Vidal,D.
Col.legi de Farmacéutics de Barcelona
Continous Education Program. Coordinator: Dr J. Bonal

INTRODUCTION AND OBJECTIVES

In October 1982, a seminar on "Clinical Pharmacy in Community
Pharmacy" was offered in Sabadell. This seminar was a part of the continuing education program that the Society of Pharmacists of Barcelona is
offering to members from 1981.

As a consequence of this seminar a working group was organized
in order to start some practical aplication of Clinical Pharmacy in community pharmacy.

The objective proposed was to study the pharmacological treatment of the patients with chronic obstructive pulmonary disease(COPD). A
ten hours previous course on pathophysiology and treatment of COPD was given to the participants in the study.

The objectives of the study designed were as follows:
- To know in   these patients.   with COPD the drugs used
  for their treatment.
- To identify the dose used of bronchodilators drugs (beta-
  - sympatomimetics and theophylline) and corticosteroids by
  this patients.
- To stimulate the development of these type of studies through
  community pharmacies.

MATERIAL AND METHOD

27 Community Pharmacists who practice their profession in the
"Vallés Occidental", area took-part in this study.

All of these had undergone a course of physiopathology and
treatment of the respiratory illness mentioned before. The project was
coordinated by a hospital pharmacist with experience in studies on drug
utilization and by a physician specialized in pulmonary care. A protocol
was designed to perform such study. The protocol included the concept of

chronic obstructive pulmonary disease, inclusion and exclusion criteria, a
questionnaire to collected data on semiology and treatment and others in
order to know the administration techniques used by patients.

The questionnaire was filled up by the community pharmacists
after a personal interview with the patients accepted for the study.

The length of the study was three months. 50 out of 56 completed questionnaires fullfil the requirements to be included in the study.

RESULTS

The characteristics of the sample were as shown in Table I.

TABLE I - CHARACTERISTICS OF THE SAMPLE							
SEX		AVERAGE	SYMPTOMATOLOGY			PATIENT CONTROLLED BY	
M	F	AGE	LIGHT	MODERATE	SEVERE	GENERAL PRACT.	SPECIALIST
32	18	53.4	13	13	24	12	38

No difference was noticed between the patients treated by general practitioners and specialists in term of severity and symptomatology.

45 patients used a beta-sympathomimetic drug, 38 used theophylline and 34 of them used both bronchodilators together.

The use of beta-sympathomimetics is show in table II.

TABLE II - USE OF BETA-SYMPATHOMIMETICS IN A SAMPLE OF 45 PATIENTS					
DRUG USED				DOSAGE	
SALBUTAMOL	OTHERS	NOT ASSOCIATED	ASSOCIATED	IRREGULAR	CONVENT:
41	4	41	4	15	30

39 of these patients used the beta-sympathomimetic by inhalation and 6 in oral form. Two patients used the beta-sympathomimetic by
both ways.

The associations of beta-sympathomimetic with other drugs in
the same dosage form were classified in 2 cathegories:

- hazardous association: those containing corticosteroids, an
tibiotics or sulphonamides.

- Not advisable associations: those containing tranquillizers,
expectorants or mucolytics.

Three patients received hazardous combination compounded
as a formula in a community pharmacy.

The use of theophylline is shown in table III.

TABLE III - THE USE OF THEOPHYLLINE					
N	USE A DRUG PRODUCT NOT ASSOC.	ASSOC.	USE TWO DRUG PRODUCTS WITH THEOPHYLLINE	ADM. TECHNIQUE IRREGUL.	CONVENT
38	13	18	7	17	21

The association with other drugs classified as hazardous or
not advisable as has been defined above, gave the following result:

Hazardous association of theophylline: 8 patients.

Not advisable association of theophylline: 17 patients.

The administratien technique have been classified as irregular
and conventional or theoretically correct. Never the less none of those 38
patients were under pharmacokinetic control.

25 out of 50 patients studied used some corticosteroid. The
use of corticosteroids is shown in Table IV.

TABLE IV - USE OF CORTICOSTEROIDS		
PATIENTS N	USE CORTICOSTEROID NOT ASSOCIATED	USE CORTICOSTEROID ASSOCIATED
25	16	9

Four of the patients took two corticosteroids simultaneously
and one of the patients received slow release one preparation by intramuscularly.

Corticosteroids by inhalation were used by 11 patients. The

use of corticosteroids associated were considered hazardous in all cases.

The self-administration of the inhalers and syrups is shown in tables V and VI.

TABLE V - THE SELF-ADMINISTRATION OF THE INHALERS						
PATIENTS	USE		INFORMATION OBTAINED THROUGH			
N	CORRECT.	INCORRECT	PHYS.	PHARMACIST	NURSE	NO ONE
41	26	15	33	1	2	5

Only 26 out of 36 patients that received information used the inhaler correctly.

TABLE VI - USE OF SYRUPS		
PATIENTS	USE SOME KIND OF MEASURE	
N	YES	NO
19	13	6

DISCUSSION

All drugs taken by the patients in the study were prescribed.

Looking at the use of beta-sympatomimetics, we can observe that drugs are relativelly well prescribed and used. However the irregular dosification of these drugs in 1/3 of the patients indicate a poor compliance with the prescriptions.

Observing the use of theophylline 25 patients received preparations of theophylline associated. In 8 of those patients this association could be ·considered hazardous association, and seven (18.4 %) out of 38 patients who were taking theophylline, used two products with theophylline simultaneously. Seventeen patients (44.7 %) took the theophylline irregularly and no pharmacokinetic control was used in any case.

The use of corticosteroids indicates a poor quality of the

prescriptions. 9 patients (36 %) received corticosteroids associated to other drugs, four patients received 2 corticosteroids simultaneously and one patient received an slow release preparation I.M. definitely dangerous in this kind of pathology.

Regarding the techniques used in the administration, 15 patients (36.6 %) using inhalers did it incorrectly despite the fact that 36 patients (87.8 %) were informed about the correct use by some health professionnal.

This indicates that this information was not enough or not well understood by the patient. Five patients (12.2 %) who were not infor med, used the inhalers incorrectly.

Is also important to point out that among the patients who used syrups, 6 of them (31 %) did not use any equipment to measure the dose which makes impossible a correct administration of such products.

CONCLUSIONS

The availability in the market of associations containing beta-sympatomimetics bronchodilators, theophylline and/or corticosteroids with other drugs induce a confusion in estabishing rational treatments in COPD.

Admitting as correct the not advisable associations, only 21 (42%) of the patients under study could be considered within recomended rational therapy at present. The remaining 58 % follows an irrational and even hazardous treatment.

This study show that there is a poor patient drug information about the self-administration of inhalers and syrups.

This study also shows the possibility to carry out similar studies through the community pharmacists. Such studies are essential to improve therapeutic habits.

The Clinical Interview: Patient Contact and
Information Gathering

I. Ponjaert-Kristoffersen, J. Klerckx (Dept of
Genetic Psychology)
H.De Clercq (Pharmacy Services), Vrije
Universiteit Brussel,
Laarbeeklaan 101 - 1090 Brussel (Belgium)

1. Introduction

It is generally accepted in behavioural sciences that all
human behaviour is function on one hand of the individual, on the other
hand of the environment. The patient (individual) is ill, which presumes
a physical disequilibrium. As a result, psychological stresses arise
such as restlessness, fear, depression, despair or agression. Additional-
ly, the patient is undergoing an unfamilar experience in a strange
environment that is governed by a strange set of customs. The hospital
setting as such has little security to offer to the patient, neither
materially (unfamiliar hospital bed, rooms and hallways that look all
alike) nor socially (nursing personnel, medical staff). This patient's
confusion can however be minimized by clearly describing the structure
of his hospital setting. This presumes, among other things, that the
patient clearly understands who of the staff is in charge of which duties.
This is fundamental to effective patient interviewing, just as clarity
is the basic rule of the clinical interview, from pharmacist to patient
as well as from patient to pharmacist.

2. Patient Contact

Patient contact is the first step in the interview. As said
before, the interviewer should be certain that positive identification
of the interview situation and of the role of the interviewing pharmacist
have been established between both participants. The interviewing
pharmacist must demonstrate, without asserting, that he knows what he is
doing and that he is in control (1).
2.1. The interview situation
2.1.1. Interviewer's identification
The interviewing pharmacist explicitely identifies himself
to the patient by indicating his name, function and assignment in the
hospital. The assignment's description is brief and to the point,
without excess of technical details and in such a manner that the
patient has a clear picture of the pharmacist's role in the structure
of medical care.
2.1.2. Purpose of the interview
The interviewer explicitly states the reason for his coming:
for instance acquisition of medication history; discussion of current
therapy; or counseling regarding proper home use of prescribed medications.
2.1.3. Length of interview time
The patient is informed of the approximate length of interview time and of the possibility to stop the interview at any time.

Furthermore, a few additional minutes should be provided at the closing
of the interview. Some patients never stop experiencing the interview
situation as threatening and won't calm down before the actual closing
of the interview. During these few additional minutes, the patients
will often provide a lot of interesting information that may well be at
least as valuable as the information aimed at during the interview.

2.1.4. Outline of the patient's future
The interviewing pharmacist guarantees the patient that, if
wanted, his drug therapy will be monitored.

2.1.5. Additional questions by the patient
After this introduction, time has come for additional
questions by the patient on the interviewer or on the design of the
interview. This is necessary in order to check whether the patient has
properly understood the interviewer's introduction.

2.1.6. Registration method
The use of a tape recorder as registration method for
information gathering is to be preferred in an explorative survey : there
is no loss of information, and this method allows the interviewer to
evaluate his own interview technique after the interviews are done. However, a double disadvantage counts against this method : for one thing
the information recorded has to be written down afterwards, for the
other the patient's spontaneity can be inhibited by the presence and
use of a tape recorder.
The written recording method saves time, but the loss of
information in explorative survey is tremendous. The interviewer usually
writes down what seems important to him, and not necessarily to the
patient.

2.2. Behaviour of the interviewing pharmacist
Clarity is the basic rule of the clinical interview. This
applies not only to the interview situation as described above, but
also to the behaviour of the interviewer in the interview situation (2).

2.2.1. Patient approach
In the interview situation, the patient can be approached in
two different ways. The first one is to regard the patient merely in
function of what is expected from the relation with the patient, for
instance when interviewing a patient in order to collect a comprehensive
medication history. Such a relation is functional and somewhat imper-
sonal, but certainly clear. Both participants know what to expect from
each other. Similar relations are very common in every day situations,
e.g. professional relations between colleagues at an office.
In the second type of relation contact, the patient is
approached as an entity with various individual aspects. Taking the
former example again, the office colleague would also be known for his
part as a father, as a husband, as a tennisplayer ...
The first, more functional type of relations is   preferred
in clinical approach to the patient; it distinctly pictures all parts
and expectations of the interview situation, and will keep probability of
role conflict to a minimum.
Should the patient insist on introducing topics out of the
scope of the interview or engage a discussion on diagnosis or prognosis,
than the interviewer ought to refer him immediately to his physician or
to the responsible members of the apropriate staff.

2.2.2. The interviewer's attitude
Professional attitude is an essential component of an effective interviewer and includes also attention to dress, hygiene,

grooming, language and behaviour.
     The attitude is reflected in both verbal and non-verbal
communication (2).
     Unexperienced interviewers may present contradictory verbal
and non-verbal attitudes; e.g. standing straight at the patient's
bedside or continously watching the clock, but all in one trying to
reassure the patient to continue quietly. Furthermore, disapproving and
critical looks or expressions should be avoided.
     2.2.3. Equality in the interview situation
     The interviewer should bear in mind that both participants,
the interviewer and the patient, are reciprocally equal in the interview
situation. This can only be achieved by an attitude that reflects concern
for the patient's position in the hospital : the hospital and its staff
are at the service of the patient and not the other way around.

3. Information gathering

     The first step in the interview is to enter in relation with
the patient; this relation is characterized by clarity and cooperation.
     The second step is the actual information gathering;
characteristics are now quantity and quality of the information obtained.
     3.1. Patient's identity.
     The interviewer posseses all necessary identification data
before entering the patient's room. Prior to any dialogue with the
patient, the pharmacist should develop a systematic approach to the
course of the interview. He should have a general idea of the questions
to be asked and their sequence; preferably, he knows the questions by
heart.
     3.2. Open and closed questions
     The phrasing of questions is a very important technique of
effective interviewing. The interviewer may use open or closed questions.
Closed questions can be answered adequately in just a few words, whereas
open questions require more than that for proper answering.
     Closed questions come in different types :
- identification type, concerning the patient's identity :
e.g. What is your name ? How long have you been working ?
Where do you live ?
- selection type, offering fixed - alternative questions in which the
patient has to select one from two or more possible responses :
e.g. Do you take MOGADON or TEMESTA ?
- questions of the yes/no type, to be answered adequately by yes or no.
e.g. If I understood you correctly, you have been admitted to the
hospital for two days now ?
     In exploring any issue, the inquiry should always start with
open, non-directive questions, reserving more direct, closed questions
to clarify ambiguities or verify facts. Clarity is the basic rule of the
interview. Therefore it is recommended to start off the interview with
open-ended questions rather than yes/no direct questions. In function
of the patient's answer, additional specific closed questions are used.
     A question or subject is finished as soon as the answer
provided is clear and to the point. This implicates full understanding
from the interviewer of all the answers as well as active listening to
what the patient is telling.
     3.3. Active listening
     A truly effective interviewer must be an " active " listener.

Listening, rather than talking, will provide the climate in which the
patient can communicate. To clarify ambiguities and in order to verify
whether he understood all answers correctly, the interviewer has
various verification techniques at his disposal :
        - Extension : a request for new information related to
something already said.
e.g. You just told me you take sleeping pills.
What is their name ?
        - Echo : An exact or nearly exact repetition by the inter-
viewer of the patient's words.
e.g. Pat. " I take only aspirin "
     Int. " Only aspirin ?"
        Echo functions as an encouragement, creating the impression
that the interviewer is interested in all the patient has to say. It
should be employed whenever one feels by the non-verbal attitude of the
patient that he has more information to offer.
        - Clarification : a direct request for information on a
vague or ambiguous prior part of the interview.
e.g. You just mentioned hypertension.
What is hypertension ?
        - Summary : a question which summarizes information pre-
viously stated.
e.g. If I understood you correctly, you have never been ill before.
Did you ever take medication before you broke your leg ?
        The summary is used to close down a subject, or as transition
from one subject to another. The summary allows the patient to order his
thoughts.
        The summary is a question of the closed type, calling mostly
for a yes.
        If necessary, the patient may insist upon a correction.
        - Confrontation : a question in which the interviewer pre-
sents the patient with an inconsistency between two or more of the
patient's statements.
e.g. You've just told me sleeping pills are harmful, but here at the
hospital you take one every night ?
        Confrontation reinforces the validity of the information,
but too frequent use of this technique irritates the patient.
        - Repetition : a question which merely repeats the question
previously asked. Repetition is necessary when the patient didn't
understand or has misinterpreted the question (which is often the result
of complicated or indistinct phrasing of the question by the interviewer).
        3.4. Interviewer's vocabulary and syntaxis
        Both interviewer's vocabulary and syntaxis reflect everyday
speech. Please no " pharmacist's talk ", but terms familiar to the
patient.
        3.5. Silences in the interview
        Silences by the patient in response to questions may embar-
ras the interviewer and thus complicate the interview   and are
attributable to a number of factors :
- they set the patient thinking if all has been said.
- they allow the patient to order his thoughts.
- they encourage the patient to continue on a particular issue.
        Brief silences of 3 to 9 seconds (3) generally reflect a
patient's attempt to recall a fact. Prolonged silence of more than 15
seconds (3) or repeated silences areoften due to faulty technique on

the part of the interviewer and may create tension in the relation.

After a brief silence, the patient will eventually continue on the same issue or else state he has nothing to add.

Proper behaviour by the interviewer is simply to wait expectantly and indicate by facial expression or verbally that he wishes the patient to continue. The interviewer may also use the summary technique or change the subject (e.g. when the patient starts crying).

Immediate interference from the interviewer may reduce the patient's spontaneity especially when the interviewer needlessly changes the subject merely to keep the conversation going.

3.6. Transition from one topic to another

The interviewer changes subject when sufficient information has been gathered, i.e. the answer responds to the purpose of the question and the information obtained is clear to the interviewer. Change of subject is also apropriate when the patient has no information to add, or if a particular subject frightens the patient. Change of subject is not used to break silences or to keep the conversation going.

To obtain fluent change of subjects, the interviewer will preferably refer to something the patient mentioned before and which is related to the next subject to be introduced. By doing so, the interviewer proves again he actively listens to the patient.

Finally, summarizing of the information previously stated is another, equally appropriate way to change subject.

3.7. Suggestive questions.

The use of suggestive questions is - in general - to be avoided because they influence the patient's response and because the question's content could reflect the interviewer's expectations. A suggestive question is based on a presumption that is not supported by sound information or experiences.

e.g. Are you happy now you don't use tranquillizers any more ?

Social desirability will force the patient to reply affirmatively although the interviewer still doesn't know whether the patient is really happy with this decision or not.

4. Closing of the interview

In bringing the interview to a close, it is good practice to give the patient an opportunity to mention anything else he may have on his mind that pertains to drug therapy. Also, if the interviewer is not clear about a particular point it may be helpful to recapitulate briefly. Occasionally, this post-interview discussion will result in some new piece of pertinent information.

When the interview is completed, the patient should be thanked for his cooperation.

In an explorative survey, e.g. when patients are interviewed to find out their educational needs on drug use, the interviewer will emphasize the importance of the information obtained that may greatly enhance the patient's well-being through proper utilization of drugs.

In a clinical interview, e.g. when patients are interviewed to obtain information on drugs taken previously, drug allergies, adverse effects and medications used at present, the interviewer will concretely agree with the patient upon close monitoring of his future drug therapy course.

5. Application

The various steps of effective patient interviewing discussed above have been applied to a study on self-medication in hospitalized patients at Brussels University Hospital (AZ-VUB). The results of this study will be published later.

6. References

(1) R.E. Froelich : " Understanding the patient : preliminaries to the interview ", in Clinical Pharmacy Practice, ed. C.W. Blisset, O.L. Webb, W.F. Stanaczek, Lea & Febiger, Philadelphia (1972) p. 89 - 96.

(2) T.R. Covington : " Interviewing and advising the patient ", in: Perspectives in Clinical Pharmacy, ed. D.E. Franke, H.A.K. Whitney, Drug Intell Publications Inc., Hamilton Ill. (1972) P. 212 - 228.

(3) H.H. Hyman : " Interviewing in social research ", The University of Chigago Press, Chigago & London (1965).

Recording outpatients drug administration

G.M.W. Konings, Y.A. Hekster, E.A.M. Helling, L.J.B. Zuidgeest and E. van der Kleijn
Department of Clinical Pharmacy, Sint Radboud Hospital,
Catholic University of Nijmegen, Geert Grooteplein Zuid no. 8,
6525 GA Nijmegen, the Netherlands

The St Radboud Hospital in Nijmegen is a University Hospital, with a total number of 965 beds, divided over 40 wards. In 1982, the total number of admissions was 25386 with 299460 hospital days and a bed occupation of 85%. Average admission duration was 12 days. Besides these clinical wards, there are 28 outpatient clinics of different specialisms. The total visits to all outpatient clinics in 1982 was: 391,693. This is an average of about 1600 patients per day.

The charging of drug costs

In the Netherlands expenses for drug costs, hospital admission, etc. are covered for about 70% of the population by Health Insurance companies under the National Health Scheme and for 30% by private insurances.

1. Inpatients

   For National Health Scheme patients the so-called "all-in" rate is used. The Health Insurance compensates a fixed amount for every hospital day related to an average costs figure, yearly determined by negotiation, and based on reference hospitals.

   For the private insured patients the "all-out" rate is used. Such patients receive their bills for the total number of hospital days, all treatments and also for the medication, based upon real costs.

2. Outpatients

   If at a regular outpatient visit, drugs are prescribed by a physician, the patient takes such prescription to his own pharmacy to be filled. In an outpatient treatment setting however, the Health Insurance compensates for some of the used medication.

   The compensated drugs include:

   a. drugs given by injection

   b. drugs not registered in the Netherlands, for which the Health

Authorities have given import authorisation.

c. incidentally prescribed drugs, that are considered not to be supplied by a community pharmacy, after permission of the pharmacist.

Development of Clinical Pharmacy Services and Drug Registra-
tion Procedures

Since 1971 the hospital has successively started with the
following elements that have been described in detail (vd Kleijn, 1976,
Hekster, Zuidgeest et al 1977).

1. Medication Monitoring System

   Every admitted patient has his own "kardexcard" on which every administered drug is registered and accounted for. This offers the possibility for a clear view of what the patient received during the
   hospital-stay. This "kardexcard" can also be used for calculation of
   drug costs for "all-out" patients. This card is sent to the Pharmacy
   after discharge of the patient from the hospital.

2. Medication-trolleys

   Drugs are placed in the medication-trolley per patient for a 24 hours
   period.

3. The Radboud Formulary

   This formulary is a restricted compulsory list of drugs to be used in
   the hospital.

4. Unit Dose System

   This system allows drug identification until administering to the
   patient.

5. Preprinted computer sheets

   This is for ordering and restocking the frequently used drugs on the
   wards.

For the organization development and maintenance of the Clinical Pharmacy
program, several pharmacy-assistants were engaged. The primary tasks of
these assistants is to control the drug supply on the wards. The activities of the "ward-service" department in those years were clearly focussed
at the medical wards. At the outpatient-clinics the only activity was
concerned with the drug control for expiration dates (once or twice a year).
Since at the outpatient clinic the use of drugs increased primarily as
a result of the increase in use of cytostatic drugs and blood fractions
in particular, it was necessary to focus attention to these outpatient

clinics for developing a new form for drug registration and accounting.
The "Kardex system" in use for inpatients was not suitable for outpatient
clinic use, mainly because of ever changing dosages of cytostatic drugs
depending on blood test results.

Routine of drug ordering

The outpatient clinics ordered their drugs in the following
way:
1. formulary drugs are requested via a preprinted computer order sheet
2. the non formulary drugs are requested via a prescription with the
   patients identification data on it, usually for immediate use.

Lists of some frequently used drugs (topics) for instance 5-fluorouracil
were prepared by the nurses. The names of the patients and the given
dosages were recorded, by date, on these lists.

Total prescription survey per patient was prepared using these lists and
dated with the day of preparing the surveys. These prescription surveys
were sent every 3 months to the pharmacy administration office for charging.

Procedure of drug charging

At the administration of the pharmacy department the following
procedure was followed:
1. calculation of the surveys
2. copying the surveys
3. filling out an outpatient-performance note for every prescription
4. sending a copy and the outpatient performance note to the hospital
   financial administration for further accounting and billing.
5. filling dates and costs on a patient-card
6. storing the original card with the total precriptions in an alphabetical sequence. This procedure was very time consuming.

Development of the outpatient medication card

At the end of 1978 a card was developed to overcome these
time consuming activities and to improve drug registration procedures.
On this card the following columns were available for recording of:
- date of administration
- which drug was administered

- the route of administration and the concentration, form and dose
- the initials of the responsible physician, and the nurse, responsible
  for preparing and administering the drug
- costs

At the right side of the card, space is available for identification of
the patient through an identity card.   Also there is space for recording the medical indication (if necessary) and the specialism of the
outpatient clinic. At the bottom a space is reserved for the responsible
physician, to sign. This card was discussed at the outpatient pediatric
oncology unit. In consultation with the physicians and nurses, a start
was made with these cards in February 1979, concomitantly with the opening of the New Pediatric Oncology Centre. Daily, a pharmacy technician
was available on the ward for giving advice how the filling of these
cards be performed. After drug administration and recording the card is
stored in a cardbox in alphabetical order on the unit. Every 3 months the
cards were collected. The pharmacy-administration-office calculated the
costs per line and totalled it. 3 copies of each card were made: two for
the hospital financial administration; one of those two copies was sent
to the Health Insurance or private companies and one remained at the hospital financial administration as a control. One copy was returned to the
outpatient clinic to keep a complete overview of the used drugs. The original remained at the pharmacy. In addition, the total drug costs per patient were shown that would stimulate the recording of all drug items used.

Extending the system

In 1979 several meetings were held with the hospital financial
administration, the Health Insurance scheme officer and the pharmacy to
evaluate the new form of medication registration for outpatient clinics.
The conclusion was positive and it was agreed to continue the system
and to extend it to all the other outpatient clinics. The introduction of
the system on the Internal Medicine outpatient-clinic, was rather difficult, and only possible after long discussions and perseverance. The
support of the new head nurse was very important. They started in June
1980. The Pediatric outpatient clinic started in September 1980, without
problems. A meeting was organized to evaluate the system with the General
headnurse of Internal Medicine, the headnurses of the various outpatient
clinics, the hospital administration and pharmacy. It could be assessed

that the outpatient medicationcard was a success.

Advantages
- the drug use per outpatient is conveniently arranged
- the information per patient is easily retrieved since the patient data
  were stored in the cardbox on alphabetical order
- orderprocedures are simplified, since all items are preprinted on
  computer ordersheets
- individual prescriptions can be omitted
- a written order of the physician is always available

Because every 3 months about 230 cards were received for charging and
since 3 copies per card were needed, the preparation of a card with 3
NCR copies was started. The card was changed to simplify the calculation
of the costs of the used drugs. The right part of the form remained the
same. At the left handside the medicationorder is recorded by a physician
with his initials; next to it (between the black lines) is the part for
the nursing staff: they are responsible for the preparation of the drugs
and they also have to record which compounds to be used for bringing the
compound in its final form. Figure 1 shows the card.

At the end of 1981 the board of directors required that at all outpatient
clinics drug use be recorded on the outpatient medicationcard.

DRUG PREPARATION

In the new outpatient clinic for Internal Medicine a decentralized unit was installed for cytostatic drug compounding under laminair
flow safety cabinet conditions. In this cabinet the nurses prepare the
"adhoc" preparations which are prescribed on the outpatient medicationcard. In addition, the safety measures such as protective clothing and
gloves are used. A training program for the nurses was organized by
pharmacy personnel.

CONCLUSION AND BENEFITS

By means of outpatient medication-cards there is a better
contact and more cooperation with the nurses of the outpatient clinics.
In addition, it allows a better knowledge of drug history per patient
since it gives a clear view of all administered drugs per patient.
There is also more influence from the pharmacy on the method of preparing
the drugs. The nurses are alerted to the care to be taken with cytostatic
drugs and less waste is produced, since the decentralization allows preparation of stock solutions.
The total amount of money that is now paid by the Health Insurance Companies have increased gradually. For 1982, this accounted for $f900.000,--$
(dutch guilders). About 90% of all drugs used at the outpatient clinics
are paid for now. This work shows the benefits of cooperation both from
an economical as a qualitative point of view.

REFERENCES

Hekster, Y.A., Zuidgeest, L.J.B., Hoelen, A.J., Bakker, J.H., and
Van der Kleijn, E., (1977). Management of Hospital Drug Distribution and
    Utilization. In Clinical Pharmacy. E. van der Kleijn and
    R.J. Jonkers (Eds). Elsevier/North Holland Biomedical Press,
    page 79-101.
Van der Kleijn, E., (1976). Methods to establish and monitor individual
    medication profiles and dosage regimens in pharmacotherapy.
    Journal of Clinical Pharmacy 1, 77-105.

IMPLEMENTATION OF THE FIRST REGIONAL DRUG INFORMATION CENTER IN SPAIN

A. Arias González
CADIME, C/. Verónica de la Magdalena, 23, Granada, Spain

G. García Molina
CADIME, C/. Verónica de la Magdalena, 23, Granada, Spain

A. García Iñesta
CINIME, C/. Valenzuela, 3, Madrid, Spain

Abstract.- Hereby there is presented the experience of the creation of the first Regional Drug Information Center (RDIC) in Spain. From the perspective of a National Drug Information Center (DIC) there was needed a more rational distribution of Drug Information (DI), according to the new political-administrative situation in Spain (Autonomous States). In essence, this RDIC has been structured in three action areas: Area of Drug Information, Education Area and Area of Management. The Area of Drug Information has the main purpose of promoting the creation of local DICs, in hospitals and pharmaceutical corporations, in order to constitute a regional network of DICs. On the other hand, the RDIC would serve as a support to the local DICs in order to solve those problems that cannot be answered by the local ones. The Education Area is directly related to the College of Pharmacy and its main purpose is giving classes and courses on DI to students and postgraduates. The Area of Management is directed to be a technical assesment, in the field of the drug, to the health authorities of the region. Within this Area, studies on use of drugs on a regional level, are included.

INTRODUCTION

Before studying the characteristics of the first RDIC in Spain, we will analyse the circumstances that influenced its creation.

On one hand, during the last years there was noted in our country a trend to the appearance of DICs, both on Hospital level and on Pharmaceutical Corporations level, but in an anarchical way, as a "spontaneous generation". Many centers appeared with the objective of having as much as bibliographical sources as possible in order to respond, above all to the questions. There was no uniformity in criteria with regard to minimum basic sources, searching and responding methodology nor a logical framework for good management. In short, there was no coordination, not even any knowledge on the existence of these centers beyond the limits of action of each one of them, hospital, city, etc. Therefore, there was missing a framework of these DICs that would involve a logical staging of the information channels.

On the other hand, the new Spanish autonomous structure facilitated an administrative-geographical framework where to develop a RDIC, in this case Andalusia, which would serve as a stimulus and support to the creation and functioning of some local DICs which would form a regional network of DICs. At the same time, this regional center could be the embryo of the future national network of RDICs.

Furthermore, we were sure, from our point of view of a DIC on a national level, that most questions which were made to and from the diverse centers, could be responded
by the consultants themselves if they have a more or less deep knowledge of the existence
and use of the basic sources of DI, for which it was fundamental to realize an educational
labour, either to last year students or to postgraduates by means of update courses and continuing education.

Finally, in such a reduced geographical field as a region is, there could be
made studies on drug use, in order to contribute to a more rational use of same and because
of that its consumption could be reduced through a coherent policy based upon adequate measures from the autonomous health authorities.

With these premises, the RDIC was structured in three areas of action: Drug
Information Center, Education Area and Pharmaceutical Management Area, which we will describe afterwards, and which logically, are interactive.

DRUG INFORMATION CENTER

In a first stage, the DIC had to be physically created with the purchase of
primary, secundary and tertiary sources necessary to develop functions and services which
would be offered and according to the initial budget we disposed of for this acquirement.

Once the material support was available, an educational program was articu-
lated for the education of the personnel of the RDIC, composed of postgraduates and doctors
in Pharmacy and Medicine, a program which was based upon the following points:

. Basics on DI.
. Study of the main bibliographical sources: primary, secundary and tertiary sources.
. Verbal and written communication techniques.
. Fulfillment and searching methodology of questions such as: Identification/Availabi-
  lity, General Information/Evaluation, Dosage/Administration, Therapeutic Use (Drugs
  of choice, Alternatives, Indications, Warnings), Clinical Situation-Drug, Adverse
  Reactions/Poisoning/Toxicology, Interactions/Incompatibilities, Drug Elaboration,
  Pharmacokinetics.

Once this period had finished, a limited promotion was started, beginning with the Pharmaceutical Services of several hospitals of the region. The reason why
we did not make a general promotion was mainly based upon the fact that we could first determine the possibilities of services of supply to the foreseen demands of questions.

We have entered in the accounts the received questions during the period
March-September 1983, except August, i.e. six months. During this time 192 questions were
answered giving an average number of 32 questions/month. This number is quite small from an
absolute point of view but relatively it is not so small, as we have to consider the short
time the RDIC was created, not having made a general promotion and also the type of questions

received: Identification/Availability 24%; Therapeutic Use (Choice, Indications, Alternati-
ves, Warnings) 19%; Evaluation/General Information 16%; Adverse Reactions/Toxicology 10%;
Interactions 6%; Clinical Situation-Drug 5%; Dosage/Administration 5%; Drug Elaboration 5%;
Others 10%.

We can observe that, although the most frequent type of question is related
to Identification/Availability, the other types which we can consider as "clinical" ones,
reach more than 60%, being Therapeutic Use and Evaluation 35% of the total amount.

Referring to the type of users, the hospital pharmacists, community pharmacists and hospital physicians made more than 75% of the questions: Hospital Pharmacists 26%;
Community Pharmacists 26%; Hospital physicians 25%; Non-hospital physicians 5%; Public Administration 9%; University 4%; Others 5%.

Due to the fact that there are no standards to measure the efficiency of the
services offered by a DIC, frequently the number of questions as a unique indication is
used and this, from our point of view, is not enough, because more value has the type of
question, its clinical character, than the absolute number of questions. We also consider
that the activities of active information such as bulletins, publications as well as educational labours, constitute the basic mainstays within the services offered by a DIC, so much
important or even more than the labour of passive information (responding questions).

On the other hand, we are developing a plan of action with the purpose to
start DICs on hospital and pharmaceutical corporation level in the diverse cities of Andalusia. The results of this project will be presented on a future occasion.

EDUCATION AREA

This is one of the activities of a RDIC, which we consider a basic one. In
our experience we have started two lines. The first one, the continuing education of postgraduate pharmacists by means of an intensive course of two weeks (more than 60 workhours)
on initiation in specialization in DI. This was the first course of this type held in Spain.
More than 40 pharmacists of whole Spain, proceeding from several media, were present at this
course: hospital pharmacists, community pharmacists, Public Administration, pharmaceutical
corporations.

In general lines, the program was based upon the following points: General
views on Documentation and DI, Sources of Information, Evaluation of biomedical literature,
Basic organization of a DIC, Practical realization of type questions, Application of computers in the health area, Information to the patient, Various topics on Drug Therapeutics,
Conferences on related subjects.

We consider the other educational line is to be concentrated on last year
pharmacy students. The sense of this program is to initiate future pharmacists into the importance their role has as drug informers, giving them basic notions on the "modus operan-
di" in this field.

MANAGEMENT AREA

Not only the active and passive information which come from a RDIC with the characteristics we are describing are enough to justify its existence. Due to its composition, its financing now and in future, as well as its institutional support, a center like this is obliged to render a technical assesment which would help the Autonomous or Regional Government to make decisions and to be at the same time   nerve   center of technical and coordinating support of the specific Areas of Management and Health Inspection. Therefore, from these initial points of view, the basic and doctrinal functions in the Area of Management are as follows:

a) Promotion of the use of information as an element of Management.

b) Promotion of the rational drug use through   objective information, which will make possible the rationalization of healthcare in the pharmaceutical fields.

c) To be the basic tool of support, which through the Documentation and Information would serve as a basis in the elaboration of technical decisions by the diverse Autonomous Governments.

On the other hand, we have started some studies on drug use, which will allow us to apply a concrete policy and some comparative studies with other regions, just like the studies made on the use of antihipertensives, anti-ulcer drugs, gammaglobulins, albumin, use of antibiotics in hospitals, etc. and in the way of connecting these parameters to the morbidity, we are making and updating a series of health indicators which can help to complete epidemiological studies of certain diseases, as well as to determine endemic diseases, both in regard to its location and its continuity and seriousness.

FUTURE ACTIVITIES

In the Area of Drug Information, we will mainly concentrate on the creation of the regional network of local DICs, in hospitals and pharmaceutical corporations of Andalusia, through a logical program of action which will be adapted to the capacities and scope of each concrete case. The RDIC will act as a support and stimulus, coordinating allied activities.

Because of being a rather small geographical area, personal contacts will be feasible with periodical meetings, for which it will be able to obtain a more flexible and active communication.

Referring to the promotion of the activities of the DIC, we have foreseen the diffusion of a handbook-leaflet for a more profitable use of this service, in which we will include a guide of basic data which the consultant has to take into account at the moment of making a question, which will facilitate the communication between the user and the DIC, and because of that, this will contribute to a better service.

Referring to the subject of publications, and within the activities of active information, we are preparing the edition of a bulletin on rational drug use. It will have an extensive diffusion, free and of easy reading, so that it can arrive to health professionals of whole Andalusia, influencing above all health professionals of rural areas, who generally lack objective information on drugs.

In the Area of Education, intimately related to the previous area, we foresee periods of short stays in the RDIC of resident pharmacists of the diverse hospitals of the region as a complement to their education.

In the second place, we will organize courses on initiation or continuing education for postgraduate pharmacists in the same line as the previous course, but carrying them out in a shorther length of time, i.e. one week, and more specifically, for instance for hospital pharmacists, community pharmacists, etc.

In the third place and within the education to postgraduates, carrying out this activity just like the previous ones together with the College of Pharmacy, we will initiate last year students of Pharmacy in basics on DI.

Finally, in the Area of Management of Pharmaceutical Health Care, we will continue our studies on drug epidemiology, which will serve as a support both for decision taking and planning and management of the health areas.

FINAL COMMENTS

1. In spite of our short experience, we think that the creation of a RDIC of these characteristics, is a viable reality and with interesting perspectives for future.

2. In our opinion, it is valid, positive and convenient to dispose of the support and connections of institutional origin (F.I.S., Andalusian Government, INSALUD, College of Pharmacy).

3. We think that in a center like this, at the very least the Areas of Information, Management and Education should be developed, for being interrelated and for being complementary to eachother.

P.S.- CADIME is a Regional Drug Information Center, at the present economically supported by the F.I.S. (Health Research Foundation of the Social Security) and institutionally supported by the Andalusian Government and College of Pharmacy of Granada.

NON COMPLIANCE MASQUERADING AS DRUG RESISTANCE

J. COOKE

Pharmacy Department, General Infirmary at Leeds,
Great George Street, Leeds

The incidence of non-compliance with drug therapy has been reported to range from 4% for a group of tuberculosis out patients (1) to 92% for a group of paediatric patients being treated for streptococcal infections (2). Failure to comply with prescribed medication may have potentially disastrous consequences such as epileptic seizures (3) or diabetic coma (4).

The economics of non-compliance are complex. In 1979 it was estimated that at least £20 million worth of drugs were lost through non-compliance (5). In addition, it could be argued that much of the resources directed towards research, development, prescribing and dispensing of pharmaceuticals are wasted if the patient does not ultimately take them.

Two cases are described here which though originally believed to be unusual drug resistance were subsequently shown to be problems of non-compliance.

CASE STUDIES

Case 1

A 27 year old woman presented with florid hyperthyroidism for which she was prescribed Carbimazole 5mg three times a day. This was gradually increased over the next six months to 45mg daily. Her thyroid function tests began to improve, she started to gain weight and her heart rate fell. However, over the next three months her symptoms re-appeared and she developed a maculopapular rash which was attributed to the carbimazole. She was changed to Propylthiouracil 150mg daily and Propranolol 30mg daily was added. Over the next six months the Propylthiouracil was increased to 800mg daily with little improvement in her thyroid function tests and despite the

addition of Potassium Perchlorate the patient remained biochemically and
clinically thyrotoxic.

During this period she insisted that she was taking her tablets but
because of the lack of response to treatment it was decided to determine whether
or not she had detectable levels of the drug in her blood. The pharmacy
laboratory developed an assay for propylthiouracil based on a modification of a
previous method (6). Estimation for serum and urinary levels of
Propylthiouracil indicated a complete absence of the drug.

On challenging the patient, she admitted to non-compliance with her
therapy. Over the next six months her condition and thyroid function tests
normalised on Propylthiouracil 300mg and Propranolol 30mg daily. However,
as she had a prominent goitre and still required drug therapy nearly three years
after her symptoms began, partial thyroidectomy was carried out and the patient
remains euthyroid two years later.

Case 2

A 42 year old lorry driver presented with a painful left calf and a
sudden onset of severe chest pain radiating down the left side. A Technetium 99
lung scan showed segmental perfusion defects most obvious in the right lung, the
appearance being consistent with pulmonary emboli. The patient was initially
anticoagulated with intravenous sodium heparin and oral warfarin. Heparin
doses were modified according to results of Kaolin Cephalin Clotting Time (KCCT)
Three days after admission the patient became increasingly breathless with chest
pain and was fitted with a caval umbrella. KCCT control was difficult to
establish and accordingly the heparin was stopped. A second lung scan on the
9th day showed improvement with resolving emboli.

It was extremely difficult to obtain a satisfactory response of the
prothrombin time, despite doses of warfarin of up to 160mg daily. A change to
Phenindione made no difference and warfarin was recommenced. It was
suspected that the patient may not be taking his tablets in spite of supervision by
nursing staff. Whilst an assay to measure blood warfarin was being developed
a fine bore nasogastric tube was inserted through which the drug was
administered. Over the next five days the prothrombin time entered the

therapeutic range on only 10mg daily. On removal of the tube the prothrombin time again fell back to the control level and remained thus despite a further increase in the warfarin dose. An assay of total plasma warfarin was performed which showed a concentration of 0.65mg L^{-1} at a time when the prothrombin time was two seconds above control.

The relationship between plasma concentrations or oral anti-coagulants and their pharmacological effects is complex. Warfarin resistance was first described as genetically determined in a human kindred when doses of 145mg of warfarin a day were required to produce a therapeutic effect [7]. At this dose a total plasma warfarin concentration of 55mg L^{-1} was recorded, whereas in a normal therapeutic group of 23 subjects all with optimal anti-coagulant control steady state warfarin concentrations ranged between 0.6 and 3.1mg L^{-1} [8]. In our patient, the warfarin concentration was appropriately near the lower limit of this range at a time when the prothrombin time was just above control. The prothrombin time response, when the warfarin was given via nasogastric tube led us to conclude that the previous and subsequent absence of response was due to non-compliance and not drug resistance.

COMMENT

Blood level estimations are routinely performed for only a relatively small number of drugs and usually because either the therapeutic range is narrow or the desired clinical response is difficult to quantify. The availability of laboratory facilities with the flexibility to estimate non-routine drugs in body fluids can provide the clinician with an important diagnostic service.

The two cases described here illustrate the serious clinical problems which can be encountered when there is a failure to comply with drug treatment. The second case is more disturbing as non-compliance occured whilst the patient was supervised as an inpatient.

REFERENCES

1. Fox. W. (1958). Problem of Self Administration of Drugs with
    Particular Reference to Pulmonary Tuberculosis. Tubercule 39:
    269-274

2. Bergman, A.B. & Weiner R.J. (1963). Failure of Children to receive
    penicillin by mouth. N. Eng. J. Med. 268 : 1334-1338.

3. Sherwin, A.L., Rob J. & Lechter M. (1973). Improved Control of
    Epilepsy by monitoring plasma ethosuximide. Archives of
    Neurology 28 : 178.

4. Miller, L. & Goldstein, J. (1972). N. Eng. J. Med. 268 : 1388.

5. Anonymous. (1979). Non-Compliance: Does it Matter?. Brit. J.
    Med. 2 : 1168.

6. McAllister, R.A. (1952). The Determination of Propylthiouracil in
    Urine with 2:6 Dichloroquinone Chlorimide. J. Clin. Path 4 : 432.

7. O'Reilly, R.A. et al. (1964). Hereditary transmission of exceptional
    resistance to certain anticoagulant drugs: First reported kindred.
    N. Eng. J. Med. 271 : 809-815.

8. Breckenridge, A., Orme, M.L.E., In Davis D.S., Pritchard N.C.
    (Eds) (1973). Biological effects of drugs in relation to their plasma
    concentrations. London, McMillan. pp 145-151.

ACKNOWLEDGEMENTS

   I would like to thank Prof. M. S. Losowsky, St James's University
Hospital and Dr P. Sheridan, Seacroft Hospital for kind advice and permission
to report their patients; Mr A. Cawood, Mr A. Crossley and Miss F Hudson in
the Pharmacy Department for measurement of propylthiouracil and warfarin and
Mrs J Walker for typing the manuscript.

PATIENT EDUCATION AND ADHERENCE TO THERAPEUTIC REGIMENS

H. F. Kabat
University of Minnesota, Minneapolis, Minnesota 55455   U.S.A.

Pharmacy is one of the learned professions that has been given a special franchise or monopoly by society. Because drug therapy must be individualized and because many drugs should only be used by patients who are under the supervision of health professionals, society has charged the pharmacist with the accountability and control of therapeutic agents.

The traditional functions of the pharmacist in our society for almost two thousand years have been the accumulation and distribution of drugs, the accumulation and distribution of drug information and the exercise of drug use control.   (Brodie, 1967)

The purpose of this paper is to examine the effect of patient education on patient adherence to therapeutic regimens.

Clinite and Kabat (1969) reported the adherence of recently discharged hospital patients to their prescribed regimens. In their sample of thirty patients visited at their home about one week after discharge from the hospital, only four patients had received all of their prescribed medication. Errors of omission and extra dose errors occurred 276 times in 1060 opportunities for an error to occur; an error rate of over 25 percent. There were 234 omissions and 42 extra dose errors. More than half of the 61 prescription orders had an error rate of over ten percent; and twelve prescription orders had an error rate above fifty percent.

Clinite and Kabat (1975) undertook another study to evaluate pharmacist/patient interaction factors which might foster adherence to prescribed regimens of self-administered drugs. Each month for four months, twenty two new patients received significantly different pharmacist interactions. They were later interviewed in their homes to assess adherence to the regimen. Group one was a control group and received

only the usual prescription label instructions. Group two patients
received a verbal review of the label instructions by the pharmacist.
Group three patients received a printed handout about drug administration,
a specific handout about their drug and the usual prescription label
instructions, but no verbal interaction. Group four received the above
handouts in addition to a verbal review of both labeled instructions and
handouts by the pharmacist.

Although group four had the highest average number of doses
per day, they had the highest level of patient adherence to their prescribed regimens. Group two (verbal review of labeled instructions)
patients had the next best adherence to their regimens. Group one
(labeled instructions only) had better adherence than group three
(printed instruction only) patients.

It was apparent that as the level or intensity of the pharmacist's interaction increased, so also did patient adherence to their prescribed regimen. Patients receiving printed instructions (patient
package inserts) were less compliant than patients who received only
labeled instructions. The "attention placebo" is unquestionably a major
factor in patient adherence to therapeutic regimens.

Grace and Kabat (1978) reported the results of a Minnesota
study designed to assess pharmacist intervention strategies in a variety
of practice settings for newly diagnosed hypertensive patients. In eight
different sites pharmacists reinforced prescribed directions, distributed
written patient education materials, took monthly blood pressures, and
reminded patients who failed to return for refills in a timely fashion.
Nationally less than one third of the diagnosed hypertensive patients are
under treatment and less than one-eighth are under adequate control. In
this study over fifty five per cent of the patients (97) introduced to
the study treatment were under adequate control and every patient who had
to drop out of the study (13) was accounted for and/or still under treatment in the study or elsewhere.

In still another Minnesota study, Beardsley, Johnson and
Kabat (1982) studied the patient characteristics of a panel of patients
receiving pharmacist initiated patient education prior to discharge from
the hospital. They found that patient drug knowledge about their drugs
and adherence with prescribed regimens were significantly correlated
with one another. However, those patients who believed that they had

some control over events that occurred in their lives (internal locus of
control) adhered to their regimens to a far greater degree than did those
patients who believed that good fortune is the result of luck or the
impact of others on them (external locus of control). Formal patient
education improved adherence to prescribed regimen, only in the internally
oriented locus of control patients. External locus of control patients
were no more compliant after patient education than if they had received
no patient education.

        Sackett and Haynes (1976) conducted a workshop on Compliance
With Therapeutic Regimens based upon their review of 300 studies of
patient compliance. They observed that 25-60 percent of patients were
non-compliant and that, while approximately one third of patients are
always compliant one third are only sometimes compliant and one third
are never compliant. They emphasized that not all compliance with
therapeutic regimens is essential. Many illnesses are self limiting;
many treatments are symptomatic so that compliance strategies need to be
coupled to treatment goals which are well defined.

        The factors determinate of adherence into several groups were
classified as follows:

1. Sociodemographic Characteristics

    Age, sex, education, social class, occupation, income, marital
    status, ethnicity, religion and family size were generally found to
    be unrelated to compliance except among the very old and the very
    poor. Residential stability was the only sociodemographic factor
    which enhanced compliance.

2. Disease Characteristics

    Frequency, severity or duration of illness, recency of attack, pre-
    vious therapy and knowledge of disease were found to be unrelated to
    patient adherence with therapeutic regimens. Patients with psych-
    iatric or personality disorders were generally noncompliant. Patients
    who had previously had the illness or where the degree of disability
    due to the illness is substantial were generally more compliant.

3. Treatment Regimen Characteristics

    Cost was found to be unrelated to adherence but complexity of regi-
    men, number of medications, number of doses, duration, safety caps,
    pain, side effects, supply and magnitude of behavioral change all
    significantly reduced compliance. Relief of symtoms and use of in-
    jections rather than oral dosage forms both were positively related

to compliance.

4. Treatment Source Characteristics

Waiting time and inconvenience are negatively related to compliance but time with provider, a long time relationship with the provider and continuity of care were all positively related to adherence with the therapeutic regimen.

5. Patient-Provider Interaction Characteristics

Providers' prediction of compliance was found to be unrelated to actual compliance. Increased supervision and/or attention, satisfaction with prescriber and clinical reports of progress were all positively related to compliance.

6. Patient Characteristics

Knowledge of disease or therapy, patient education, intelligence, and personality factors were unrelated to compliance with therapeutic regimens. Residential instability and social isolation were found to be negatively related to compliance while stable supportive families, prior compliance, positive feedback and the patient's perception regarding the seriousness of the illness, personal susceptibility to the disease, efficaciousness of therapy and desire to treat are all positive correlates to adherence with the regimen.

Among the tested strategies which they found to be effective are: alteration of treatment, affect a behavioral change, reduce complexity of regimen, increase efficiency and convenience, increase level of supervision and increase patient satisfaction.

Adherence to therapeutic regimens in one patient behavior while noncompliance is many different patient behaviors. The problem of noncompliance is further confounded because patient behavior is not necessarily consistent, that is, the patient may adhere to the regimen while the disease is fulminating but become noncompliant when he becomes asymptomatic. Further, time does not always permit the pharmacist to give the patient the attention that is necessary, so it is probably best to select high risk groups of patients where the treatment outcome is predictable, for example, patients with diabetes, hypertension, schizophrenia and streptococcal infections in children and then to utilize enabling factors where they are likely to be positive influences on adherence to prescribed regimens. Increase the level of supervision and satisfaction and foster the use of physician providers who do so also.

Reference List

Brodie, D. C. (1967). Drug Use Control. Drug Intell.
1, 63-65.
Clinite, J. C. and Kabat, H. F. (1969). Errors During Self-
Administration. JAPhA NS9, 45-47.
Clinite, J. C. and Kabat, H. F. (1975). Improving Patient
Compliance. JAPhA NS16, 74-76.
Grace, M. and Kabat, H. F.(1978). Pharmacist Intervention,
Apoth. 2, 20-21.
Beardsley, R., Johnson, C.A., and Kabat, H. F. (1982). Drug
Self Administration, Cont. Pharm Prac. 5, 156.
Sackett, D. L. and Haynes, R. B. Compliance With Therapeutic
Regimens, Johns Hopkins University Press, Baltimore, MD, U.S.A.

WORKING GROUP ON PATIENT EDUCATION

Coordinator: Altimiras, J.

Authors: Almeda,M.; Andrés,A.M.; Bartroli,M.; Bassons,T.; Bo-
net,R.; Cabanes,J.; Carmona,A.M.; Castejón,A.; De Quadras,E.; Eritja,R.;
Escribano,M.R.; Fité,B.; Gascón,M.P.; Gonzalez,M.B.; Gudiol,T.; Llambi,F.
Roca,M.; Serrano,M.F.; Serrat,M.

Col.legi de Farmacéutics de Barcelona

Continous Education Program. Coordinator: Dr J. Bonal

INTRODUCTION

Continuing education courses oriented to community pharmacists
are developed in the Society of Pharmacists of Barcelona from 1981. These
courses had been promoted by an education committee constituted by hospital and community pharmacists. This committee defined the philosophy of
the program and supervised its development. At the same time a coordinator of the program is responsible for the planning and execution of all
the courses and activities according to the objectives of the committee.

The objectives of this program are to put the pharmacists up
to date with pathophysiology, pharmacology and applied therapeutics and
to reorient and change the mentality of professional practice towards
clinical pharmacy practice.

Until now more than 600 pharmacists have taken some of these
courses, most of them several.

In May and Setember of 1982, workshops on "Clinical pharmacy
in community pharmacy" were offered to discuss the concept and philosophy
of clinical pharmacy and its practical application. Some of the participants
were established. One of these groups is working on patient education
programs.

This paper shows the method and first results of this group.

OBJECTIVES OF THE GROUP
- To update on all subjects selected for patient education.
- To study methods and techniques of patient education.
- To prepare printed information about drugs and health
  education to the patient.
- To motivate other community pharmacists of Barcelona to

distribute the printed material.

WORKING METHOD

- One hospital pharmacist, who was one of the teachers at the mentioned workshop, and with experience in patient education, acted as coordinator of the working group and supervised the text.

- At the begining, the first meetings of the group established its priority: the most used drugs and basically those that are used as selfmedication or those that are frequently object of consultations in community pharmacy. That means, drugs that are usually bought without prescription (laxatives, drugs for flu, antidiarrheals, etc...).

- Later the group was divided in three smaller groups and one subject was assigned to each one.

- The steps followed by each group were:

a) To collect bibliography with the colaboration of the coordinator.

b) To write an up-to-date monograph on the selected subject

c) To select the information that has to be given to the patient.

d) To design the patient information booklet.

- Review of the produced material by the coordinator.

- To submit the materials to the board of the Barcelona Pharmacists Society, through the education committee in order to be printed and distributed among the community pharmacists.

RESULTS

As a result of this work until now monographs and patient education booklets have already been printed on drugs for flu, laxatives and ectoparasites. The society of pharmacists is giving its financial support.

The scheme of the monographs that will be distributed to all the community pharmacists are as follow.

DRUGS FOR FLU

- Aetiology and definition of the flu. Differences respect to common cold and allergic rhinitis.

- Definition of drugs for flu. Composition. Action.

- Drug interactions.
- Cautions and side effects.
- Prophylaxis of the flu.
- Practical advice.

LAXATIVES
- Definition.
- Usual constipation and secondary constipation.
- Types of laxatives.
- Practical advice on the use and abuse of laxatives.

ECTOPARASITES
- Definition.
- Different types.
- Treatment of scabies.
- Treatment of pediculosis.
- Prophylaxis.

Figure 1. Booklets already printed

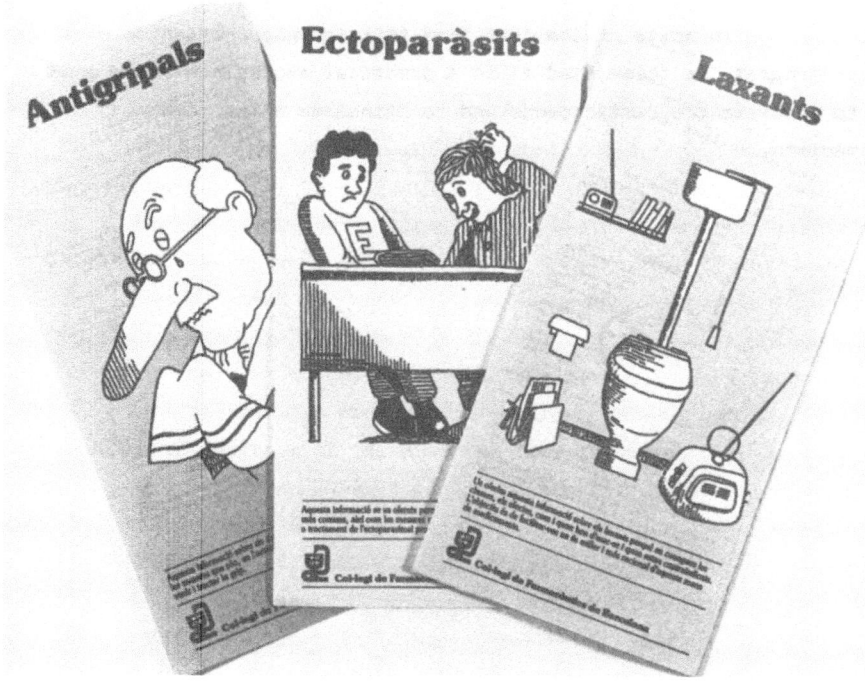

Other materials are going to be finished on subjects like antidiarrheals, cough preparations and antiemetics.

CONCLUSIONS

- The need for changing the professional practice of community pharmacists is recognized and one of the ways is patient education.

- We realize that the acquisition of the knowledge is mandatory. In this sense the cooperation between hospital and community pharmacists, has been very positive.

- The dynamics of the group, working together to study a theme and to apply the knowledge to a practical objective, is an efficient method of selfeducation.

- The work of this group is in agreement with philosophy of the continuing education program of the Society of Pharmacists of Barcelona.

- This experience shows a high degree of interest from community pharmacists to improve their profesional practice through serious and constant work. The interest of the Pharmacists Society to promote and support these activities is also evident.

- In spite of the fact that this is only initiation of a larger program, we think that it is a practical experience and a good way to motivate the participants and to stimulate other community pharmacists.

PICTOGRAPHS - A USEFUL AID FOR THE RIGHT ADMINISTRATION OF
MEDICINES TO THE PATIENT

A.W. Lenderink
Hospital Pharmacy, Tilburg, The Netherlands

After the introduction of unit-dose packaging in our hospital
- some fifteen years ago - the number of mistakes made in the
administration of medicines has decreased.
Unit-dose packaging prevents many mistakes because every unit
(e.g. tablet, capsule, suppository, syringe/ampoule) can be
identified by its own label.
On this label several data are printed such as the name of the
preparation, the strength and mostly a date of production. In
a computerised system there is also an articlenumber and sometimes - especially when the preparation is not stable - there
is a date of expiration.
With unit-dose packaging it is possible that each patient gets
the correct medicines.
But it is not only important that the patient gets the right
medicine. He should also take the preparation at the right
time.
Most of the prescriptions of the physician or specialist state
the frequency of administration. A definition of the exact
time at which the medicine has to be taken is mostly absent.
In a hospital the times of administration often coincide with
the times at which meals are given, so it is very important to
know whether the preparation should be taken, before, during
or after the meal, because the time of administration will
have effect on interactions with the food, rate of absorption,
bio-availability etcetera.
Nowadays facts become known about administration of certain
drugs at a specific time of the day, because of the diurnal variation of metabolism (chronopharmacology).
Sometimes it is not the time of the day that is most important

but a certain period of life; some preparations should not be
administered during the first trimester of pregnancy or during
lactation.

Another aspect which is important - especially with oral medication - is a correct way of administration.

If you chew an enteric coated tablet, there will be no protection of the stomach-wall.

This is an increasing problem because of the still increasing
number of forms for oral use.

In former times one had pills and powders, nowadays there are
tablets that have to be sucked and tablets that have to be swallowed as a whole. Also there are capsules that have to be taken
orally and capsules for inhalation by means of a rota-haler.
And even more new forms are introduced: dosule, chewing-gum.
From the nurse it cannot be expected that she knows all the
facts about the correct time and way of administration for
every medicine. So, in one way or another the hospital-pharma-
cist has to see that the nurse is provided with the necessary
information. Although, there are several ways by which this information can be given (e.g. booklet, label on the box in which
the drugs are brought to the ward), I think that a description
of how and at what time, these specific dosage forms should be
taken, must be present at the time of administration. This can
be achieved if the information is printed on the unit-dose
label.

In many cases the information is little, and there is not a
great problem to print it on the label (e.g. i.v., i.m. and
s.c. for the parenteral forms), but with oral preparations the
space left on the label for the necessary information is too
small.

By using pictorial symbols or pictographs we can show in a simple way the right time and method of administration. In this
way the pictographs will help the nursing personnel to recognize
those medicines for which they have to be alerted with regard
to the right time and method of administration.

UNUSED DRUGS IN THE HOME - INDICATION OF NONCOMPLIANCE
OR POOR PRESCRIPTION HABITS

H. Turakka, K. Vainio and H. Enlund
Department of Social Pharmacy, University of Kuopio,
P.O.B. 6, SF-70211 Kuopio, Finland

Unwanted leftover drugs in the home are a potential health
hazard because they can:
    *increase the misconceptions in drug taking
    *lead to unnecessary self medication
    *be ineffective or even more toxic than the original drug
     when the active components have aged and deteriorated
    *form a risk for intoxication, especially among children
    (Abuse...1976, Allen 1977, Crooks & Christopher 1979)
The relation between the size of home drug stock and intoxication
freouency is not clear (Basavaraj & Foster 1982), but because drugs are
one of the most common form of unintentional poisoning, their availability
and accessibility can be a predisposing factor (Poikolainen 1977, Eskola
1981, Mahdi et al. 1983). In any case, unused drugs form a waste of financial resources both to the individual and to society through reimbursement
systems.

    There are few reliable analyses of people's habits in storing
drugs at home (e.g. Dunnell & Cartwright 1972, Hays et al. 1976, Allen
1977, Skinner et al. 1978, Crooks & Christopher 1979). A more comprehensive picture of the magnitude and reasons for drug hoarding can be
obtained from compliance studies involving home interviews but also these
have been only seldomly published (e.g. Law & Chalmers 1976, Turakka &
Enlund 1978). Information about people's own opinions of unnecessary drugs
have been obtained from some reports about drugs returned to community
pharmacies or during dump-campaigns, but these, unfortunately, have been
primarily interested in organizational aspects as well as weight and/or
prices of returned drugs (Irtizaali 1974, Homer & Rawlings 1974, Bradley
& Williams 1975, Sixsmith & Smail 1978). Some Swedish studies also have
analysed other aspects as well, such as the age of different types of
drug, possible reasons for returning each drug and socio-demographic

background of returners (Eklund & Wessling 1975, Boethius & Möller 1979, Roos 1979).

The purpose of this study was to gather information about the number, type, quality and age of unused drugs in the home and, furthermore, to evaluate reasons for their accumulation.

MATERIAL AND METHODS

Study material. A two-day dump-campaign for unused leftover drugs was arranged in 1980 in the town Porvoo (19.000 inhabitants) in Southern Finland, in collaboration with the health centre, hospital and the two pharmacies in the town. Our department analysed the drugs returned during these days to the pharmacies. Approximately 3 % (N=185) of the households in the town returned a total of 2835 packages, i.e. on average 15 per household.

Methods. The persons who brought the drugs were asked for the reasons for returning by a short interview which also included demographic data of the patient whose drugs were returned and his right for partial or full reimbursement for drug from Sickness Insurance. Afterwards data on drug, strength, dosage form, expiry date, amount and date of dispensing, price and amount left were recorded from the packages. Each package was counted separately. As one drug item we counted each portion of a specific drug dispensed at the same time, regardless in one or more original standard packages. This information is available on the type-written instruction label attached to each package in the pharmacy. (In Finland it is required that the drugs must be dispensed in standard manufacturers' packages).

As the comparison we used the Finnish sales statistics for drugs sold to community pharmacies in 1979.

RESULTS

Amount and type of returned drugs. The typical form that drug return took was the return of only a few packages; 55 % had less than 11 packages. On the other hand, 10 % of the total number of people brought about one third of all the returned drugs. The highest number per single person was 68 items and 4 persons (2 %) each returned more than 55 items.

The percentage distribution of returned drugs according to therapeutic class paralleled the patterns of sales statistics in Finland. Noteworthy exceptions were cardiovascular and gastrointestinal drugs

which were over-represented in returned drugs and cough medicines which
were under-represented (Fig. 1).

Age of returned drugs. The average age of the drugs was 8
years, the oldest package being over 40 years old (Fig. 2). Over-the-
counter (OTC) drugs had been stored significantly longer than prescription
drugs (Fig. 3). Of the prescription drugs, the symptomatic ones, i.e.
those designed to be taken when necessary, were systematically older
(p<0.001) than those for continuous use or for short-term treatment
schedule (e.g. antibiotics).

Amount of drugs left unused. On average, 60 % of the contents
of packages were unused. The different drug groups did not differ significantly from each other, e.g. of antibiotics 53 %, cardiac drugs 62 %,
analgesics 60 % and respiratory drugs 55 % were left in the packages.
Sixteen per cent of all packages were totally unopened. Of the different
dosage forms suppositorias were least preferred. On average, 71 % of
their contents were left and 29 % of these packages (N=96) were unopened.

Value of unnecessary drugs. The value of these unwanted drugs
(90 % could be priced) was 33.200 FMK (7350 USD) , i.e. about 40 USD per

Fig 1. Proportions of returned medicines compared with
proportions sold in Finland in 1979

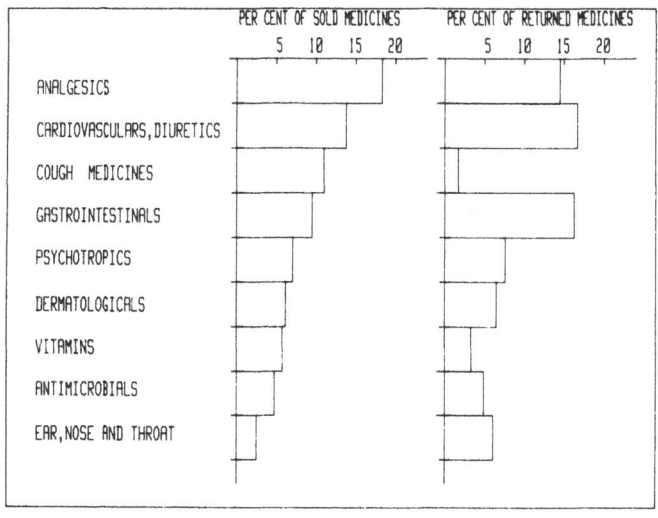

Fig. 2. Age distribution of returned medicines

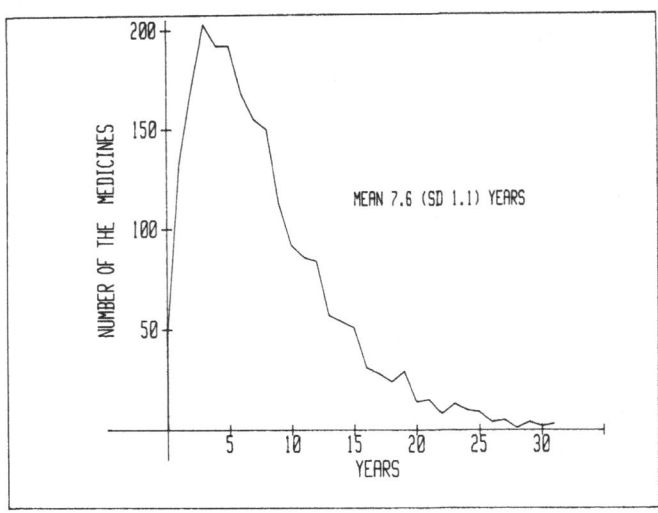

Fig. 3. Age distribution of prescribed and OTC medicines

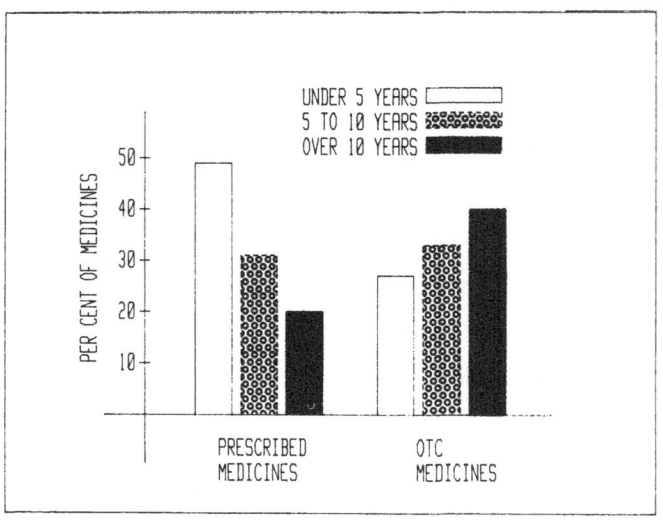

household. The highest value per single person was about 290 USD and per family about 360 USD, but 2/3 of households returned drugs amounting to less than 45 USD.

The highest value of different drug classes was that of cardiovascular drugs (Fig. 4). These are generally reimbursed totally by the National Sickness Insurance. The greater amount of newer packages among cardiovascular drugs than on average is clearly demonstrated in the figure.

Reasons for returning. The reason for returning the drug was given by the patient himself for only 125 packages. These were: got well 40 %, side effects 22 %, don't need the drug 18 %, did not help 14 %, doctor changed 12 % and other reason 19 %. More than half were returned by some other person than the patient. In most of the cases where the patient returned his own medicines, the answer was that he could not remember because the drug had been stored for such a long time. Many patients even did not have any idea what was the rationale of the medication. About 20 % of the drugs were returned because the patient had died.

Fig. 4. Cost distribution of the returned medicines according to drug groups

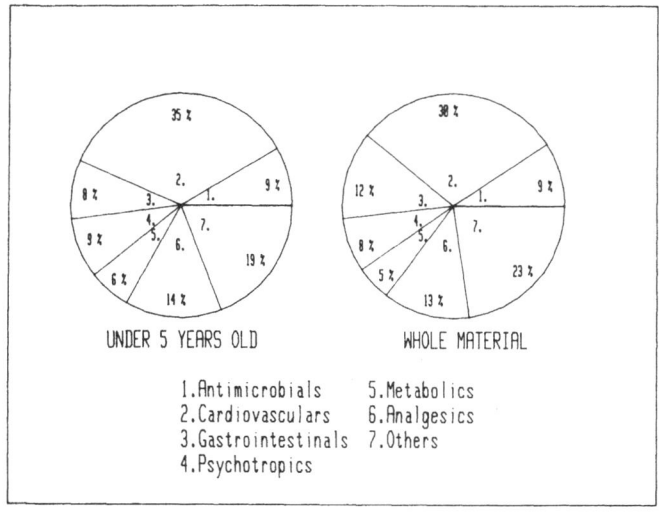

UNDER 5 YEARS OLD   WHOLE MATERIAL

1.Antimicrobials   5.Metabolics
2.Cardiovasculars   6.Analgesics
3.Gastrointestinals 7.Others
4.Psychotropics

WIFE

Date of dispensing	Brand	Amount dispensed	Amount returned
Sept. -75	Truxal (chlorprotixen)	3 x 100	100
Nov. -75	Indocid (indomethacin)	2 x 30	30
Jan. -76	Truxal	2 x 100	128
March -76	Indocid	2 x 30	30
July -76	Kalium Duretter	250	250
Apr. -77	Diabinese (chlorpropamid)	2 x 100	200
Aug. -77	Nobrium (medazepam)	100	94
Sept. -77	Diabinese	2 x 100	192
Dec. -77	Moduretic (amiloride + hcl-thiazide)	100	100
Dec. -77	Dibein (glibenclamid)	100	5
Apr. -78	Cardiosedan ("cardiotonicum")	2 x 100	100
Apr. -78	Moduretic	100	39
Apr. -78	Nobrium	100	100
July -78	Cardiosedan	2 x 100	100
Aug. -78	Doxal (doxepine)	30	26
Aug. -78	Moduretic	100	96
Oct. -78	Fluanxol (flupentixol)	2 x 100	32
Jan. -79	Nitroglycerin	100	100
Apr. -79	Fluanxol	2 x 100	100
Apr. -79	Aspam (diazepam + aspirin)	2 x 30	60
Aug. -79	Temesta (lorazepam)	2 x 100	18
Aug. -79	Valium (diazepam)	100	20
Oct. -79	Temesta	2 x 100	100
Oct. -79	Truxal	100	72
Oct. -79	Fluanxol	2 x 100	200
Nov. -79	Temesta	2 x 100	100
Nov. -79	Akineton (biperiden)	50	50
Jan. -80	Tolvon (mianserin)	90	7
Jan. -80	Tolvon	90	90
March -80	Cardiosedan	2 x 100	200

Price ab. 230 USD

MAN

Date of dispensing	Brand	Amount dispensed	Amount returned
March -75	Bellergal	100	77
Oct. -76	Mogadon (nitrazepam)	2 x 100	91
Feb. -77	Betnovate crem.	30 g	30 g
March -77	Betnovate crem.	30 g	30 g
March -77	Locacorten crem.	30 g	30 g
Jan. -78	Nose-drops	50 ml	25 ml
Apr. -78	Caprysin (clonidine)	100	100
July -78	Sennapur (sennosid)	3 x 100	200
Jan. -79	Sennapur	2 x 100	200
Feb. -79	Valium	100	27
March -79	Nose-drops	50 ml	20 ml
May -79	Nitroglycerin	100	100
June -79	Delmeson acnefoam	40 g	30 g
Aug. -79	Delmeson acnefoam	40 g	40 g

Price ab. 110 USD

+ 10 BRANDS OF OTC DRUGS

Date of dispensing	Brand	Amount dispensed	Amount returned
June -74	Lanoxin novum (digoxin)	x 100	100
June -74	Lanoxin novum	1 x 100	100
Nov. -74	Lanoxin novum	1 x 100	43
March -75	Lanoxin 0.25 mg	1 x 100	100
July -75	Lanoxin 0.25 mg	1 x 100	100
Dec. -76	Furix (furosemide)	2 x 100	153
	Digoxin 0.25 mg	x 30	3
	Visken (pindolol)	x 100	89
	Edecrin (etacrynic acid)	x 100	60
	Cardiosedan ("cardiotonicum")	x 100	60
	Visken (pindolol)	x 100	28
	Medamor (amiloride)	x 50	21

CASE III: A WOMAN'S MEDICINES, RETURNED BY THE HUSBAND. REPORTED THAT THE PHYSICIAN HAS BEEN CHANGED AND THE NEW TABLET STRENGTH 50 MG

Date of dispensing	Brand	Amount dispensed	Amount returned
March -79	Cloxan 100 mg (chlorprotixen)	2 x 100	100
June -79	Cloxan 100 mg	2 x 100	100
Oct. -79	Cloxan 100 mg	2 x 100	100
Jan. -80	Cloxan 100 mg	1 x 100	100
May -80	Cloxan 100 mg	1 x 100	47

Table 1. Sample: drugs returned from three typical households

Table 1. gives some examples of returned drugs and partly illustrates why they were unused. Case I represents polypharmacotherapy which was particularly common in cases where cardiovascular disorders were combined with a need for sedative medication. Case II is a good example of noncompliance of a patient with specific and totally reimbursed drugs in chronic treatment. Case III had diminished by herself the dosage because she felt it too high. She, still however, regularly received the entire prescription (free of charge) from the pharmacy. After changing the doctor, her own dosing schedule was approved. This is an example of lack of patient-doctor communication. A middle-aged woman returned an aged bottle of tetracycline capsules and complained that these did not ease her stomach pains, in fact they made them worse. The reason why she believed them to be GI-drugs was that she had stopped the antimicrobial treatment several years earlier because of GI-symptoms, and had written on the label "stomach pain". Afterwards she misinterpreted her own "instructions" as the indication, not as side effects.

DISCUSSION

It seems that noncompliance is one factor resulting in the accumulation of leftover drugs in the home. However, the overrepresentation of returned drugs used in chronic diseases, and antimicrobial packages which were left more than half full (the disease being presumably cured), points even more to overprescribing. A remarkable part of the returned drugs belonged to totally reimbursed drugs for which the doctor does not have to consider the patient's ability to pay for the treatment. The patient often obediently fetch these free of charge drugs even though he does not feel the need to use them. There is some evidence that drugs that are fully reimbursed are more readily obtained in larger quantities than those which incur the patient's own financial liability, as is the case with the consumption of other health services (Newhouse et al. 1981).

The finding that the percentage distribution of returned drugs, with few exceptions, paralleled the distribution of total drug sales is interesting. This correlation was even clearer in our earlier study (Turakka et al. 1981). This proves that a rather constant proportion of prescription drugs remain unused regardless of type of medication. This study, however, does not allow one to draw conclusions on how large the proportion of all purchased drugs are unnecessary.

An important factor influencing the storage time seems to be

the nature of the medication. Prescription drugs are discarded earlier
than OTC-drugs, even though some prescription drugs are regarded suitable
for self-medication even later (e.g. GI-drugs). On the contrary, the attitude towards medication for the heart is more cautious, because these
drugs were overrepresented and also newer than others. This suggests
that people respect more prescription drugs and are more anxious with
those drugs they consider to be most potent. A general belief is that
cardiac drugs are more potent compared with many other prescription drugs.
The fact, that also antimicrobials were newer than on average proves that
these are considered more as occasional drugs and that information concerning the ineffectiveness of old antimicrobials has had some effect
(but not the information that the whole course has to be taken). On the
other hand, OTC-drugs often are purchased to be stocked and to be taken
when needed. They also are personally purchased by the patient at his
own expense which may influence their longer storage. In addition, their
rationale is known, because it has to be given according to the official
rules on the manufacturer's label. On the contrary, dosing instructions
and indication never are given on the manufacturer's label of prescription
drugs.

The knowledge of proper use of the drugs stored at home seems
to be inadequate. Problems occur with which drugs are to be taken on a
regular basis and which drugs when needed. Also the suitability of different drugs for "self-medication" and, particularly, how long a time the
drugs can be used after they have been purchased apparently is a problem
for lay people. This is partly due to deficiences in given instructions
by the health professionals,e.g. indication and to be taken when needed
may be missing from the attached instruction label, even though it is
required in official guidelines (Turakka & Enlund 1978). Partly this is
also an indication of the need for general drug education, beginning
already from primary school level.

The mechanisms of accumulation of OTC-drugs and prescription
drugs differ from each other. Unused prescribed drugs easily are considered as an indication of patient noncompliance which is true in part
of the cases. However, there are many other reasons partly due to the
organization, partly due to the unsatisfactory activities of health care
personnel. The doctor, of course, can prescribe a wrong medicine but
apparently a more common reason is overprescribing, appearing particularly as unnecessary polypharmacotherapy. Also prescribed packages can be

too large in countries where original manufacturers' packages are required, e.g. in Finland. The pharmacies willingly deliver as large portions
as legally permissible. The reimbursement systems can favor excessively
high purchases. Often the drug has to be changed, or one drug becomes unnecessary because of cure, referral to institutional care or death. When
no common destruction system exists for drugs which should be considered
as risk waste, these form a problem for the household.

Our initial proposal for solving the problem of leftover
drugs in the home is immediate action to organize a clearing system, both
for environmental reasons and for insuring patient safety. In the longer
term, we suggest actions should be taken to avoid the accumulation of
unwanted drugs by:

*better and more critical prescribing habits

*reassessment of the reimbursement criteria

*a less commercial and more patient- and problem-oriented
 pharmacy attitude

*closer cooperation between health personnel in solving the
 drug problems of the patient.

REFERENCES

Abuse of Medicines (1976). Report by a Working Party. Council of Europe,
        European Public Health Community. Drug Intell. Clin. Pharm.,
        10, 17-33, 94-110, 172-178.
Allen, A. (1977). Chemist & Druggist, 258-260.
Basavaraj, D.S. & Foster, D.P. (1982). J. Epidemiol. Comm. Health,36,
        31-34.
Boethius, G. & Möller, B. (1979). Svensk Farm. Tidskr.,83, 539-542.
Bradley, T.J. & Williams, W.H. (1975). Pharm.J.,215, 542,547.
Crooks, J. & Christopher, L.J. (1979). In Self-Medication, ed. J.A.D.
        Anderson, pp. 31-39. Lancaster: MTP Press Ltd.
Dunnell, K. & Cartwright, A. (1972). Medicine Takers, Prescribers and
        Hoarders, London: Routledge and Kegan Paul.
Eklund, L.H. & Wessling, A. (1975). Svensk Farm. Tidskr.,79, 499-503.
Eskola, J. (1981). In Progress in Clinical Pharmacy III.eds. H.Turakka &
        E.v.d. Kleijn,   pp. 127-132. Amsterdam: Elsevier/North-
        Holland Biomedical Press.
Hayes, P. et al. (1976). Med.J.Aust.,1, 235-236.
Homer, W.J. & Rawlings, F.H. (1974). Pharm. J.,214, 324,326.
Irtizaali, S.R.A. (1974). Pharm. J.,214, 323-324.
Law, R. & Chalmers, C.(1976). Br. Med. J.,1, 565-567.
Mahdi, A.H. et al. (1983).Epidemiol. Comm. Health,37, 291-295.
Newhouse, J.P. et al. (1981). N. Engl. J. Med.,305, 1501-1507.
Poikolainen, K. (1977). Scand. J. Soc. Med.,5, 115-121.
Roos, K. (1979). Oförbrukade läkemedel i hemmen (en förundersökning).
        Stencile, Länstyrelsens reprocentral, Uppsala.
Sixsmith, D.G. & Smail, G.A. (1978). Health Bull.,36, 88-90.

Skinner, R.F. et al. (1978). Pharm. J., 218, 326-327.
Turakka, H. & Enlund, H. (1978). J. Clin. Pharm.,3, 103-112.
Turakka, H. et al. (1981). Suom. lääk. l.,36, 1463-1466.

EVALUATION OF THE DOSAGES OF SPANISH PHARMACEUTICAL
SPECIALITIES

Acevedo P.
Drug Information Center. Valenzuela 5. Madrid-14. Spain

García Iñesta A.
National Institute of Health. Alcalá 56. Madrid-14. Spain

The Drug Data Bank contains all pharmaceutical specialities
marketed in Spain.

It has therapeutical, pharmacological, economical,
technological and administrative data of each speciality. Among this data
there are the minimum and maximum dosages of each speciality.

Within the quality control of the information contained in
the above mentioned Data Bank we have initiated a revision of the
reliability of the data collected on dosages with the object of being able
to use these dosages in studies about drug consumption of 1000 inhabitants
per day.

This will serve as comparison of drug usages within the
country and with other countries and as a comparison of the cost per
treatment day.

MATERIAL AND METHODS

Type of sample

a) We chose therapeutic subgroups with specialities with one
active ingredient.

b) We chose the active ingredients of the subgroup that are in
the biggest number of marketed specialities.

c) We considered oral, parenteral and rectal routes of
administration.

The group of specialities with these characteristics was the
sample of the study. As source of information we took the prospect of each
speciality and the Drug Data Bank ESPES. The information contained in the
Data Bank comes from the information forms that are filled out by the
respective laboratories.

This form contains the minimum and maximum dosages which refer according to the content of the container to the minimum and maximum total number of administration units recommended for an adult weighing 70 kg. In pediatric forms the dose refers to the oldest children for which the drug is indicated.

The sample of study has one hundred and thirty four specialities belonging to the following therapeutic subgroups: oral antidiabetics, antimycotics and antirheumatics non-steroids plain and contain the active ingredients indicated in table 1 administered by oral, parenteral and /or rectal route of administration.

CHARACTERISTICS OF THE SAMPLE

Therapeutic groups	Drugs	Number of pharmaceutical specialities	Routes of administration
Oral Antidiabetics	Chlorpropamide Glibenclamide Tolbutamide	23 Pharmaceutical specialities	Oral By mouth (only antimycotics) Intramuscular
Antimycotics, excl. Griseofulvin	Amphotericin Nystatin Ketoconazole	14 Pharmaceutical specialities	Intravenous Rectal (only antirheumatics)
Antirheumatics Non steroids plain	Phenylbutazone Indomethacin Ketoprofen Naproxen	97 Pharmaceutical specialities	
3 Therapeutic groups	10 Drugs	134 Pharmaceutical specialities	5 Routes of administration

Table 1

First, we compared the dosage indicated by the Drug Data Bank with the one indicated by the prospect and we observed three different cases:

1. The data coincide, when both minimum and maximum dosages coincide.

2. The data doesn't coincide, when one of the two data doesn't coincide.

3. Incomplete data, when:
   - one or both were missing in the prospect
   - one or both were missing in the Data Bank
   - the prospect was missing

Secondly, we compared the dosages indicated by the prospect of specialities with the same drug, same concentration and same route of administration.

We took the mode values and calculated the degree of coincidence given in percentage. In other words, the number of specialities that had the same dosages. We established the range of coincidence and represented the values in a frequency histogram.

Thirdly, we compared these mode values with the dosages recomended by the following sources: Martindale, Ama, Goodman and Gilman, Florez and Vidal.

DRUG DATA BANK-PROSPECT

Total results

Coincidence of data	43,3%
Non coincidence of data	38,8%
Incomplete data	17,9%

Table 2

RESULTS DRUG DATA BANK - PROSPECTS

	Antimycotics	Oral antidiabetics	Antirheumatics
Coincidence...........	57,2%	8,7%	49,5%
Non coincidence.......	21,4%	65,2%	35,0%
Incomplete data.......	21,4%	26,1%	15,5%

Table 3

RESULTS AND DISCUSSION

Table 2 shows the results obtained by comparing the dosages
of the Drug Data Bank with the dosages indicated in the prospects.

The following table reflect the partial results by
therapeutic subgroups. The highest degree of coincidence is in
antimycotics: 57,2% and the lowest in oral antidiabetics: 8,7%. In
antirheumatics the coincidence was 49,5%. (see table 3).

When we compared the dosages indicated by the prospect of
specialities with the same composition and route of administration, we
took the data which presented the highest incidence and calculated the
number of specialities that had these dosages expressed in percentage.

In an analysis by therapeutic subgroups, we observed that the
range of coincidence of minimum dosage was in the three cases from 50% to
100%, this is to say that at least in half of the specialities the
prospect recommends the same minimum dosage. In regard to maximum dosage
the dispersion of data is greater (except in antimycotics).

In the antirheumatics subgroup, there are ten values which
correspond to ten groups of comparable specialities. In six of these
groups there is an unanimity in minimum dosage but in maximum dosage only
in one group is there unanimity.

In the antimycotics subgroup the frecuency histogram of
minimum dosage and maximum dosage are identical, and in the oral
antidiabetics again there is a great dispersion of data in both, maximum
and minimum dosage. (see figure 1).

When we compared the mode values of dosages indicated by the
prospects with the sources of information, we observed that the
coincidence was about 60% corresponding to the following active
ingredients: indomethacin, ketoprofen, naproxen, ketoconazol and
glibenclamide.

CONCLUSIONS

The Drug Data Bank's data and the prospect's data don't coincide even in 50% of the sample studied, which indicate that the laboratory don't always adjust the minimum and maximum dosages to those indicated by the prospect of the speciality.

There are few prospects in which minimum and maximum dosages appear clearly specified.

There is more agreement in establishing minimum dosages than maximum dosages.

In order to make comparative studies of consumption referred to dosage per 1000 inhabitants and cost treatment per day, it is necessary that minimum and maximum dosages data as given by Drug Data Bank be reliable and homogeneus. That is to say 1) that prospect's information and Drug Data Bank coincide, 2) that prospect of preparations with the same quali and quantitative composition contain the same dosage data and 3) that these data coincide with the accepted international dosages.

These circumstances have appeared in the drugs of the sample that had standard prospects according to the bulletin of the PHARMACY ADMINISTRATION DEPARTMENT. In these cases we observed that the degree of coincidence neared 100%. Consequently we think that the inclusion of standard doses based on objective data should be increased as it has been done with some drugs in some routes of administration.

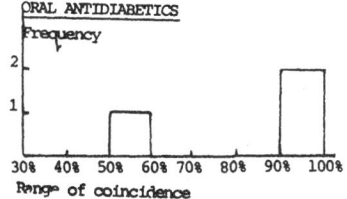

ORAL ANTIDIABETICS

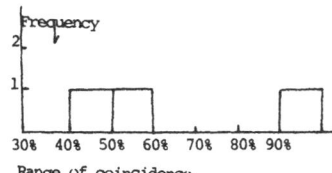

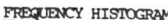
FREQUENCY HISTOGRAM

Figure 1

STABILITY OF HIGH-DOSE METHOTREXATE SOLUTIONS

E. Cantalapiedra, D. Garcia Rodriguez, M. Anaya,M. Ceña,
B. Megia
Pharmacy Service. Centro Especial Ramon y Cajal. Madrid

The demonstration by Farber et al in 1948 that temporal remissions could be obtained in acute leucosis in children with the use of aminopterin constituted a fundamental advance in chemiotherapy of cancer. Subsequent studies revealed that amethopterin or methotrexate (MTX) had a higher therapeutic index and a better chemical stability, generalising its use in the treatment of acute lymphoblastic leukemia, choriocarcinoma, cancer of the breast, of the lung, carcinoma of the head and neck,

The toxicity produced in the attempts to increase the dosage of MTX to improve the therapeutic results proved to be an obstacle.

The first attempt to modify the toxicity produced by MTX by the use of the citrovorum factor or folinic acid was published by Schouebach et al (1950) but the works of Goldin (1978) have been far more decisive in this field. The effect obtained was named "folinic acid rescue" and, since then it has been used extensively in clinical practice.

In the hospital pharmacy solutions of sodium MTX reconstituted in sodium chloride 0,9% injection are prepared.

The purpose of this work is the study of the stability of this solution with time, conserved refrigerated and protected from light.

METHODOLOGY
Reconstitution of the vials

The vials of sodium MTX, 500 mg, preservative-free preparation, are reconstituted in an horizontal laminar air flow bench with 10 ml of sodium chloride, 0,9% injection, the contents of the vials are then transferred to viaflex bag, being filled to capacity with sodium chloride injection 0,9% in such a way that the concentration of MTX is 1%.

Study of the stability of the methotrexate by means of ultraviolet spectrophotometer

Samples are taken from the bag at the moment of preparation and every seven days for two and a half months. Using the Beckman model 24 Spectrophotometer the absorbance of the aliquotes is measured with MTX concentration of 10 microg. ml^{-1} in HCl 0,1N, and a wavelength of 303 nm, all measurements obtained are measured against sodium chloride 0,9% injection diluted in HCl 0,1 N.

Study of the stability of MTX by means of high pressure liquid chromatography (HPLC) in USP XX.

Standard preparation: Dissolve a suitable quantity of USP
MTX RS in Mobile phase to obtain a final solution having known concentration of about 100 microg/ml.

Assay preparation: Transfer an accurately measured volume
of MTX sodium solution, equivalent to about 25 mg of MTX, to a 250 ml
volumetric flask, dilute with Mobile phase to volume, and mix.

By means of a sampling valve introduce equal volume (about 10 microl) of the assay preparation and the standard preparation into
a HPLC, Perkin Elmer 601, operated at room temperature and a flow
rate of about 1,5 ml/min.

Measure the peak responses at identical retention times
obtained with the assay preparation and the standard preparation, and
calculate the quantity, in mg, of $C_{20}H_{22}N_8O_5$ in the portion of MTX taken by the formula:

$$250(C/V)(P_u/P_s)$$

In wich C is the concentration in mg. ml^{-1}, of USP MTX RS
in the standard preparation, V is the volume, in ml, of solution taken, and
P_u and P_s are the peak response obtained from the assay preparation
and the standard preparation, respectively.

RESULTS

Study of the concentration of MTX by means of ultraviolet
spectrophotometer from the moment of preparation to two and a half
months later.

The absorbance of the samples of MTX diluted in HCl 0,1N
are measured in the ultraviolet spectrophotometer with a wavelength
of 303 nm. In table I are shown the concentrations obtained using the
formula:

$$C_2 = C_1 \frac{A_2}{A_1}$$

Table I. Time course of MTX concentration

Time (Weeks)	Absorbance (Wavelength=303nm)	Concentration (Microg. ml^{-1})
0	590	10,00
1	601	10,18
2	560	9,49
3	596	10,10
4	558	9,45
5	569	9,64
6	605	10,25
7	599	10,15
8	602	10,20
9	588	9,96

Where C_2 is the final concentration, C_1 the initial concentration, A_2 the final absorbance and A_1 the initial absorbance.

Comparison of the problem with the standard USP RS:

The ultraviolet spectrum of standard MTX is shown with that of two samples of MTX in Figure I, one, a week after its preparation (A), and the other, two and a half months after its preparation (B).

As can be seen the same peaks of maximum absorption were obtained in the samples and in the standard.

Figure I: Ultraviolet spectra of MTX sodium (10 microg. ml^{-1})

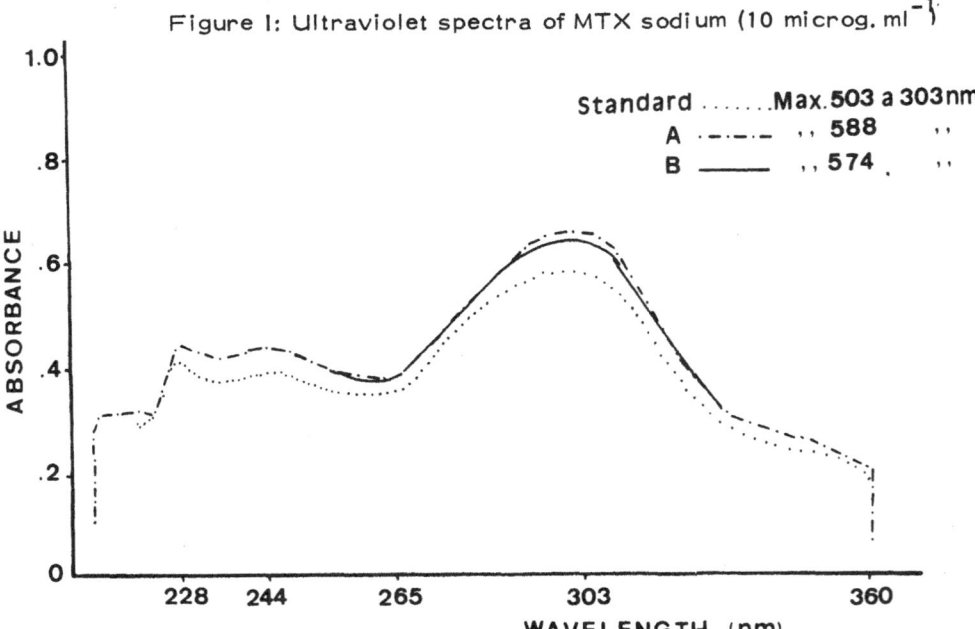

Standard ....Max. 503 a 303nm
A .—.—.—   ,, 588   ,,
B ———   ,, 574 .   ,,

Determination of MTX sodium concentration by means of HPLC in USP XX:

Against the possibility that certain products of MTX hydrolisis have the same absorbance at the same wavelength as that of MTX, the concentration of MTX was determined by means of HPLC according to USP XX.

The chromatographic properties of MTX solutions fresh prepared (A), prepared two and a half months (B) and five and a half months (C) in advance were compared to those of a standard solution of MTX fresh prepared. (Table II).

The results shown here indicate that commercially available MTX behaves in the same way as standard one (Figure II) and it seems to be stable high-dose MTX solution in sodium chloride 0,9 % injection throughout the period of time studied.

Table II. Time course of MTX stability assayed by HPLC

Sample	Retention time (sg)	Peak area (mm^2)	Methotrexate (mg. ml^{-1})
Standard	68	7670	
	73	4459	
	181	128573	9,67
A	54	2480	
	69	8988	
	181	157822	10,9
B	59	3225	
	68	4626	
	182	140672	10,4
C	57	2282	
	69	3301	
	182	149618	10,7

Figure II. Chromatogram of standard MTX (A) and MTX solution in sodium chloride 0,9% injection five and a half mönths in advance. (C).

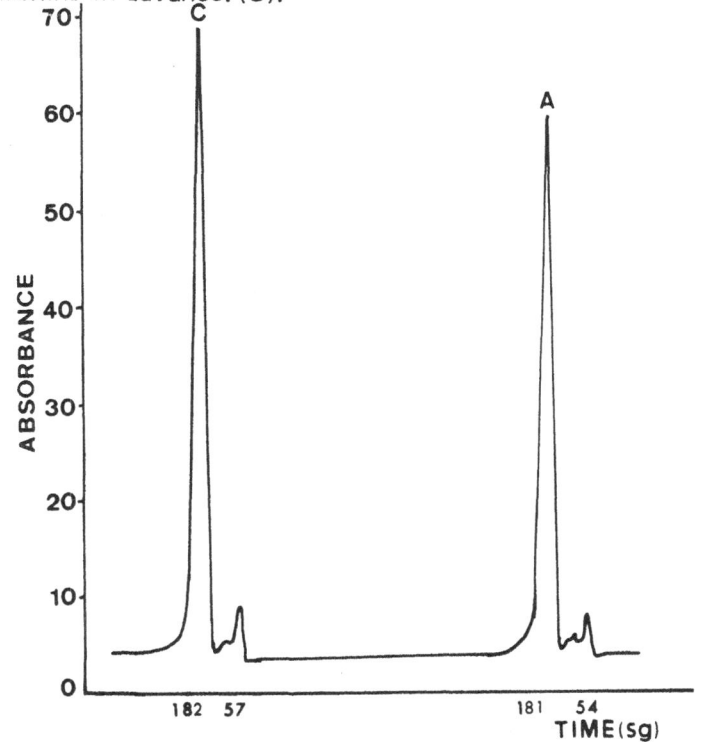

CONCLUSION

From these results can be inferred the possibility that the
solution 1% of MTX in sodium chloride injection, stored and refrigerated and protected from light may be used five and a half months
after its preparation, provided it has been prepared and conserved
in completely sterile conditions.

REFERENCES

Anon: The United States Pharmacopeial Convention, 20th
rev (1980). Inc; Rockville, Maryland, 508.

Cradock, J; Kleinman, L; Rahman, A. (1978) American Journal
of Hospital Pharmacy, 35.

Farber, S; Diamond, L. K; Mecer, R D et al (1948). N. Engl.
J. Med. 238 ;787-793.

Frei, S; Freireich, E; Gehan, E (1961). Blood, 18 , 431

Goldin, A. Cancer Treat. Rep, 62 , 307-312 (1978).

Hignite, C. E; Shen, D; Azarnoff, D (1958). Cancer. Treat. Rep
62 , 13-18.

Morrison, R. A; Oseekey, K. B; Fung, H. O (1978). American
Journal of Hospital Pharmacy, 35 , 18.

Schouenbach, E. B; Greenspan, E. M; Colsky, J. (1950). J. Amer
Med. Assoc . 144, 1558.

PROBLEMS WHICH ARISE IN THE CONTINUOUS INFUSION OF HIGH DOSES
OF FLUOROURACIL

BACHILLER MP, ARRIZABALAGA MJ, CARRASCO ME,
RODRIGUEZ-SASIAIN JM.
SERVICIO DE FARMACIA. R.S. "NTRA. SRA. DE ARANZAZU"
SAN SEBASTIAN (SPAIN)

5-fluorouracil (5-FU) is an antineoplastic agent which acts
as an antimetabolite to uracile. Its nucleotide interferes with the syn
tesis of DNA by blocking the cellular enzyme thymidylate synthetase; and
producing the inhibition of cellular growth (Calabresi & Park, 1982).
The drug is used for the palliative treatment of certain malignant neo-
plasms, especially those of the gastro-intestinal tract, breast, bladder,
ovary and head and neck.

American Society of Hospital Pharmacists states that the usual
dose by intravenous injection is 12 mg/kg/day for four consecutive days.
If there is no evidence of toxicity, it may be continued with 6 mg/kg on
alternative days up to a total of twelve. The cycle may be repeated every
thirty days.

At present there is a school that recommends the use of this
agent at higher dosages: 1000 mg/m^2/day by means of continuous infusion,
affirming that this therapy allows an increase in the number of remissions
and a decrease in the adverse effects. This rule, when applied to head and
neck tumors, consists of utilizing bolus cis-platinum (100 mg/m^2); taking
the usual precautions; 5-FU continuous infusion for 120 hours at a concentration of 1 mg/ml in 5% glucose up to the total dose. Bleomycin is likewise used (Al-Sarraf et al 1981; Decker et al 1983; Hong & Bromer 1983).

The drug product Fluorouracil Roche, used to prepare the aforementioned infusions, presents its drug in the form of a solution buffe-
red with TRIS in order to maintain a pH range of 8.6-9.0 to prevent the
decomposition of 5-FU. It is therefore fair to ask if the drug keeps stable during the long infusion period, at the high concentration used and
in a 5% glucose solution whose pH ranges between 4-5 in this drug product
on the Spanish market. Trying to discover how long a prepared 5-FU solution can be kept in the aforementioned concentrations, it was found that

information on this data does not coincide; King (1973) states that decomposition does not take place in 24 hours, and so does Trissel (1980),
but Morris states that the mixture is stable for only 6 hours. This paper
is an attempt to find out if 5-FU solution at a concentration of 1 mg/ml
in 5% glucose solution is stable for 48 hours.

METHODS

Two experimental sets were prepared composed of 5 vials each
with 500 ml of 5% glucose; in each two Fluorouracil ampoules of 250mg
were injected reaching a final concentration of 1 mg/ml. One of the experimental sets was protected from light while the other one was left exposed. Every two hours a sample was taken to determine the 5-FU, the last
one 48 hours after having added the drug. 5-FU was measured using the
USP spectrophotometric method at 266 nm by beans of a double-beam spectro
photometer. All the determinations were made in duplicate.

RESULTS

The values of absorbance obtained at different times for the
5-FU solutions in 5% glucose at the concentration 1 mg/ml are shown in
the table I.

TABLE I

Time (hours)	Vials protected from light	Vials exposed to light
0	0.557	0.563
2	0.565	0.575
4	0.563	0.580
6	0.567	0.563
8	0.542	0.551
10	0.550	0.563
12	0.564	0.566
24	0.564	0.566
48	0.563	0.561

No statistically significant differences are observed between the antineoplastic concentration just after the solution was added, and that after
48 hours; either in the set protected from light or in the set exposed to
light.

DISCUSSION

The appearance of new norms on the dosification and administra
tion of 5-FU puts in doubt its stability in acid solutions and at high
concentrations, a question that cannot be solved by resorting to sources
of information on intravenous mixtures available, since there is still
some uncertainty about this question from publications that issue contra
dictory conclusions. As can be seen from the results of this paper, it
seems clear that the product is sufficiently stable and would not present any problems if the solution were kept for 48 hours, even if special
precautionary measures regarding exposure to light were not taken (Milovanovic & Nairn 1980). This information is similar to that obtained by
Hardin et al (1982), who proved that 5-FU is stable for 48 hours in solutions for parenteral nutrition with glucose. It should also be pointed
out that these authors used another analytical method to determine 5-FU,
such as high pressure liquid chromatography. They have also proved that
fixation to glass or plastic is not produced. The conclusions of these
authors coincide with that of this work.

The setting out of preparation norms by the pharmaceutical
service can be the key to this specific case: and in this way it is possible to store 5-FU solutions for relatively long periods of time instead of having to prepare the mixture every 6 hours, as would be the case
if the stability was that indicated by Morris. Both the asepsis of the me-
-thod and the advantage of not having to change the vials, imply that continuous administration for a period of 24 hours can safely achieved.

REFERENCES

Al-Sarraf, M.; Drelichman, A.; Peppard, S. et al (1981). Adjuvant cis-
         platinum and 5-fluorouracil 96 hour infusions in previously
         untreated epidermoid cancers of the head and neck. Proc ASCO,
         22, 428.
American Society of Hospital Pharmacists. American Hospital Formulary
         Service. Washington: American Society of Hospital Pharmacists.
         Perpetual edition.
Calabresi, P. & Parks, R.E. (1982). Quimioterapia de las enfermedades neo
         plásicas. En: Goodman Gilman A, Goodman LS, Gilman A eds.:
         Las bases farmacológicas de la terapéutica. 6ª edición. Buenos
         Aires:Panamericana.1249-51
Decker, D.A.; Drelichman, A.; Jacobs, J. et al (1983). Adjuvant chemothe-
         rapy with cis-diamminodichloroplatinum II and 120-hour infu-
         sion 5-fluorouracil in stage III and IV squamous cell carcino-
         ma of the head and neck. Cancer. 51,1353-5.
Harding, T.C.; Clibon, U.; Page, C.P.; Cruz, A.B. Jr (1982). Compatibili-
         ty of 5-fluorouracil and total parenteral nutrition solutions.

J Parent Ent Nut. 6,163-5.
Hong, W.K. & Bromer, R. (1983). Chemotherapy in head and neck cancer. N Engl J Med. 308, 75-9.
King, J.C. (1973). Guide to parenteral admixtures. St. Louis:Cutter Laboratories. Inc.
Milovanovic, D. & Nairn, S.G.(1980). Stability of fluorouracil in amber glass bottles. Am J Hosp Pharm. 37, 164-5.
Morris, M.E.(1981). Intravenous drug therapy manual. 5th edition. Ottawa General Hospital.
Trissel, L.A. (1980). Handbook on injectable drugs. 2nd edition. Washington: American Society of Hospital Pharmacists. 223-5.

DISSOLUTION "IN VITRO" OF SOME SLOW-RELEASE THEOPHYLLINE PREPARATIONS AND COMPARISON WITH "IN VIVO" RESULTS

Mangues, M.A.*; Cáliz,A**; Pujol, F.* and Bonal,J.*

Hospital de la Santa Creu i Sant Pau. *Pharmacy Service. ** Respiratory Service. Barcelona. Spain

The purpose of the present study is to test "in vitro" release characteristics of the sustained release Theophylline products that are already or will be marketed in Spain in the near future, as well as the "in vivo" disposition of the commercially available products.

MATERIAL AND METHODS

Four slow-release Theophylline preparations were assayed (Table I). For the "in vitro" dissolution test, the apparatus 1 described in the USP XX/NF XV was used, which was slightly modified by adding a stirring element.

TABLE 1. ASSAYED FORMS.*

TRADE NAME	DRUG	MANUFACTURER	DOSE	LOT	PREPARATION
THEOLAIR[R]	THEOPHYLLINE	ABELLO, S.A.	250 MG	T_1 T_2	SCORED TABLETS
			175 MG	T_1	
THEO-DUR[R]	THEOPHYLLINE	ANTIBIOTICOS, S.A.	300 MG	B-1	SCORED
			100 MG	B-1	TABLETS
EUFILINA RETARD[R]	AMINOPHYLLINE	ELMU, S.A.	350 MG	282861=E_1 NA6092=E_2	SCORED TABLETS
THEOPHYLLINE DIFFUCAPS	THEOPHYLLINE	EURAND, S.A.		6E 9E	BEADS FOR FILLING CAPSULES

* All the assayed forms were kindly supplied by the manufacturers.

The composition of the dissolution medium was: KH_2PO_4 0.05 M HAc 0.05 M, Tween 80 0.05%, HCl q.s. pH 2 and H_2O q.s. 1 litre. First, the pH of the medium was kept at 2; then it was increased to 5,6.3 and 7 at 1, 1.5 and 4 hours, respectively, after the begining of the assay. That was done by adding NaOH 4 N to the medium. The dissolution medium had a volume of 900 ml when we started the assay. Every 15 minutes a sample of 4 ml was taken by means of a syringe and filtered. Each sample was replaced

by an equal volume of the medium. The length of the assay was 8 hours.
Each assay was repeated 3 times. The concentration of Theophylline in the
samples was determined by measuring the UV absorption at 270 nm. The pro
file of dissolution of every form assayed was plotted and the dissolution
rate (% Dose/time) was calculated as the slope of the least squares regression line of the percentage of amount dissolved vs time.

Theolair[R] and Theophylline diffucaps were used for the "in vi
vo" study. Twenty asthmatic non-smoking patients from the Respiratory Ser
vice of our Hospital participated in it. Twelve of them, 1 male and 11 fe
male, with ages ranging from 23 to 52 years received Theolair[R] and eight,
1 male and 7 females, with ages ranging from 33 to 61 years received
Theophylline diffucaps. None of the patients had gastrointestinal, hepatic,
renal or cardiovascular disturbances. Prior to the study, all patients we
re receiving plain tablets of Aminophylline at 6 hour intervals. Serum
concentrations were measured at 4, 5 and 6 h from the administration of
the drug. The individual elimination half-life (t ½) was calculated. If the
serum concentrations obtained were not in the therapeutic range of
Theophylline, a new total daily dose was calculated for the slow release
preparation in order to achieve an average steady-state serum concentration of 75 mcmol/l , assuming that linear elimination occurs and in accordance with the dosage possibilities of each form. Patients received the
slow-release Theophylline preparation for at least three days at 12 hours
intervals. Then, blood samples were obtained every 2 hours during a dosage interval. Theophylline was measured in serum by enzyme immunoassay
(EMIT[R]). Fluctuations in serum concentration during a dosage interval for
each patient were determined from the differences between the highest
(C max) and the lowest (C min) values during that dose interval, and expressed as a percentage of C min.

RESULTS AND DISCUSSION
Although the "in vitro" study shows that the four assayed
forms had a slower release of Theophylline in relation to the plain tablets, the dissolution profiles are different for each form. Differences
between lots and even between different dosages of one product have also
been found, except for Theolair[R] (Fig. 1) Further studies are needed to
evaluate the clinical importance of this fact.

For Theolair[R] we found a pH-dependent release pattern. The dissolution rate was found to be higher when the pH of the medium increased at 6.3 (Fig. 1). That is in agreement with the results obtained by Jonkman with this form (Jonkman, 1981,a). Hence, it is possible that the rate of Theophylline absorption from this slow-release product might be altered in the presence of food, antiacids and H_2-histamine antagonist. Jonkman et al. (Jonkman, 1981,b) found "dose dumping" in a few subjects taking Theolair[R] on an empty stomach with a full glass of water. In our study, 10 out of the 12 patients treated with Theolair[R] showed Theophylline plasma levels within the therapeutic range, while the other two (P_1 and P_2) achieved very high C max values and fluctuations, wich were aberrant according to the Chauvenet criteria (Chauvenet 1959   ). That might be attributed to the phenomenon called "dose dumping" (Fig. 2).

FIGURE 1. "IN VITRO" RELEASE OF THEOPHYLLINE FROM THE ASSAYED FORMS. MEAN ± SD VALUES ARE SHOWN.
——————— PLAIN TABLETS OF THEOPHYLLINE.

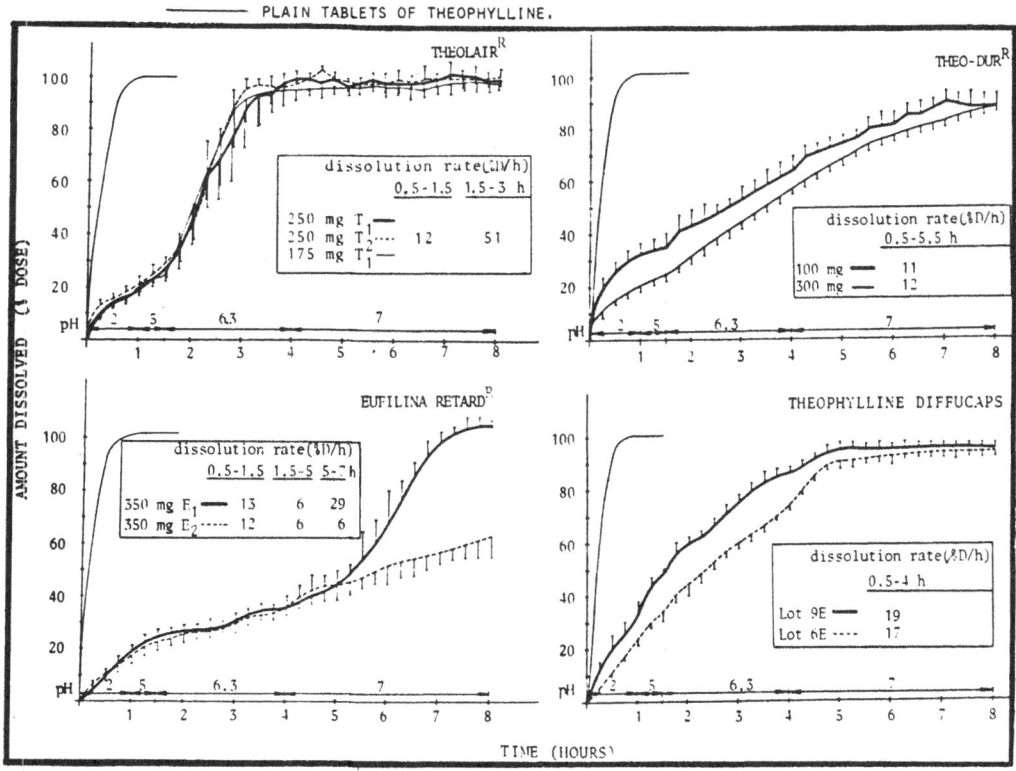

Very different dissolution profiles were obtained from the two lots assayed of Eufilina Retard[R] (Fig. 1). Möller (Möller, 1981) carried out studies of dissolution with this form, marketed in Germany, and he assumed that the dissolution of the Aminophylline from the matrix was also pH-dependent, because at pH 5 or over, polyacrylates, where the drug is embedded, underwent strong swelling and a quicker release was to be expected at that point. It seems that the Lot E_2 did not developed this phenomenon. Variations in the pH of the medium do not seem to affect the release of the other assayed forms. Hendeles establishes (Hendeles, 1983) that, ideally, absorption of slow-release preparations should be constant, i.e., zero order. Therefore, it would be desirable that dissolution was also constant. Out of the assayed forms, only Theo-Dur[R] and Theophylline diffu caps fulfil this uniformity in the dissolution, although the first one has a slower dissolution rate than the second one (Fig. 1).

Plasma levels within the therapeutic range were obtained in all patients treated with Theophylline diffucaps (Fig. 2). Table 2 shows the main pharmacokinetc parameters attained in the "in vivo"study. Note that the time at which maximum plasma concentrations were achieved (Tmax), was shorter for Theolair[R] than for Theophylline diffucaps. This is in accordance with the "in vitro" dissolution rate of both products (Fig.1).

FIGURE 2. STEADY-STATE PLASMA THEOPHYLLINE CONCENTRATIONS FOLLOWING THE ADMINISTRATION OF TWO SLOW-RELEASE PREPA-RATIONS. MEAN± SEM VALUES ARE SHOWN. PATIENTS P_1 AND P_2 TAKING THEOLAIR ARE NOT INCLUDED IN THE AVERAGE.

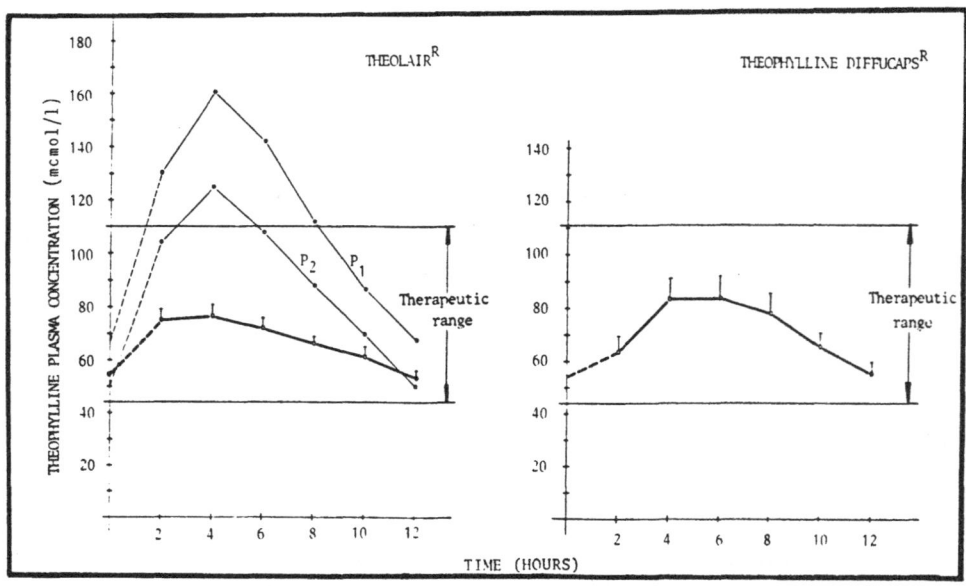

Fluctuations in plasma concentrations (Table 2) are function of the rate of absorption of the product, the rate of elimination of the drug from the patient and the dosing interval selected. Since the width of the therapeutic range of Theophylline, fluctuations must be less than

100% to maintain the plasma level within the therapeutic range throughout each dosing interval (Hendeles, 1983). For 10 of the patients treated with Theolair[R], the fluctuation was 57.4 $\pm$ 8.4%. The two patients with toxic levels had fluctuations of 134.3 and 145.6%. For Theophylline diffucaps the mean value was 67.0$\pm$ 8.4%.

Most of our patients had long half lives of elimination (Table 2) and it is not surprising to obtain low fluctuations at dosing interval of 12 hours. Good fluctuations could probably be obtained in these patients by administering plain tablets at 8 hours intervals. The slow release formulations had special therapeutic advantage in patients with short half lives of elimination because the fluctuations in plasma concentrations between doses of a rapid release formulation can be excessive, even at dosing intervals as short as six hours. In the study using Theophylline diffucaps, three patients with half lives shorter than 5 h were included. All three maintained therapeutic levels over 12 hours intervals. It seems that this product has a slow enough absorption rate to allow maintenance of plasma concentrations within the therapeutic range, with 12 h dosing intervals, in patients with rapid elimination, but a bigger number of patients would be necessary to support this assumption.

TABLE 2. PHARMACOKINETIC PARAMETERS OBTAINED IN THE "IN VIVO" STUDY.

	DOSE (MG/KG/DIA)	T 1/2 (H)	CMIN (HCMOL/L)	CMAX (HCMOL/L)	T MAX (H)	PERCENT FLUCTUATION (CMAX-CMIN/CMIN)x100
THEOLAIR [R]						
MEAN±SEM:	10.9±0.4	10.5±0.9	53.7±2.3	82.4±3.7	3.9±0.6	57.4±8.4
RANGE:	(9.6–13.5)	(6.7–15.0)	(43.5–64.0)	(69.0–104.6)	(2.0–6.0)	(19.7–100.6)
P1	13.0	4.7	68.5	160.5	4	134.3
P2	12.7	8.6	51.0	125.3	4	145.6
THEOPHYLLINE DIFFUCAPS						
MEAN±SEM:	11.7±1.1	6.8±1.1	55.0±4.4	91.6±8.0	5.8±0.6	67.0±8.4
RANGE:	(8.9–18.7)	(3.0–12.6)	(38.0–72.8)	(53.3–121.0)	(4.0–8.0)	(22.8–102.9)

REFERENCES

Chauvenet (1959), In Documenta Geigy. Tablas científicas. 5th Edition,p.43
        Basle: Ciba-Geigy Ltd.
Hendeles, L & Weinberger, M. (1983). Pharmacotherapy,3, 2-44.
Jonkman, J.H.G. et al (1981a). In Proceedings of the 1st European Congress of Biopharmacy and Pharmacokinetics, Ed. Aiache & Hirtz, pp 182-191. Paris: Tecnique et documentation.
Jonkman, J.H.G. et al (1981 b). Int. J. Pharmaceutics, 8, 153-6.
Möler, H. (1981). In Proceedings of the 1st European Congress of Biopharmacy and Pharmacokinetics, Ed. Aiache & Hirtz, pp 316-325. Paris: Tecnique et documentation.

A COMPARATIVE STUDY OF THE SECONDARY EFFECTS OF THREE VARIATIONS OF BROMP-TON SOLUTION

Torres Pons, M.D.; Gamundi Planas, M.C.; Ribot Roca, A.;
Aguas Compaired, M.; and Barba Boada, M.
Quinta Salud La Alianza. Pharmacy Service
Barcelona. Spain

The techniques employed to relieve pain and potenciate analgesia have always been a cause of concern for both the physician and the pharmacist. Within the last few years Brompton solution has been used in Spain for the treatment of chronic pain, especially in the treatment for terminal cancer. The prescriptions used in preparation of Brompton solution are quite different. No variation of Brompton solution has suppressed the secondary effects of morphine; that is to say, until the present, the ideal formula of Brompton solution has not been achieved.

In this communication we present a study carried out in two of our hospitals to determine which variation of the prescription produces minimal secondary effects.

Material and methods:

Among the many variations of Brompton solution which exist, we chose three at random. The formulas used were:

FIGURE 1. FILE OF DATA

Solution "A": Morphine; Simple syrup 2,5 ml; Gin 2,5 ml; Distilled water q.s. 10 ml.

Solution "B": Morphine; HCL 10% 0,2 ml; Ethanol 25% 2,0 ml; Distilled water q.s. 10 ml.

Solution "C": Morphine; Cocaine 10 mg; Simple syrup 2,5 ml; Gin 2,5 ml; Distilled water q.s. 10 ml.

In the three formulas the concentration of morphine was increased as necessary according to the progression of the disease.

The subjects in the study were hospitalized or ambulatory oncology patients. They were selected because no other analgesic was administered in their actual treatment.

Each participating patient was identified in a separate file (figure 1) along with the following data: responsible physician, diagnosis allergies and possible secondary effects which the patient might present because of treatments administered before the use of Brompton solution.

The concentration of the morphine used was noted in the file as well as the dates of the initiation and termination of the treatment.

The secondary effects studied were: nausea, vomiting, anorexia, constipation, diarrhea, confusion, perspiration, dry mouth, sensation of hot flashes, vertigo, bradycardia, palpitation, sedation, miosis, insomnia.

The analgesic power of the formulas tested was evaluated directly by the patient.

The results were collected by a hospital pharmacist directly from the patient, family members. In some isolated cases in which, no interview was possible, because of the patients condition, the information was obtained from the nursing staff.

Results:

The study was carried out with a total of 43 patients (30 males and 13 females), distributed according to the following groups: A, 13 patients; B, 18 patients and C, 12 patients.

TABLE 1. DURATION OF TREATMENT WITH THREE VARIATIONS OF BROMPTON SOLUTION

DURATION TREATMENT	A		B		C		TOTAL	
	Nº cases	%	Nº cases	%	Nº cases	%	Nº cases	%
0 - 1 week	6	46,20	7	38,88	5	41,66	18	41,86
1 - 2 weeks	2	15,30	1	5,55	3	25,00	6	13,95
2 - 4 weeks	2	15,30	4	22,25	3	25,00	9	20,94
4 -12 weeks	2	15,30	3	16,66	1	8,34	6	13,95
+ 12 weeks	1	7,90	3	16,66	——	——	4	9,30

The ages of the patients ranged from 30 to 80 years; 78,66% of the patients were over 50 years of age.

' The duration of the treatment is indicated in table 1. The treatment was administered for less than one week in 41,86%of the subjects and lasted more than three months in only 9,3% of the cases. In 48,83 % treatment was given one week to three months.

To value analgesia we did the following classification:. Insufficient, good and no value   according to the need of the patient. It was ·considered as no value in cases when the patient couldn't give the information.

The evaluation of the results of the analgesia is indicated in table 2.

- There were no significant variations among the three formulas tested.

- The effective initial doses was from 60 mg/day (10 mg/4h.)

- The sufficient analgesia is with 180 mg/day (30 mg/4 h).

The secondary effects of the three variations are listed in table 3. Although there are several, they are quantitatively and qualitatively different. In it, the secondary effects that patiens was before the treatment wich Brompton solution, it was not mentioned.

The more frequent secondary effects tested were: constipation, confusion, palpitation, dry mouth, hallucinations e insomnia. It was distribute in:

TABLE 2 . ANALGESIC VALUATION

DOSE-	VALUATION	A N° cases	B N° cases	C N° cases
30 mg/day	Insufficient	——	3	1
	Good	1	3	1
	No valuation	3	3	3
60 mg/day	Insufficient	2	4	3
	Good	5	4	3
	No valuation	1	—	—
120 mg/day	Insufficient	1	1	2
	Good	4	3	2
	No valuation	—	2	—
180 mg/day	Insufficient	1	—	—
	Good	2	3	2
	no valuation	—	—	1

Solution "A" : Confusion and palpitation

Solution "B" : Dry mouth

Solution "C" : Hallucinations and insomnia

The constipation occured in approximately the some proportion with all three formulas.

The solution C presented lesser sedation than A and B. We think it was due to the cocaine.

Conclusions:

- All the variations tested caused secondary effects.

- The secondary effects tested in the formula B were the minor importance.

- The more frequent effects secondary found were:

Solution "A" : Confusion and palpitation

Solution "B" : Dry mouth

Solution "C" : Hallucinations and insomnia

- The analgesic power was similar in all three groups

- The effective initial doses was from 60 mg/day (10 mg/4 h)

TABLE 3. PERCENTAGE THE ADVERSE EFFECTS

A		B		C	
Symtons	%	Symtons	%	Symtons	%
Constipacion	38,40	Dry mouth	55,50	Other	58,00
Confusion	38,40	Constipacion	38,40	Constipacion	33,00
Palpitation	38,40	Sedation	27,70	Dry mouth	33,00
Other	38,40	Hallutination	11,00	Hallutination	25,00
Sedation	30,00	Confusion	11,00	Nausea	25,00
Dry mouth	30,00	Nausea	11,00	Perspiration	25,00
Perspiration	30,00	Palpitation	11,00	Confusion	16,00
Hallutination	15,00	Hot flashes	11,00	No side effects	16,00
No side effects	15,00	Perspiration	11,00	Vertigo	16,00
Hot flashes	15,00	Other	11,00	Vomiting	16,00
Anorexia	15,00	Bradycardia	5,50	Bradycardia	8,00
Bradycardia	7,90	Vertigo	5,50	Palpitation	8,00
Vertigo	7,90	Anorexia	0,00	Sedation	8,00
Vomiting	7,90			Anorexia	8,00

REFERENCES:

Castro, I.; Aliaga, L.; (1981). Use of the Brompton   mixture in cancer
    patients. Boletin A.E.F.H. <u>6</u> (22)

de la Concepción, N.; Sant, M.; Oller, I.; (1981) Statibility of Bromp-
    ton's mixture. Boletin A.E.F.H. <u>6</u> (22)

Hillier, E.R.; (1983) "Oral narcotic mixtures". British Medical Journal.
    <u>281</u>, 701-702

Howrie, D.L.; (1981). Brompton's mixture for pain relief. J. Pediatr.
    (Letter). 666-7

Mount, B.N.; and col. (1976). "Used of the Brompton mixture in treating
    the chronic pain of malignant disease". CMA Journal. <u>115</u>, 122-
    124.

Palle B. Neumann; Hans Henrikren and col. (1982)."Plasma morphine concen-
    trations during chronic oral administration in Patients with
    cancer Pain". Elsevier Biomedical Press. <u>13</u>, 247-252

Pardo, C.; Mas, M.P.; Alberti, R. and Triquell, L.; (1980). Participación
    del Farmacéutico en la asistencia de los pacientes neoplásicos
    terminales hospitalizados y en regimen ambulatorio. XXV Con-
    greso Nacional de la A.E.F.H.

Melzack, R.; Ph D. and col. (1976) The Brompton mixture: effects on pain
    in cancer patients. CMA Journal. <u>115</u>, 125-128

Rosatti, P.; (1981) Tractement de la douleur de cancereux par la morphi-
    ne. Medicine et Hygiene. <u>39</u>, 3880-3881

Masters, N.I. (1979). The Brompton cocktail (Letter). The Lancet. <u>2</u>

SERUM AND SPUTUM CONCENTRATIONS OF AZLOCILLIN, CEF-
TAZIDIME AND CEFOPERAZONE IN PATIENTS WITH CYSTIC
FIBROSIS

N. Martini, L. Castellani, G. Scroccaro and L. Bozzini
Hospital Pharmacy Service - Borgo Roma - Verona, Italy

G. Mastella, M. Agostini and G. Barlocco
Regional Cystic Fibrosis Center - Verona, Italy

INTRODUCTION

This study was carried out to evaluate the serum pharmacokine
tics and sputum concentrations of Azlocillin (AZLO), Ceftazidime (CAZ)
and Cefoperazone (CEF) in patients with cystic fibrosis.

MATERIALS AND METHODS

- Patients' data and drug dosing (all values are reported as mean $\pm$ S.D.;
range is given in brackets)

	AZLO 5 PATIENTS	CAZ 6 PATIENTS	CEF 6 PATIENTS
Age (yrs)	14.4 ($\pm$ 6.9) (5–23)	13.6 ($\pm$ 3.8) (7–18)	13.5 ($\pm$ 3.6) (10–20)
Weight (Kg)	29.8 ($\pm$ 12.6) (14.2–45.4)	27.8 ($\pm$ 9.3) (18.0–44.5)	29.6 ($\pm$ 14.8) (19.0–57.0)
Sex M F	2 3	3 3	6 0
Dose (mg/Kg/day)	400	200	200
Rate of administration	i.v. infusion over 30'	i.v. infusion over 30'	i.v. infusion over 30'
Dosing interval (h)	8	8	8

- Assay method: serum and sputum samples were determined by microbiological plate assay using Proteus Morganii NCTC 235 as test-organism and An
tibiotic Medium N. 1 (Merck) as the test medium. Standard concentrations were prepared using a pH-7 phosfate buffer. The presence of beta-
lactamases in all sputum samples was assayed with Nitrocefin 87/312 method.

- Blood sampling: serial blood samples were drawn following the first dose of the multiple-dose treatment at 0, 0.5, 1, 2, 4, 6, 7.5 hours after
the end of the infusion and were stored at -20°C until assay.

- Sputum sampling: during the five days of therapy, a complete postural
  drainage of sputum was obtained four times a day at 10 A.M., 12 A.M., 2
  P.M., and 4 P.M. The sputum samples were homogenated and stored immedia-
  -tely at -20°C until assay.

-kinetic analysis: two-compartment open model infusion was used for esti
  mating the single-dose kinetic variables of CAZ and CEF, while for
  AZLO, one-compartment open model was used.

RESULTS

TABLE I: Mean serum-level-time concentrations for AZLO, CEF and CAZ (the
administered doses were: AZLO 133 mg/Kg, CEF and CAZ 66.7 mg/Kg)

TIME AFTER INJECTION	MEAN SERUM CONCENTRATION (± S.D.) (mg/1)		
(h)	AZLO	CEF	CAZ
0.0	531.0 (± 167.2)	422.0 (± 222.0)	222.0 (± 84.7)
0.5	329.0 (± 195.4)	192.0 (± 33.5)	111.1 (± 37.0)
1.0	200.6 (± 70.6)	126.0 (± 35.7)	62.4 (± 23.1)
2.0	86.0 (± 16.7)	71.0 (± 16.7)	27.4 (± 7.4)
4.0	32.5 (± 15.7)	20.8 (± 5.0)	10.8 (± 1.9)
6.0	6.3 (± 4.1)	7.6 (± 2.4)	3.0 (± 0.9)
7.5	3.0 (± 2.0)	4.4 (± 1.4)	1.8 (± 0.8)

TABLE II: Results on the sputum

	SPUTUM SAMPLES		
	TOTAL N°	ANTIBIOTIC FOUND IN: N° %	ANTIBIOTIC CONCENTRATIONS (range : mg/1)
AZLO	100	0 0	0 - 0
CEF	120	47 39.2	0.06 - 1.7
CAZ	118	118 100	0.2 - 5

Beta-lactamases: beta-lactamases were found in nearly all spu
tum samples (90.5%). As regards CAZ and CEF, the antibiotic level measured in the sputum, did not appear to be influenced by the presence of beta-lactamases; in fact, no correlation between the antibiotic sputum con-

centrations and the corresponding beta-lactamase activity was demonstrated.

TABLE III: Estimated kinetic parameters (all values are reported as mean
($\pm$ S.D.); range is given in brackets).

	AZLO	CAZ	CEF
Cl (ml h^{-1} Kg^{-1})	176.5 ($\pm$ 60.2) (113.2–242.6)	232.3 ($\pm$ 57.1) (155.7–299.4)	164.3 ($\pm$ 71.3) (116.1–306.6)
Vd$_{area}$ (ml/Kg)	245.2 ($\pm$ 66.7) (145.2–311.4)	465.2 ($\pm$ 140.2) (224.5–597.7)	317.4 ($\pm$ 126.1) (171.1–540.7)
t$\frac{1}{2}$ß (h)	0.98 ($\pm$ 0.16) (0.83–1.20)	1.40 ($\pm$ 0.39) (1.00–2.12)	1.35 ($\pm$ 0.22) (1.02–1.65)
t$\frac{1}{2}$$_\alpha$ (h)		0.25 ($\pm$ 0.04) (0.19–0.31)	0.22 ($\pm$ 0.13) (0.08–0.46)
K$_{12}$ (h^{-1})		0.84 ($\pm$ 0.29) (0.59–1.31)	1.53 ($\pm$ 1.51) (0.30–4.51)
K$_{21}$ (h^{-1})		1.23 ($\pm$ 0.46) (0.57–1.81)	1.80 ($\pm$ 1.21) (0.74–4.05)
K$_{10}$ (h^{-1})		1.25 ($\pm$ 0.31) (0.85–1.74)	1.41 ($\pm$ 0.88) (0.74–3.04)
Vc (1/Kg)		0.20 ($\pm$ 0.07) (0.11–0.26)	0.11 ($\pm$ 0.07) (0.02–0.21)

CONCLUSIONS

These main conclusions can be drawn from this pharmacokinetic
study:

- the clearance of AZLO, CAZ and CEF in CF patients is higher than in nor
  mal subjects and that is in accordance with previous studies on CF popu
  lation (Bergan 1979, Blumer 1983);

- the commonly-used dosing guidelines for these antibiotics may be inappropriate when CF patients are to be treated;

- antibiotic concentrations in the sputum are low and seem to be only one
  of the multiple factors influencing the clinical outcome of therapy.

REFERENCES

Bergan T, Michalsen H. Pharmacokinetics of azlocillin in children with cy
stic fibrosis. Arzeneimittelforschung 1979; 29: 1955-7.

Blumer JL. Ceftazidime in cystic fibrosis: pharmacokinetic evaluation and
therapeutic efficacy in patients with multiple drug-resistant
Pseudomonas (Abstract). Symposium on: "Ceftazidime in clinical practice", Glaxo Research LTD, London. 1983.

A "SMART" PORTABLE INFUSION PUMP FOR AUTOMATIC COMPUTATION
AND DELIVERY OF LIDOCAINE INFUSION REGIMENS

W.F. Nicholson, M.D. and R.W. Jelliffe, M.D.
Laboratory of Applied Pharmacokinetics, Section of Clinical
Pharmacology, University of Southern California School of
Medicine, Los Angeles, CA, USA

Immediate achievement and subsequent maintenance of a stable
and effective serum lidocaine level is therapeutically desirable. Efficacy can be better achieved and assessed clinically, arrhythmias controlled with less breakthrough, and toxicity avoided.

With conventional lidocaine therapy, usually given as a bolus
loading dose followed by a constant infusion at a fixed rate, one sees an
early drop in the serum level because of lidocaine's 2-compartment behavior. Frequently, breakthrough arrhythmias occur during this period of
low serum levels. These are usually treated with extra boli which raise
the serum level back toward an effective level.

The cause of this early fall in levels is the distribution of
drug from the central (serum) compartment into the peripheral compartment
without adequate replacement back into the central compartment of drug
which is lost to the peripheral comparatment. With such conventional
therapy, serum levels then usually climb slowly later on over 12-24 hours
until equilibrium is finally achieved between the central (serum) and
peripheral (all the rest) compartments.

To really achieve and maintain a stable serum level from the
beginning, the initial loading dose must instead be followed by a tapering infusion regimen during the distribution phase. This tapering
infusion regimen properly replaces the drug lost to the peripheral compartment during distribution and maintains a constant serum level throughout. Only after distribution is complete and equilibrium is achieved
can one then give the final fixed-rate maintenance infusion which replaces the drug as it is metabolized and/or excreted.

In the past, computation of such tapering infusion regimens
required a large time-shared computer. Furthermore, the actual delivery
of such regimens was difficult because the changing infusion rates required frequent manual resetting of the infusion apparatus.

Our laboratory has now developed a "smart" portable infusion
pump for automated computation and delivery of such lidocaine regimens.
As shown in Figure 1, it consists of an IVAC volumetric infusion pump
which is controlled by a Hewlett-Packard HP-41CV programmable handheld
calculator with clock function and integral magnetic card reader.

The calculator prompts the user to enter the patient's age,
sex, weight, estimated cardiac output, and the desired serum lidocaine
level. It then calculates a multistep, tapering infusion regimen, adjusted to the patient's clinical factors, using an a priori 2-compartment
model based on population parameter estimates. The calculator then controls the infusion pump and delivers the entire infusion regimen automa-

tically, instructing the pump to change the rate of infusion at the
appropriate times.

APPLICATION OF THE SUPERPOSITION PRINCIPLE
In the past, when a patient's response to a chosen serum level
was not satisfactory, the time-shared program was run again.   The past
lidocaine therapy was entered, a new serum level goal was chosen, and a
new tapering infusion regimen was computed to take the patient's serum
level from the old value to the new goal and to maintain it there continuously. This new regimen was then downloaded into the smart pump and
automatically delivered.
However, the kinetic behavior of many drugs can be described
as linear, time-invariant, multicompartment systems. This is generally
true for lidocaine. Because of this, the superposition principle for
linear systems can be used to achieve and maintain upward adjustment of
serum lidocaine levels for patients who are kinetically stable. The
superposition principle permits this upward adjustment at any time simply
by superimposing a certain percent of the original regimen upon itself,
starting at the desired time. The clinical problem of increasing the
serum level is now greatly simplified. The calculations now can be automatically performed within the smart pump itself, at the bedside, without
recourse to the time-shared computer.

OPERATION OF THE SMART PUMP
This smart pump is presently developed for calculating and
delivering these tapering lidocaine infusion regimens. It prompts the
operator to enter the patient's age, sex, estimated cardiac output, (as a
clinically estimated percent of normal) and the desired serum level goal.
It then calculates a nine-step tapering infusion regimen individualized
to that patient. The first step is the loading infusion. It is given not
as a bolus, but as a short infusion of the loading dose over three
minutes. This is followed by seven tapering steps which optimally approximate an exponentially tapering infusion. The ninth and last step is
the final maintenance infusion rate. Once computed, the regimen can be
reviewed and checked by the operator before administration. The apparatus is then started up, and the above regimen is automatically delivered.
If, after a period of observation, the patient has not responded to the
initial serum level goal, the infusion may be interrupted and the smart
pump instructed to achieve a higher serum level using the superposition
principle described above.
Serum levels, drawn at appropriate times, can then be entered
into the time-shared computer when the results become available, along
with the infusion regimen actually delivered, to find improved and more
specific estimates of the patient's pharmacokinetic parameter values.
-Using these new parameter estimates, the time-shared computer then recon-
structs and plots the time course of his lidocaine levels over all past
therapy, for better comparison with his clinical behavior during that
period. It then develops a new infusion regimen for further therapy.
This regimen can be downloaded into the smart pump either by direct
connection or by magnetic card.   The smart pump then delivers the new
tapering regimen automatically, just as before.

OTHER CLINICAL USES FOR THE SMART PUMP
This "smart" infusion apparatus, with additional programming,

is capable of automatic computation and delivery of pharmacokinetically designed infusions for several other drugs. Examples are theophylline, procainamide, quinindine, aminoglycosides, cardiac glycosides, and anesthetic and analgesic agents. For each of these drugs, it is then possible to review, evaluate, and adjust, if necessary, the goals and patient parameters which had been entered, and to develop new regimens for further therapy. Other schedules of drug and fluid delivery, such as intermittent infusions or timed infusions can also be entered into the smart pump for automatic delivery. This can allow the nurse to hang a 24-hour supply of IV antibiotic and have the appropriate doses delivered automatically at the proper times by the smart pump, with significant cost savings in the tubing and other apparatus usually associated with each individual dose.

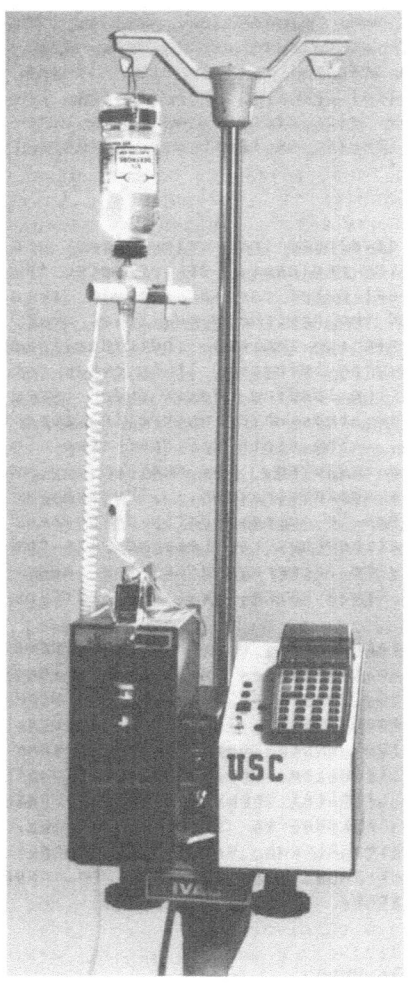

Several utility functions could be programmed into this apparatus, for example, to record the times at which serum levels were drawn or when other important interventions were made. Also, for each patient, the record of prior infusions of a particular drug, the present status of the pump, and other related information could be written onto a magnetic card. This would allow this information to be easily transfered between these smart pumps or to be entered into hospital information systems for further storage and analysis.

This "smart" pump should significantly enhance the reliability, precision, and safety of intravenous therapy with many drugs. Its battery power and portability permit its easy use in the field, the emergency room, the intensive care unit, or coronary care unit, thus greatly simplifying the task of delivering intelligent, pharmacokinetically designed drug dosage regimens to achieve and maintain clinically selected serum level goals.

Figure 1. "Smart" infusion pump in which an HP41CV hand calculator with computer interface (right),starts and controls an IVAC volumetric infusion pump (left), with its own interface (center), computing and automatically delivering infusion regimens of lidocaine and other drugs.

DIGITALIS THERAPY: THE CASE FOR DIGITOXIN

R.W. Jelliffe, M.D.
Laboratory of Applied Pharmacokinetics, Section of Clinical
Pharmacology, University of Southern California School of
Medicine, Los Angeles, CA, USA

Digoxin became a popular drug because of its relatively
short duration of action, its rapid excretion, and its resulting relatively rapid escape from toxicity. This was thought to reduce the
threat to life of an episode of digitalis toxicity.
However, deaths from digitalis toxicity usually occur within
the firsat 12 hours after the problem is recognized, and late deaths are
not described, thus reducing the impact of that argument. Furthermore, it
is well known in other situations that rapidly acting, rapidly excreted
drugs must be monitored more often in order to achieve safety in therapy.
This reasoning, well known for nitroprusside, has not been
rigorously extended to the case of digitalis therapy, although Moe, for
example, long ago advocated the use of digitoxin because of its greater
stability (1). With digitalis, just as with nitroprusside, while it is
good to get out of toxicity rapidly, it is dangerous to get into it
rapidly.
The cumulation of drugs and their approaach to a new steady
state following any change in dosage or renal function takes place by the
mirror-image of their decay, and is essentially complete in 5 drug half-
times. Because of this,drugs such as digoxin (and ouabain) have a more
rapid approach to a new steady state, and have more rapid accumulation
following a decrease in renal function than do drugs with longer half-
times, such as digitoxin, which have greater pharmacokinetic stability as
a result, just as stated by Moe.
The ability to evaluate pharmacokinetic stability as the bedside is poor for digitalis therapy where, except for the control of
ventricular rate in atrial fibrillation, our ability to perceive clinical
response to a certain total body concentration of glycoside, or to a
certain serum level, is poor. However, the pharmacokinetic behavior of
both digitoxin and digoxin has been well characterized by many studies by
many investigators over many years. Such pharmacokinetic models are well
known, and the influence of altered renal function upon these models is
also well known.

CLINICAL SIMULATIONS
Simulations in our laboratory with such models, using the
clinically-oriented USC*PACK time-shared computer programs for digitoxin
and digoxin therapy, employing both the older 1-compartment models of
digitoxin and digoxin (2) and the newer 2-compartment models (3,5), have
shown that in order to observe patients at an equal degree of change in
their total body glycoside concentration, a patient on digoxin (t1/2 =

1.5 days) must be observed and evaluated 4 times as often as a similar patient receiving digitoxin (t1/2 = 6 days) when his renal function is normal and creatinine clearance is 100 ml/minute, simply because the half-time of digoxin is 1/4 that of digitoxin. An anuric patient receiving digoxin (t1/2 = 4.5 days) must be monitored twice as often as a similar patient receiving digitoxin (t1/2 = 9 days), as his half-time is 1/2 that of digitoxin.

These simulations have shown that the accumulation of digoxin occurring 1 day after a fall in creatinine clearance from 100 to 75 ml/min is 8.4 times greater than the similar accumulation of digitoxin. It is 5.7 times greater for a fall in creatinine clearance from 75 to 50, 3.9 times greater for a fall from 50 to 25, and 3.3 times greater for a fall from 25 to 0 ml/min.

SLOWER ONSET OF TOXICITY WITH DIGITOXIN
Because of this, the total body concentration (and serum levels) of digitoxin are much less altered by day-to-day changes in a patient's physiology than are those of digoxin. This results in a much slower onset of toxicity, with smaller changes in total body glycoside concentration between observations and consequent earlier detection (at equal frequencies of observation). This permits toxicity to be detected when it poses less of a threat to the patient's life before the problem is recognized.

OTHER FACTORS
In addition, the better bioavailability of digitoxin, its lesser renal sensitivity, and its greater lipid solubility with greater CNS uptake and perhaps fewer cardiac manifestations of toxicity, all suggest as well that therapy with digitoxin may well carry less threat to life than therapy with digoxin. Examination of the relative incidence of digitalis toxicity with either drug also shows a definite tendency for a lower incidence of toxicity with digitoxin therapy (largely in Europe) than with digoxin therapy (largely in the USA). These combined pharmaco-kinetic and clinical facts strongly suggest that digitoxin is probably the safer and preferred glycoside for general use.

1. Moe GK, and Farah AE: Digitalis and Allied Cardiac Glycosides, in Goodman LS, and Gilman A: The Pharmacological Basis of Therapeutics, 4th edition, Macmillan Co., New York, 1970, p 700.

2. Jelliffe RW, Buell J, and Kalaba R: Reduction of Digitalis Toxicity by Computer-Assisted Glycoside Dosage Regimens. Ann Int Med., 77:891-906, 1972.

3. Jelliffe RW, Bechtol LD, and Crabtree R: The Bioavailability of Digitoxin. Clin Pharmacol & Ther., 27(2): p261, 1980.

4. Reuning RH, Sams RA, and Notari RE: Role of Pharmacokinetics in Drug Dosasge Adjustment. 1. Pharmacologic Effects, Kinetics, and Apparent Volume of Distribution of Digoxin. J Clin Pharmacol., 13:127-141, 1973.

5. Jelliffe RW, Schumitzky A, D'Argenio DZ, Rodman JH, and Forrest A: Improved Two-Compartment Computer Programs For Feedback Control of Digitoxin and Digoxin Therapy. Submitted for consideration for presentation at the 54th Scientific Sessions of the American Heart Association Meeting, Dallas, Texas, November 15-19, 1981.

CLINICAL AND PHARMACOKINETIC STUDY IN PATIENTS WITH OSTEOSAR-
COMA OF THE LONG BONES TREATED WITH DOSE METHOTREXATE

C.Valverde Mordt
Orthopedic Surgery Service.General Sanjurjo Hospital.Valencia

I.Font Noguera
Pharmacy Service. General Sanjurjo Hospital. Valencia.SPAIN

N.V.Jiménez Torres
Pharmacy Service. General Sanjurjo Hospital. Valencia.SPAIN

ABSTRACT. Four patients affected with Osteosarcoma of the long
bones and treated with Amputation en Adjuvant Chemotherapy Protocol that included High Dose Methotrexate (HDMTX) with Citrovorum Factor Rescue (CFR) were subjected to strict clinical,
biochemical, radiological and pharmacokinetic studies, during
time periods ranging from ten to nineteen months. The results
showed that, after giving HDMTX from 7.5-12 $g.m^{-2}$ doses, the
plasma levels, 24 and 48 h after the IV infusion was completed,
were placed at around 1.80 and 0.34 $mcmol.l^{-1}$, respectively.
On the other hand, two out of the four patients developed
symptoms of oropharyngeal mucositis with a necrotic ulcer in
one of them. A forearm blister appeared in the second one. In
one patient a platelet count depression with hematemesis followed Cyclophosphamide infusion. Two patients showed electrocar-
diographic changes after receiving Adriamycin. Disease free
survival at present is four years six months and three years
one month respectively in two patients. The other two died,one
and two years, respectively, after the start of chemotherapy.

I) INTRODUCTION

High Dose Methotrexate (HDMTX), alone or in conjunction with
other chemotherapeutic agents, has been used successfully in the treatment
of Osteosarcoma (OS). In fact, since the studies of ROSEN et al (1,2),
HDMTX has begun to be widely used in the pre- and postoperative phases of
OS. Of the different established therapeutic protocols, the greatest response with this kind of tumour has been obtained with the T_7 and T_{10} (3).

In this paper, we intend to inform on the clinical results
obtained with four patients affected by OS and undergoing clinical pharmacokinetic follow-up.

II) PATIENTS AND METHODS

II.1) Patients, Surgical and Chemotherapy treatment

The cases involved two males and two females 7,8,17 and 22
years old, respectively, and tumour situation in distal femur, proximal

tibia (two cases) and distal tibia. Three of the tumours were "classical"
OS and one a telangiectatic OS. All patients were admitted in hospital as
emergencies. This constitutes an unfavourable prognostic factor (4). All of
them were free from metastases at the time of diagnosis. On admission, a
radiological study was carried out, as well as an analytical examination.
The four patients have been treated with radical surgery.

In Table 1, the doses of MTX, length of treatment type of chemotherapeutic protocol are shown for each patient. In all cases, treatment
including HDMTX, preceded by Vincristine, hydration and alkalinization of
urine. Two hours after MTX, calcium folinate (citrovorum factor) was given
IM 9-12 mg every 6 h up to 12 doses.

II.2) Pharmacokinetic follow-up

The number of pharmacokinetic follow-ups carried out was 6
complete and 1 partial. Before beginning treatment, we opened a record
card for each patient (Figure 1) including the identification data of the
patient and his pharmacotherapeutic profile. The determination of MTX was
carried out through the method of enzyme immunoassay (EMIT^{TM}).

III) RESULTS

III.1) Plasma levels and Toxicity

The curve of plasma levels obtained through the mean values
found (n=4) at each of the previously established times, is represented in
Figure 2. The percentage of the variation coefficient varies from 17.84 to
47.06 for 0 and 48 h after IV infusion, respectively.

The administration of MTX was very frequently followed by vomiting. There was a constant but reversible alopecia. In one case two weeks

TABLE 1.-Chemotherapy protocols used for different patients

Patient	Dose MTX/ course $(g.m^{-2})$	No.cour-ses MTX	Total dose MTX/patient (g)	Treatment duration (months)	Protocol
YM	6.0	18	108.0	12	EORTC post
AV	7.5	9	67.5	12	ROSEN T_5 pre.post.
VB	7.5-8.0	16	180.4	10	ROSEN T_5 pre.T_7post.
ILL	7.5-12.0	18	212.3	19	ROSEN T_4 post.

after a HDMTX course a large forearm blister appeared.Two patients developed on two occasions orophargyngeal mucositis with a necrotic ulcer, which
subsided after 15 days with hydration, antibiotherapy and calcium folinate
mouthwashes. In no case did this symptomatology oblige us to stop treatment.
However, these situations, except that of alopecia, were not detected in
the patients undergoing pharmacokinetic follow-up (Figure 2).

As far a biochemical and kidney and liver function follow-up is
concerned,we found no abnormal values which might have supposed changes in
the initial situation of the patients after MTX treatment.

Figure 1.- Model of record card for clinical pharmacokinetic follow-up of MTX.

Clinical Pharmacokinetic Laboratory   R.S.G.S.

    PHARMACY SERVICE   Valencia

FOLLOW-UP CARD FOR METHOTREXATE (MTX)

Patient ....Patient´s number .....Date of birth.....Dpt-bed......

Weight ....Height ........S.C...... Diagnosis ....Treatment.................

HYDRATION: IV infusions given ....

           Volume given before MTX ....and after MTX ....
ALKALINIZATION: ⊂ Oral: Dose..................
                ⊂ IV: Volume given ....

Urine (ml)	pH urine	Date	Time	Urine (ml)	pH urine	Date	Time
Before infusion MTX				During and after infusion MTX			

INFUSION MTX: ...... $g.\bar{m}^2$ ....g total ....begins ....ends.

LEUCOVORIN: Dosage..................

Concomittant medication ....

SAMPLE TAKEN (BLOOD).   Date   Time   PL (mcmol l⁻¹)

   1st- 0 hour after IV infusion   ....

   2nd- 6 "   "   ....

   3rd- 12 "   "   ....

   4th- 24 "   "   ....

   5th- 36 "   "   ....

   6th- 48 "   "   ....

RESULTS

Time from start of MTX infusion	24 h	48 h	72 h
Toxic PL (mcmol.l⁻¹)	10	1	0.1
Theoretical PL (extrapolation)(mcmol.l⁻¹)			
Plasma clearance $(l.h.\bar{m}^2)$			

PHARMACOKINETIC COMMENTARY

III.2)   Therapeutic Response and Survival

An objective response could be observed only in one case in which the patient had a biopsy and was given a preoperative T_5 protocol, and the anatomopathological study of the surgical specimen after knee disar ticulation showed a decrease in the size of the tumour, with extensive ne crosis and very few areas of viable tumour, as well as decrease of the radiological image of the tumour.

Two cases , 7 years old, distal tibia and 8 years old, proximal tibia, respectively, are surviving free from metastases, four years six months and three years one month, respectively; actually they have comple ted their chemotherapy protocol. The other two died, one and two years, respectively, after the initiation of chemotherapy.

IV)   DISCUSSION

We may state that the preoperative protocols are effective when the primary tumour is diagnosed early, as an objective individual res ponse is evident in the decrease in size and extensive necrosis of the

FIGURE 2.-Plasma levels of MTX after IV infusion

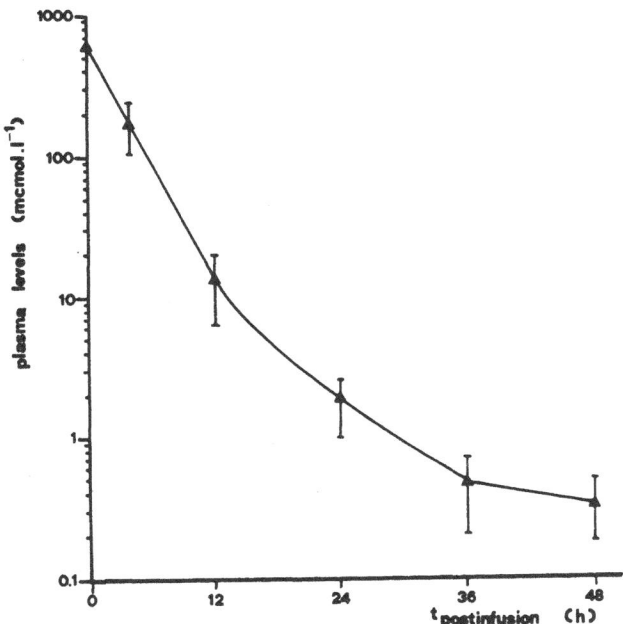

tumour. A metastases free survival is also achieved.

The average PL reached in our patients at the end of IV infusion of MTX was 623.67 ± 111.27 mcmol.l^{-1}. These values are comparable with those obtained by other authors with similar treatment(5)Differences of up to 37.5% (4.5 g.m^{-2}) in the range of IV doses used ($7.5-12$ g.m^{-2}) have had no consequences on the PL values at zero time.

V) REFERENCES
1) ROSEN,G. et al. (1975) The rationale for multiple drug chemotherapy in treatment of osteogenic sarcoma. Cancer,35, 936-45
2) ROSEN,G. et al.(1979) Primary osteogenic sarcoma.The rationale for preoperative chemotherapy and delayed surgery. Cancer,43, 2163-77
3) ROSEN,G. et al. (1982) Preoperative chemotherapy for osteogenic sarcoma: selection of postoperative adjuvant chemothepy based on the response of the primary tumor to preoperative chemotherapy. Cancer,49, 1221-30
4) BROSTROM,L. (1979) On the natural history of osteosarcoma: aspects on diagnosis, prognosis and endocrinology. Acta Orthopaedica Scandinavica. Suppl.183. Munksgaard.Copenhagen.
5) ISACOFF,W.H. et al. (1974) Pharmacokinetic of high dose methotrexate with citrovorum factor rescue. Cancer Treat Rep, 61,1665-74

PHARMACOKINETICS OF NETILMICIN IN CHRONIC LIVER DISEASE

M.O.Rodrigues[*],M.F.Marques[*], J.A.Morais[***], A.P.Correia[**]
M.E.Camilo[**], J.Pinto Correia[**].Departments of Pharmacy[*]
and Medicine II[**], University Hospital of Santa Maria;
Faculty of Pharmacy[***], Lisbon, Portugal

We present preliminary results of an undergoing stu
dy conducted in an Intensive Care Unit of Gastroenterology in
order to evaluate Netilmicin pharmacokinetics in patients with
liver cirrhosis and high risk of renal dysfunction.

Material and Methods

From April to September 1983, we studied six male
patients with hepatic cirrhosis, with ages ranging from 39 to
65 years (mean: 53). Reasons for Netilmicin therapy were:
sepsis 1, infected ascites 2, urinary or respiratory infections in 3 patients. Netilmicin was administered by intravenous
infusion during 30 minutes. The daily dosage was determined
according to the body weight. Serum samples were drawn twice
daily, starting 48 hours after the beginning of treatment: the
first immediately before infusion and the second 30 minutes
after end of infusion. Levels in serum and whenever possible
in ascitic fluid were measured in order to determine elimination curve. Additionaly serum creatinine and urea concentra -
tions were evaluated.

Netilmicin concentrations in serum and in ascitic
fluid were determined by E.M.I.T.. Pharmacokinetics analysis
was performed assuming the one-compartment open model.

Results and comments

A progressive increase of the minimum daily concentration was observed in 3 patients. In these patients a highly significant correlation between the minimum daily serum levels of Netilmicin and the creatinine levels was found(Fig.1)

In the remaining 3 patients the minimum daily serum concentrations were stable into the normal range, as well as the renal function.

The maximum concentrations were determined only in five patients. There was no significant increase during the treatment, without any correlation with the change of creatinine levels.

The patients were divided according to their clinical liver situation: group 1 - critically ill (sepsis and infected ascitis in chronic liver disease)and group 2 - stable chronic liver disease. The following Netilmicin pharmacokinetic parameters were considered in each patient: constant of elimination rate, half-life and clearance.

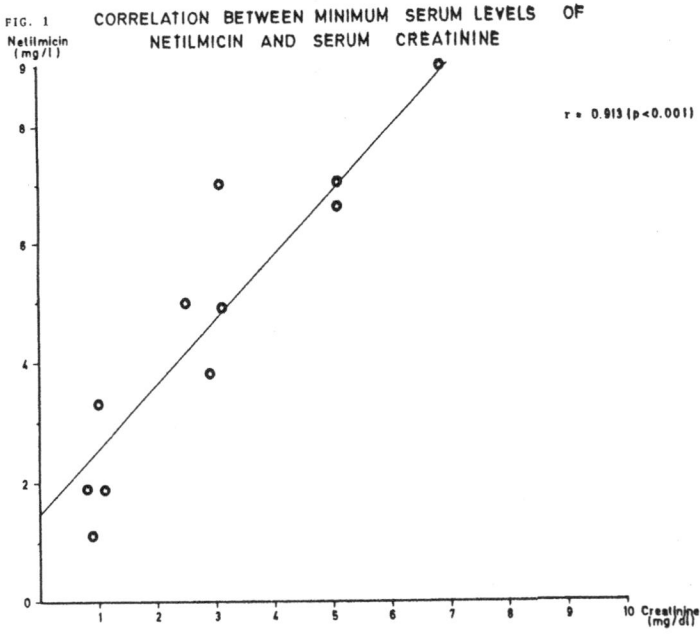

FIG. 1   CORRELATION BETWEEN MINIMUM SERUM LEVELS OF
           NETILMICIN AND SERUM CREATININE

$r = 0.913 \ (p < 0.001)$

In every patients of group 1 (table 1) the values
of all the pharmacokinetic parameters were different in begin
ning and at the end of Netilmicin therapy. We can also see
that the deterioration of renal function (measured by creatinine levels) was accompanied by an increase of Netilmicin half
-life.

TABLE - 1 PHARMACOKINETIC PARAMETERS
(Group of critically ill liver patients)

Patients	Ke (hr.$^{-1}$) start	end	T1/2 (hr.) start	end	Cr(mg /dl) start	end	Cl (ml/min) start	end
F.L.	0.085	0.044	8,1	15,7	1.4	3.4	17,8	9.3
V.S.	0.169	0.129	4,1	5,3	0.8	1.3	46	35
A.H.	0.144	0.105	4,8	6,5	1.0	1.6	48.2	35.1

On the other hand, in the stable group (table   2)
the different parameter values remained stable through   the
therapy period. So the determination of a mean value was possible. No change in the renal function was observed.

TABLE - 2   MEAN PHARMACOKINETIC PARAMETERS
(Group of stable liver patients)

Patients	Ke (hr^{-1})	$T_{1/2}$ (hr)	Cl (ml/min.)
J.P.	0.191	3.6	48
A.S.	0.171	4.0	43
A.L.	0.255	2.7	85.1

In one patient with ascites, serum and ascitic fluid
levels of Netilmicin were determined concomitantly every hour
or every two hours between 2 consecutive administrations (Netilmicin 150 mg b.i.d.). Elementary pharmacokinetic analysis
of the serum data using semilogarithmic plot (Fig. 2) suggests
the possible existence of a two compartment open model. This
might be explained by the presence of a significant ascites.

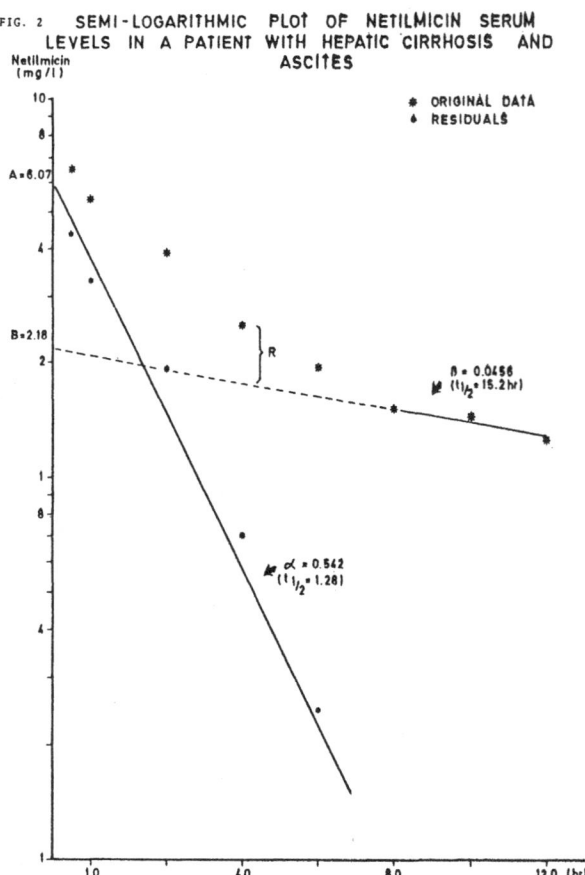

FIG. 2   SEMI-LOGARITHMIC PLOT OF NETILMICIN SERUM
          LEVELS IN A PATIENT WITH HEPATIC CIRRHOSIS AND
          ASCITES

The corresponding equation is shown in Fig. 3, and the value is very low yielding a very high terminal half-life, 15 hours. As shown ascitic fluid levels were constant and within in the therapeutic range of serum. The detailed treatment of data in ascitic fluid obviously needs study of more patients, which is now in progress.

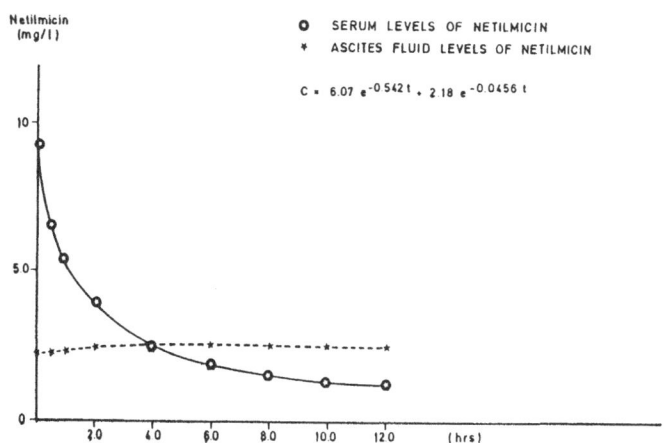

FIG. 3 SERUM AND ASCITIC FLUID LEVELS OF NETILMICIN IN HEPATIC CIRRHOSIS PATIENT, WITH ASCITES DURING DOSAGE INTERVAL (150 mg b.i.d.)

O SERUM LEVELS OF NETILMICIN
* ASCITES FLUID LEVELS OF NETILMICIN

$C = 6.07\,e^{-0.5421\,t} + 2.18\,e^{-0.0456\,t}$

In conclusion, our preliminary results suggest that: 1) the minimum daily concentrations are more reliable than peak concentrations for pharmacokinetic parameters and dosage adjustment. It presents a good correlation with renal function. 2) Critically ill liver patients seem more vulnerable to toxic effects of Netilmicin therapy. So they demand close monitoring of serum levels.

References

Burkle, W.S. (1981). Comparative evaluation of the aminoglyco
    side antibiotics for systemic use. Drug Intell.Clin.
    Pharm., 15: 847-862
Guay, D.R.P. (1983). New drug evaluations - Netilmicin. Drug
    Intell.Clin.Pharm., 17: 83-91
Jelliffe, R.W. (1973). Creatinine clearance - Bedside estima-
    te. Ann.Intern.Med., 70: 604
Ristuccia, A.M. et al (1982). The aminoglycosides - Symposium
    on Antimicrobial Therapy. Medical Clinics of North
    America 66: 302-312
Rowland, M. et al (1981). Clinical Pharmacokinetics; Lea et
    Febiger, Philadelphia
Winter, M.E. (1981). Basic Clinical Pharmacokinetics,Applied
    Therapeutics Inc., S.Francisco

TIMESHARED COMPUTER PROGRAMS FOR M.A.P. BAYESIAN ADAPTIVE CONTROL OF DOSAGE REGIMENS OF AMINOGLYCOSIDES, LIDOCAINE, DIGOXIN, DIGITOXIN, PROCAINAMIDE, AND QUINIDINE

R.W. Jelliffe, M.D., A. Schumitzky, Ph.D., D.Z. D'Argenio, Ph.D., D. Katz, Ph.D., W.F. Nicholson, M.D., J.H. Rodman, Pharm.D., A.K. Hurst, Pharm.D., A. Forrest, Pharm.D., T.M. Gilman, Pharm.D., and F.J. Goicoechea, M.D.
Laboratory of Applied Pharmacokinetics, Section of Clinical Pharmacology, University of Southern California School of Medicine, Los Angeles, CA, USA

E. Kolb, M.D.
Community Hospital of the Monterey Peninsula, Carmel, CA, USA

This Laboratory has developed time-shared computer programs for adaptive control of dosage regimens of the above drugs. In all the programs, parameter values of an a priori 1 or 2-compartment model of the drug are adjusted to important patient characteristics to develop an initial regimen to achieve and maintain desired therapeutic goals. In addition, an optimal strategy for therapeutic drug monitoring is computed so that serum levels, usually a carefully selected series of pairs of levels, can be obtained, within clinical constraints, at optimal times for greatest accuracy in computing the patient's own pharmacokinetic parameter values when the results subsequently become available (1).

The model is then fitted to the patient's serum level data using a Maximum A-posteriori Probability (M.A.P.) Bayesian fitting procedure (2). The fitted model is then used to reconstruct the pharmacokinetic behavior of the drug over all of his past therapy, for comparison with his past clinical behavior. Using clinical judgement and the above reconstruction, a therapeutic goal is again chosen, and the fitted model is used to compute the new adjusted dosage regimen. This regimen is also converted into practical advice for administration such as flow settings for infusion apparatus and diagrams of how the syringe or bottle should empty during the infusion. Lastly, a new optimal strategy for subsequent monitoring of the new therapy with the fitted model is computed.

Programs from other centers have generally analysed data obtained only during a single dose interval. When patient factors affecting excretion change, such programs discard all previous serum data and must begin all over again with totally new data in some new, and again single, dose interval. This has resulted in inefficient, suboptimal, and costly use of serum level data.

DESIGN OF THE PROGRAMS
The present programs, in contrast, compute the intercept and slope of the relationship between the elimination rate constant of the drug and either creatinine clearance or cardiac output, depending on the program. Because of this, the programs can analyse serum level data which have been acquired over many different dose intervals, even if the rate constant for excretion has been changing greatly during that time. Because of this design, when renal function changes, for example, one does not have to discard previous serum data. Instead, it can usually be kept and integrated with more selectively ordered new data, which need not be so extensive as to constitute starting all over anew. This has resulted

in much more optimal and economical use and ordering of serum levels, and
in more cost-effective patient care.
        The M.A.P. Bayesian fitting procedure is designed to find the
mathematical "best match", or fit, between what is known about the
pharmacokinetic parameter values in the general population on the one
hand, and on the other, the data of serum levels (either plentiful or
sparse) found in that particular patient. This blend of these 2 sets of
data has usually resulted in improved prediction of subsequent serum
levels compared to predictions resulting from least-squares fitting procedures. In addition, the fitted models in these programs are usually
also "more informed", as they are usually based on more serum level data
points, usually taken at optimally chosen times, than are models based on
fitting data obtained only during a single dose interval. Such a fitted
model is usually better able to "thread its way" through random variations in parameter values that can appear from one dose interval to
another due to laboratory error, dosage error, and the many other errors
that occur in such clinical situations, to find the most accurate parameter values and therefore the most accurate next dosage regimen to achieve
the chosen goals.

THE AMINOGLYCOSIDE PROGRAMS
        The aminoglycoside programs allow one to plan, monitor, and
adjust therapy with gentamicin, tobramycin, netilmycin, amikacin, kanamy-
cin and streptomycin for adult patients, and with gentamicin for newborns
(under 2 weeks old). Since the programs operate in the presence of changing renal function, they allow one to manage therapy even for adult
patients who must undergo hemodialysis. For such patients, we have found
that one can represent an episode of hemodialysis by entering a "dose" of
zero, a value of creatinine clearance for that "dose" which is the patient's baseline value plus an extra 50 ml/min of apparent creatinine
clearance for dialysis of aminoglycoside with modern apparatus (or 25
ml/min for older apparatus), and by entering a "dose interval" which is
the duration of hemodialysis. After dialysis, another dose of zero may be
entered, if needed, using his baseline value of creatinine clearance and
a dose interval from then until the next dose was given.
        With regard to monitoring, one can obtain a peak aminoglyco-
side level shortly after a dose and couple it with other pre- and post-
dialysis levels of aminoglycoside (and creatinine, to estimate his baseline creatinine clearance with another computer program, using the rise
from a post- to a pre- dialysis creatinine level), and can make intelligent and useful fits to serum level data even for hemodialysis patients.
In our experience to date, reconstructions made from such data have shown
that patients generally have tended to receive aminoglycoside doses after
having been dialysed, rather than when they often actually needed doses
to achieve and maintain desired peak and trough serum levels. The present
programs help to understand and manage these patients.
        One clinical study with these programs analysed all patients
receiving gentamicin therapy who were evaluated by the drug therapy
consult service of the Los Angeles County-University of Southern California Medical Center from October 1978 through June 1979, who had a total
of at least 10 serum levels drawn. Ten such patients were found. In these
patients, serum levels of gentamicin were both prospectively predicted
and subsequently achieved with essentially equal precision in the 6
patients with significantly changing creatinine clearance as in the 4
patients whose renal function was stable (3).

For the aminoglycosides, optimal times to obtain serum levels for monitoring appear to be shortly after the peak with the first dose of a new regimen, and at an optimal time in the latest subsequent dose interval one is willing to wait for, depending on the clinical situation and the urgency to know the result of the second level. The later one can wait to obtain the second level, up until a steady state has been reached, the more accurate will be the estimates of the patient's pharmacokinetic parameter values resulting from the data(1).

The procainamide and quinidine programs are similar in concept to the aminoglycoside programs.

THE LIDOCAINE PROGRAM

Lidocaine is a flow-limited, hepatically metabolized drug. It is therefore important to estimate hepatic blood flow. One can do essentially this by utilizing data of the effect of age upon cardiac output and by making a clinical estimate of a patient's cardiac output as a percent of normal for his age. In this way, one can convert clinical data of a patient's age, history, and physical findings into a reasonable a priori value for the elimination rate constant of lidocaine. This program is designed to operate in the presence of changing cardiac output, just as the other programs operate in the presence of changing creatinine clearance.

Lidocaine requires a 2-compartment pharmacokinetic model. Achievement and maintaince of a stable serum level during the distribution phase of the drug requires an initial loading infusion, analogous to a bolus, followed by a tapering infusion protocol during the distribution phase, and, after equilibration, a final fixed rate maintainance infusion. The present program develops such regimens.

A randomized prospective study compared the achievement and maintenance of therapeutic serum levels with such computer-assisted (CA) regimens compared to conventional therapy (CT). A separate audit of clinical outcome was also conducted. CA regimens provided significantly more effective serum levels, especially in the first hour (2.65 ug/ml), than did conventional therapy (1.5 ug/ml, $P < 0.05$). In the audit of outcome, this was reflected in the findings that ventricular fibrillation occurred in only 2 of 78 CA patients, compared to 8 of 78 CT patients. Extra bolus doses or infusion adjustments were required in 33 of the 78 CT patients but only in 2 of the 78 CA patients, a significant difference ($P < 0.001$). Regimens developed with this program thus improved therapeutic precision, suggestively reduced the incidence of ventricular fibrillation, and significantly reduced the need for dosage adjustments to control breakthrough arrhythmias (4).

For lidocaine, optimal times to obtain serum levels are at the end of an initial 5 minute loading infusion (analogous to a bolus), approximately 15 and 70 minutes later, and at the latest possible time consistent with the clinical urgency to know.

THE DIGOXIN AND DIGITOXIN PROGRAMS

These programs use a 2-compartment model with central (serum) compartment and peripheral (inotropic effect) compartment (5,6). There is no need to wait 8 hours before obtaining a serum level. The sampling strategy to characterize the central compartment optimally is actually to obtain a peak level at 1.5-2.0 hours after the first dose in a regimen, and a trough level in the latest subsequent dose interval one is willing to wait for on clinical grounds. For characterization of the peripheral compartment, preliminary computations suggest that levels at 0.5 and 7.0 hours after the first dose may optimally monitor the distribution phase.

When serum levels become available, the 2-compartment model is fitted to them, and the reconstructed central and peripheral data are plotted for comparison with the patient's clinical behavior. New goals may be chosen. Using the fitted model, a new regimen is then calculated. These oral dosage regimens are developed to achieve and maintain not serum levels, but rather a chosen peak total body glycoside concentration in the peripheral compartment. This regimen is then then apportioned into appropriate doses for each day of a typical week, using the chosen available tablet size. A forward simulation then plots probable central and pereipheral data which should result from that regimen, helping visually to understand the important clinical relationships that exist between the central and peripheral compartments, and to see what the probable serum levels will be.

The programs appear to date to improve the abililty to achieve and maintain rate control for patients with atrial fibrillation, and to shorten hospital stay. They also aid greatly in modeling the effect and magnitude of the digoxin-quinidine interaction in patients, not only the elevation of serum levels, but also the reduction of peripheral uptake and inotropic effect seen with the interaction.

The programs are accessed with conventional remote terminals and are used by community and teaching hospitals over an international time-sharing facility (7). Its network has local telephone numbers for access in the USA, the UK, France, Holland, West Germany, and Belgium. The GTE TELENET network can also be used for access from Spain, Italy, and other countries, including the Far East.

REFERENCES

1.   D'Argenio DZ: Optimal Sampling Times for Pharmacokinetic Experiments. J. Pharmacokinetics and Biopharmaceutics, 9(6): 739-755, 1981.

2.   Sheiner LB, et al: Forecasting Individual Pharmacokinetics. Clin. Pharmacol. Ther., 26:294-305, 1979.

3.   Forrest A, Gilman T, Rodman J, and Jelliffe RW: A Time-shared Computer Program for Adaptive Control of Aminoglycoside Therapy. Clin Pharmacol & Ther., 27(2): p 254, 1980.

4.   Rodman JH, et al: Clinical Studies with Computer-Assisted Initial Lidocaine Therapy. Archives of Internal Medicine, in press.

5.   Reuning RH, Sams RA, and Notari RE: Role of Pharmacokinetics in Drug Dosasge Adjustment. 1. Pharmacologic Effects, Kinetics, and Apparent Volume of Distribution of Digoxin. J Clin Pharmacol., 13:127-141, 1973.

6.   Jelliffe RW, Bechtol LD, Crabtree R: The Bioavailability of Digitoxin. Clin Pharmacol Ther, 27(2): p 261, 1980.

7.   Comshare, Inc., (Mr. Suda). 3325 Wilshire Boulevard, Suite 500, Los Angeles, California 90010. (213) 387-1177.

PHARMACOKINETIC BEHAVIOUR OF HIGH DOSE METHOTREXATE

I.Font Noguera
Pharmacy Service.General Sanjurjo Hospital.Valencia.SPAIN

N.V.Jiménez Torres
Pharmacy Service.General Sanjurjo Hospital.Valencia.SPAIN

ABSTRACT.-Because of the low therapeutic index of MTX,it necessary to monitor its plasma   levels in order to prevent its
toxicity, since the clinical parameters are not sufficiently
effective for such an aim. The objective of the present work is
to study the behaviour of MTX under two aspects: on the one
hand, the prospective identification of patients with high toxicity risk, and on the other, to succeed in establishing ranges
of doses for IV infusion, so that its plasma   levels are
situated within the established ranges. The results found using
the EIA technique in five patients subjected to doses of
$7.5\text{-}12$ g.m^{-2} during 4 h of IV infusion,permit the establishment
of the following pharmacokinetic parameters and constants for
MTX in these conditions: $t_{1/2}\alpha$ and β 1.96 ± 0.27 and 10.21 ± 1.52 h
respectively; Clp,0.17 ± 0.06 l.h^{-1}.Kg^{-1}; V_β ,2.50 ± 0.89 l.Kg^{-1};
K_{12},0.008 ± 0.004 h^{-1}; K_{21},0.073 ± 0.015 h^{-1} and K_{13},0.350 ± 0.055 h^{-1}

I) INTRODUCTION

Methotrexate (MTX) has a low therapeutic index due to the
fact that its toxicity is conditioned principally by the plasma concentration and by the time of contact with the tissues, it is necessary to determine the plasma levels (PL) (1). In this way, it is possible to reach a
pharmacokinetic model which controls the variation of its concentration in
function of the characteristics of the patient and the dose given. And this
must be so, insofar as with this kind of drug it is not, in general, possible to correlate PL with clinical response (2).

Thus, the aim of the present work is, on the one hand, to iden-
tifify in advance those patients at high risk from toxicity, and, on the
other hand, to establish a range of doses for IV infusion, so that the PL
come within the established intervals (at 24 h, 10 mcmol.l^{-1} and at 48 h
1 mcmol.l^{-1}).

II) PATIENTS AND METHODS

II.1) Patients and chemotherapeutic protocols

Table 1 reports on the chemotherapeutic protocols with cytostatics (3,4) and on the dose given and duration of treatment in five patients with an average age of 15.4 (8 to 22) years and an average weight of 42.3 (35-52) Kg. The total treatments carried out with pharmacokinetic follow-up was ten.

The IV hydration was established 24 h before the start of MTX treatment, at a velocity of 125 ml.h^{-1} of 5% Glucose and 0.9% NaCl in equal parts. To guarantee the pH of urine being equal to over 7, 250 ml NaCO$_3$H 1/6 M were given simultaneously.

The MTX was infused IV for 4 h with doses of 4.5-12 g.m^{-2}. A variable period of between 7 to 30 days elapsed between the sequential application of each MTX course. Two hours after MTX infusion, calcium folinate was given IM at doses of 9-12 mg every 6 h for 72 h .

II.2) Samples taking and analytical method

The extractions (2ml of blood) were made at 0,4,6,8,12,24,36 and 48 h after MTX infusion. We used the technique of enzyme inmunoassay (EMIT^{TM}) which determines the total MTX with a coefficient of variation less than 10%.

II.3) Pharmacokinetic analysis

The pharmacokinetic study of the postinfusion phase was carried out according to LOO and RIEGELMAN's method (5) for a two-compartment open model. In order to calculate the constants and parameters which define the pharmacokinetic model followed by the MTX, we have used the established methods (6).

III) RESULTS

Table 2 shows the plasma   half-life of phase α and β ($t_{1/2}\alpha$ and $t_{1/2}\beta$) of MTX in each patient. All these values are of $p<0.05$ with respect to the mean value. One case (VM) was excluded because this condition was not fulfilled. This table includes plasma clearance (Clp) and the apparent volume of distribution of the phase β (V_β). In these values a great intra- and interindividual variation can be seen. The transfer rate constants K_{12},K_{21} and K_{13} obtained for the MTX are also shown in this table.

On correlating Clp with infusion rate (Ko) we observe that there is no linearity ($r=0.210$,$p>0.1$). This situation is also found on correlating V_β and Ko (r=0.229,p>0.1). These facts are in complete accordance with the excellent linearity found with Clp versus V_β(r=0.916,p<0.001) That is, the $t_{1/2}$ is independent of the dose.

None of the patients in the ten pharmacokinetic follow-up treatments carried out, presented clinically perceptible toxic effects, which fact coincides with the PL at 24 h and 48 h being under 10 and 1 mcmol.l^{-1}, respectively.

TABLE 1.-Chemotherapy protocols used for different patients

Patient	Dose MTX/ course $(g.m^{-2})$	No.cour- ses MTX	Total dose MTX/patient (g)	Treatment duration (months)	Protocol
AV	7.5	9	67.5	12	ROSEN T_5 pre.post
VB	7.5-8.0	16	108.4	10	ROSEN T_5 pre.T_7post
ILL	7.5-12.0	18	212.3	19	ROSEN T_4 post.
TS	8.0	7	62.0	7	ROSEN T_7 post.
VM	4.5-8.8	11	93.5	8	ROSEN T_7 post.

TABLE 2.- Pharmacokinetic constants and parameters of MTX after intravenous infusion

Patient	Dose $(g.m^{-2})$	Ko $(g.m^{-2}.h^{-1})$	$t_{1/2}\alpha$ (h)	$t_{1/2}\beta$ (h)	Clp $(1.h^{-1}.kg^{-1})$	V_β $(1.kg^{-1})$	K_{12} (h^{-1})	K_{21} (h^{-1})	K_{13} (h^{-1})
VB	8.0	1.3	1.74	10.12	0.21	3.01	0.010	0.071	0.386
ILL	7.5	1.4	2.11	10.34	0.12	1.82	0.009	0.069	0.317
ILL	7.5	1.9	2.26	7.26	0.18	1.88	0.018	0.105	0.281
AV	7.5	1.9	1.90	10.88	0.14	2.19	0.004	0.065	0.360
VB	8.0	2.0	2.30	12.87	0.09	1.73	0.003	0.055	0.298
TS	8.0	2.0	1.52	10.86	0.28	4.39	0.009	0.065	0.447
TS	8.0	2.0	1.78	9.76	0.15	2.16	0.005	0.072	0.384
ILL	12.0	3.0	2.08	9.04	0.21	2.78	0.005	0.078	0.327
$\bar{x}$	8.3	1.9	1.96	10.21	0.17	2.50	0.008	0.073	0.350
$\pm$SD	1.5	0.5	0.27	1.52	0.06	0.89	0.004	0.015	0.055

IV)   DISCUSSION

With doses of 7.5-12 $g.m^{-2}$, the PL reached are similar in their evolution in time. On the other hand, the pharmacokinetic constants calculated (Table 2) fultil the required conditions for a two-compartment model. This behaviour of MTX has been reported by various authors (7), independently of the dose and of how it is given. However, mono-, tri- and multi-compartmental models have also been proposed (8,9).

The V_β obtained for our patients is 105.75$\pm$37.65 l . This high value suggests that the MTX is situated in "third spaces" which function as deposits. However, the relationships K_{12}/K_{21}=0.11; K_{12}/K_{13}=0.02 and K_{21}/K_{13}=0.26, show that MTX is a drug which tends to disappear rapidly from the organism (10). The mean value of Clp, 119,9 $ml.min^{-1}$,(77.6-162.2) suggests that the MTX is eliminated primarily through renal excretion (11).

In the group of patients studied, we have observed no influence of the age of patient on the Clp and $t_{1/2}$ of the MTX; a fact also pointed out by other authors (12).

A global analysis of the $t_{1/2}$,K_{12},$K_{21}$and K_{13} and Clp and V_β , obtained for our patients, would seem to support the idea that the latter are more prone than the former to be influenced by the technical conditions found on giving MTX and by the clinical situation of the patient (13). This observation leads us to admit that a modification in the degree of balance of MTX is produced between the central and peripheral compartment and important intra- and interindividual variations are found in the value of V_β (Table 2).

However, in some patients with a high V_β value, the $t_{1/2}\beta$ may be increased in the course of MTX treatment. This situation involves establishing PL-Time criteria to identify in advance those patients with potential MTX toxicity (14). Consequently, it would not seem to be viable to estimate PL theoretically, as inherent factors in the method of administration and the clinical situation of the patient influence the pharmacokinetics.

REFERENCES

1) BLEYER,W.A. (1978) The clinical pharmacology of methotrexate Cancer,41,36-51.
2) CROM,W.R. et al. (1981) Methotrexate: therapeutic use serum concentration monitoring. In Individualizing drug therapy. Practical applications of drug monitoring, ed.W.J.Taylor &

A.L.Finn.Vol.1,pp.150-73.New York:Gross,Townsend,Frank,Inc.
3) ROSEN,G. et al. (1975) The rationale for multiple drug chemotherapy in treatment of osteogenic sarcoma. Cancer,35,
   936-45.
4) ROSEN,G. et al. (1979). Primary osteogenic sarcoma.The
   rationale for preoperative chemotherapy and delayed surgery.
   Cancer,43, 2163-77.
5) LOO,J.C. & RIEGELMAN,S. (1970) Assessment of pharmacokinetic
   constants from postinfusion blood curves obtained after IV
   infusion. J Pharm Sci,59, 53-5
6) GIBALDI,M. & PERRIER,D. (1975). Pharmacokinetics.New York:
   Marcel Dekker Inc.
7) STOLLER,R.G. et al. (1975). Pharmacokinetics of high dose
   methotrexate (NSC-740). Cancer Chem Rep,part 3,6,19-24.
8) ROBERTS,D. et al. (1979). Serum levels of methotrexate by
   the ligand-binding assay after high dose therapy for osteosarcoma. Cancer,44,881-90
9) BISCHOFF,K.B. et al. (1971). Methotrexate pharmacokinetics.
   J Pharm Sci,60,1128-33.
10)PLA,J.M. & POZO,A. (1974). Manual de iniciación a la bio-
   farmacia. Barcelona: Romargraf,S.A.
11)PITMAN,S.W. et al. (1975). Clinical trial of high dose methotrexate (NSC-740) with citrovorum factor (NSC-3590).
   Toxicologic and therapeutic observations. Cancer Chem Rep,
   part 3,3, 43-9.
12)EVANS,W.E. et al. (1979). Pharmacokinetic monitoring of
   high dose methotrexate early recognition of high-risk patients. Cancer Pharmacol, 3, 161-6.
13)ISACOFF,W.H. et al. (1974). Pharmacokinetics of high dose
   methotrexate with citrovorum factor rescue. Cancer Treat
   Rep,61, 1665-74.
14)NIRENBERG,A. et al. (1977). High dose methotrexate with
   citrovorum factor rescue: predictive value of serum methotrexate concentrations and corrective measures to avert
   toxicity. Cancer Treat Rep,61,779-83.

INFLUENCE OF DIFFERENT FACTORS ON PHENOBARBITAL AND DIPHENYLHYDANTOIN
PLASMA   CLEARANCE IN CHILDREN: POSOLOGIC IMPLICATIONS

Ron* L.; Martinez-Pacheco** R.; Vila-Jato** J.L.; Graña* I.; Tojo* R.

* Pediatric Departament
** Pharmaceutical Service
Hospital General de Galicia. Santiago de Compostela. (Spain)

The main goal of this comunication is to evaluate the influence
of age, sex, nutritional index, dose and type and lengh of treatment on
the plasmatic clearance of phenobarbital (PhB) and diphenylhydantoin
(DPH) in children and to stablish the posologic repercussions of these
factors.

METHOD

Patients-. The study was carried out on the 107 children- 55
males and 52 females- whose ages ranged from 2 to 14 years. Of these, 30
were given monotherapy with PhB while the rest were treated with both
drugs. The doses ranged from 1.38 to 8.82 $mg.Kg^{-1}.day^{-1}$, in the case of
PhB and from 2.54 to 8.33 $mg.Kg^{-1}.day^{-1}$ in the case of DPH. The duration
of the treatment ranged from 10 months to 8.5 years.

Procedure-. The following data were obtained for each patient:
sex, weight, eight, type of treatment, dosage and plasma level of the
drug or drugs administered. Monitoring of the plasma levels of the two
drugs began as soon as the steady-state had been reached (Pippinger 1978)
Blood was extracted half-an-hour prior to the administration of the following dose. The EMIT system (Syva 1981) was the analytical procedure used
in all cases.

Estimation of plasma clearance-. The plasma clearance of PhB
and DPH was stimated as being the quotient obtained between the dose administered and the observed steady-state plasma level.

Statistical treatment of data-. The effect of factors studied
on the plasma clearance of PhB and DPH were analyzed according to a linear
multiple regression program designed for a HP-85 computer (Llabres 1981)

RESULTS

The mean plasma concentration values of PhB and DPH are 15.32
$mg.l^{-1}$ (2.75-55.0) and 3.76 $mg.l^{-1}$ (0-20.0).

Phenobarbital-. Those factors having a significant effect on PhB plasma clearance were identified by means of the regression program; only two factors- age and administration of DPH- were found to be signifiant, as shown by the regression ANOVA in Tables 1 and 2.

Source of variation	d.f.	sum of squares	F	α
Regression	1	178.4	10.9	< 0.01
Residual	105	1956.4		
Total	106	2034.8		

TABLE 1-. Regression ANOVA of PhB plasma clearance versus age

The effect of age is expressed quantitatively by the equation:

$$\text{Plasma clearance of Phenobarbital} = 11.41 - 0.32. \text{Age (years)} \quad (\text{ Eq. 1 })$$

Source of variation	d.f.	sum of squares	F	α
Regression	1	66.5	3.47	0.05-0.01
Residual	105	1986.3		
Total	106	2034.8		

TABLE 2-. Regression ANOVA of PhB plasma clearance versus administration with DPH

Administration of the two drugs reduced PhB clearance and this effect is expressed by the equation:

$$\text{Plasma clearance of Phenobarbital} = 8.88 + 1.77. \ (\ 0;1\ ) \quad (\text{ Eq. 2 })$$

In which 1 corresponds to PhB monotherapy and 0 to the administration of the two drugs. The above effect is show graphically in Figure 1

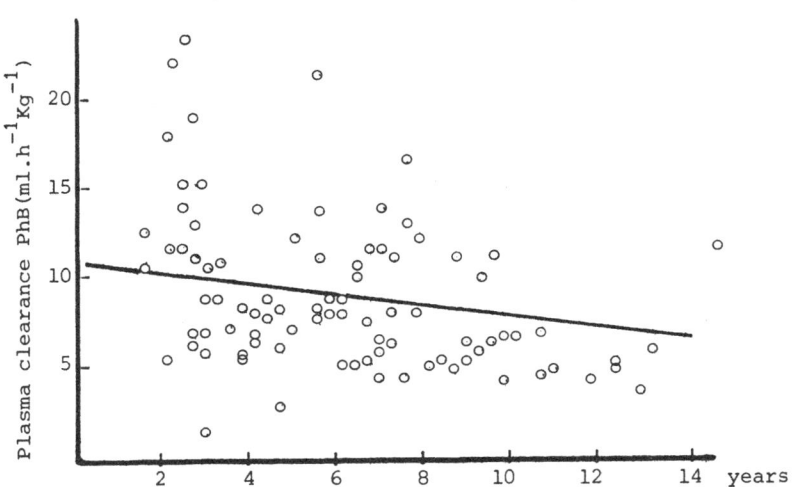

FIGURE 1-. Influence of age on the PhB plasma   clearance

diphenylhydantoin-. The analysis of those factors affecting the plasma clearance of DPH is limited by the fact that data relating to DPH monotherapy are not available; the results, therefore, correspond to the administration of PhB and DPH.

As the regression ANOVA shows (Table 3) only age was found to have any effect on the plasma clearance of DPH

Source of variation	d.f.	sum of squares	F	α:
Regression	1	5911.4	10.88	< 0.01
Residual	41	22278.0		
Total	42	28190.4		

TABLE 3-. Regression ANOVA of DPH plasma clearance versus age

The regression ANOVA gives the following mathematical expression:

Plasma clearance of DPH = 89.3 - 4.0. Age (years) (Eq 3)

The above effect is shown in Figure 2

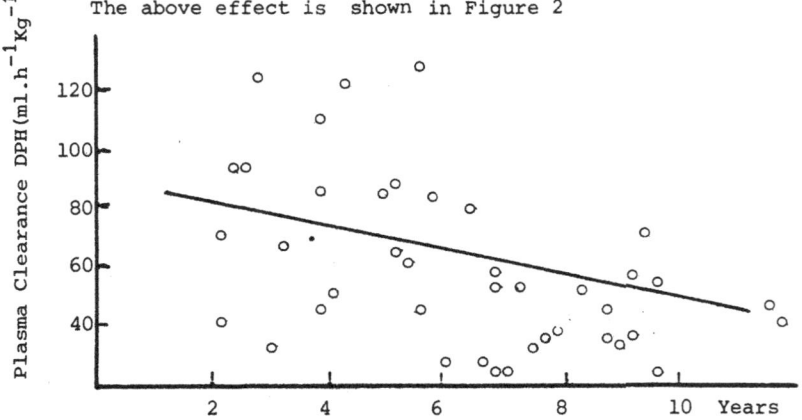

FIGURE 2-.Influence of age on the DPH plasmatic clearance

DISCUSSION-.

Phenobarbital-. The decrease in the value of clearance produced by age has already been observed by numerous authors and the results obtained are similar to those found here (Svensmark et al. 1964; Eadi 1977; Hooper 1973). Equation 1 enables one predict the annual decrease in clearance value. However, this approximation may not be a practical one for a posologic purpose since it ignores the possibility of a critical age where a radical change take place; clearance values corresponding to the different age sub -groups were compared. The results obtained showed 3 to be the critical age. In this respect, the regression ANOVA- introducing age as a false variable is quite eloquent. Table 4 shows the mean values observed for the two age sub-groups in question.

Source of variation	d.f.	sum of squares	F	α
Regression	1	352.2	19.7	< 0.01
Residual	105	1682.1		
Total	106	2034,3		

TABLE 4-. Regression ANOVA of PhB plasma clearance versus age
(Critical age: 3 years)

Diphenylhidantoin-. The effect of age on clearance values has
already been described in several publications (Van Dijk 1980); Berlet
1975) where similar changes are reported. As in the case of PhB age ranges having the same clearance were looked for. Here, the results also proved to be conclusive, showing a strong decrease in clearance value from 6
years onwards. The regression ANOVA (Table 5) shows these differences
quite clearly.

Source of variation	d.f.	sum of squares	F	α
Regression	1	10125.3	23.0	< 0.01
Residual	41	18064.6		
Total	42	28189.9		

TABLE 5-. Regression ANOVA of DPH plasma clearance versus age
(Critical value: 6 years)

Posology-. The plasma clearance of both drugs is independent of
the model and the observed effects can be easily related to individual posologic requirements. Thus we have:

$$\text{Maintenance Dose} = C_{ss}.Cl_p \qquad (\text{ Eq. 4 })$$

Where C_{ss} is the mean steady-state concentration considered as
optimum. Taking in account Eq.4 the following doses for PhB are proposed
when C_{ss} value is the mean value of all observed plasmatic levels:

Monotherapy   Children over 3 years = 3.39 $mg.Kg^{-1}.day^{-1}$
                Children under 3 years= 5.05 $mg.Kg^{-1}.day^{-1}$
With DPH   Children over 3 years = 3.20 $mg.Kg^{-1}.day^{-1}$
                Children under 3 years= 4.85 $mg.Kg^{-1}.day^{-1}$

In DPH two sub-groups having different posologic requirements
were stablished:

Children under 3 years = 8.61 $mg.Kg^{-1}.day^{-1}$
Children over 3 years = 5.26 $mg.Kg^{-1}.day^{-1}$

The posology here suggested leads us to one other important
point, namely that, in the administration of PhB and DPH, the optimum dose
of both drugs changes radically according to the patient´s age, as the

data shows:

Children under 3 years: PhB/DPH = 56/100

Children between 3-6 years:PhB/DPH = 37/100

Children over 6 years: PhB/DPH = 60/100

This individualized posology should greatly facilitate the ajustement of the steady-state concentrations of both drugs. However, this would have to be confirmed by means of a clinical study similar to the one carried out and using the proposed guide-lines. This clinical study is already under way.

REFERENCE LIST

Berlet H. (1975). Serum levels of Phenytoin in children. In Schneider, Janz, Gardner-Thorpe, Meinardi and Sherwin Eds: Clinical Pharmacology of Antiepileptic Drugs. pp 63-69. Berlin. Springer-Verlag

Eadie J.M. et al. (1977).Factors influencing plasma Phenobarbitone levels in epileptic patients. Brit. J. Clin. Pharmacol. 4. pp 541-547

Hooper W.D.& Eadie J.M.& Tyler J.H.(1973).Plasma Diphenylhidantoin levels in Australian children. Aust. N.Z. J. Med. 4. pp 456-461

Llabres M & Vila Jato J.L.& Martinez R. (1981) RLIN: A linear multiple regression program:V Congreso de la Asociacion Española de Farmacologos. Salamanca (Spain)

Pippenger C.E. (1978).Monitoring of Antiepileptic Drugs.In Baer D.M. and Dito W.R. Ed. Technical Improvement Service. Volum. 111. American Soc. of Clinical Pharmacologists

Svensmark O.& Buchthal F. (1964).Diphenylhidantoin and Phenobarbital (serum levels in children). Am. J. Dis. Child. 108. pp 82-87

Syva (1981). EMIT: Technical Rapport of Syva. Barcelona

Van Dijk A.& Uges D.R.A. (1980). Analytical and Pharmacokinetic aspects of Phenobarbital, Phenytoin, Primidone and Carbamazepine. In The serum concentration of Drugs. Merkus F.W.H.M. pp 65-78. Amsterdam. Excerpta Medica.

INDIVIDUALIZATION OF PHENYTOIN DOSAGE

G. C. Muscas, G. Zaccara, G. Arnetoli, R. Zappoli
2nd Neurological Institute, University of Florence, Italy

A. Messori, G. Donati-Cori, C. Manfriani, E. Tendi
Hospital Pharmacy, USL 10/D, Florence, Italy

T. Valenza
Clinical Analysis Laboratory, USL 10/D, Florence, Italy

Over the past few years, numerous reports have been published regarding individualization of phenytoin (PHT) dosage for treatment of epileptic patients (Ludden et al. 1976; Mullen 1977; Mullen & Foster 1979; Vozeh et al. 1981; Graves et al. 1982; Messori et al. 1983 a,b). Considerable effort has in fact been devoted to devising and testing methods to predict the PHT dose required to achieve a given steady-state target plasma concentration. It is agreed that, in most patients, optimal seizure control can be obtained with plasma PHT concentrations ranging from 10 to 20 mg/L. On the other hand, serious toxicity is known to result from plasma concentrations above 25-30 mg/L.

Nonlinearity of PHT kinetics complicates the problem of calculating individualized dosage regimens. The nonlinear kinetics of PHT can be described through the Michaelis-Menten model. Hence, the relationship between the daily dose and the corresponding plasma concentration at steady-state (Css) in a given patient is defined on the basis of two kinetic parameters: the maximum elimination rate (Vmax) and the plasma concentration at which the elimination rate is half-maximum (Km). These two parameters undergo wide intersubject variability: ten-fold and five-fold variations have in fact been demonstrated for Km and Vmax, respectively (Bauer & Blouin 1982).

The kinetic procedures that have been proposed for individualizing the dosage of PHT use different theoretical approaches to account for the nonlinearity of PHT kinetics. Most of these procedures share the purpose of calculating individual values of Km and Vmax from the Css-D data pairs that are known for the patient concerned. Once these

parameters have been estimated, the PHT dosage capable of producing the
desired Css value can easily be determined.

Obviously, the more Css-D data pairs are known, the more
reliable is the estimation of individual values of Km and Vmax and the
subsequent prediction of the optimal dosage. Nevertheless, the clinical
usefulness of these kinetic techniques in individualizing dosage depends
upon the capability of reliably estimating individual kinetic parameters
from limited plasma level data. As a result, the most important clinical
application of these techniques is the calculation of individualized
dosage regimens of PHT in those cases where only a few Css-D data pairs
(e.g. one or two data pairs) are known for a given patient.

When only one Css-D data pair is known, the population
clearance (PC) method offers the best compromise between the conflicting
needs to increase the dose and avoid the risk of toxic levels of plasma
PHT concentration (Messori et al. 1983 a). It has been estimated (Muscas
et al., unpublished observations) that a very low percentage (approximately 5 percent) of those patients who require upward dosage adjustments
will achieve plasma PHT concentration above 20 mg/L, if a desired Css
value of 15 mg/L is selected in using the PC method.

When two Css-data pairs are known, a number of kinetic
techniques (Ludden et al. 1976; Mullen 1977; Mullen & Foster 1979; Vozeh
et al. 1981) have been proposed for individualizing PHT dosage. Some of
these techniques (Ludden et al. 1976; Mullen 1977; Mullen & Foster 1979)
adopt a linear transformation of the Michaelis-Menten equation to
estimate individual values of Km and Vmax from the plasma level data. An
important drawback to these techniques is that they are heavily affected
by those factors (such as variations of compliance, intraindividual
variations of PHT kinetics) that deviate PHT kinetics from the ideal
behaviour defined by the Michaelis-Menten model. On the other hand,
other techniques, such as the Bayesian feedback (BF) method (Vozeh et al.
1981), use a different approach because they appropriately exploit all
relevant population information previously available regarding PHT

kinetics as well as the Css-D data which are available for the patient
concerned. As stated by Vozeh, "the individual response (Css) information
is most valuable for predicting future dosage, but prior (population)
information is also of value, and should not be ignored". Indeed,
preliminary findings support the view that the BF method should be
preferred for clinical use when two Css-D data pairs are known.

When three Css-D pairs are known, individual PHT kinetics
can be well characterized on the simple basis of the measured Css-D data.
In such a case precision of the calculated Michaelis-Menten parameters
appears to be satisfactory, particularly if a nonlinear least-squares
technique is employed for parameter estimation (Messori et al. 1983 b).
A nonlinear unweighted least-squares procedure for estimating Km and Vmax
(Messori et al. 1983 a,b) has recently been programmed onto a hand-held
calculator so that this procedure can easily be applied in routine
clinical practice. As shown by Ruffo et al. (unpublished observations),
use of a weighted nonlinear least-squares procedure for calculating PHT
kinetic parameters offers no advantage over the unweighted approach
proposed by Messori et al.

Since individual PHT kinetic parameters can be reliably
determined from the measured Css-D data when three data pairs are known,
use of population data for estimating Km and Vmax in this case has been
questioned in a recent study (Messori et al. 1983 b). While, at present,
no conclusion can be drawn about this problem, we nevertheless believe
that the Bayesian approach may not be very accurate in dealing with drugs
(such as PHT) that demonstrate a very wide intersubject variation of
kinetic parameters. Indeed, the data from our laboratory show that the
intersubject standard deviations of Km and Vmax are larger than the
values, reported by Vozeh et al. (1981), which are incorporated into the
calculator program designed for application of the BF method. Our data do
not therefore support the hypothesis, proposed in a recent report (Yuen
et al. 1982), that the BF method is applicable to a patient population
other than the one from which the population parameter estimates were

were derived. On the other hand, we feel that the performance of the
BF method can be improved considerably if specific population data are
obtained through the NONMEM computer program (Sheiner et al. 1979) and
used as input variables of the calculator program proposed by Vozeh et
al. (1981).

REFERENCES

Bauer L.A. & Blouin R.A. (1982). Age and phenytoin kinetics in adult
        epileptics. Clin.Pharmacol.Ther.,$\underline{31}$,301-4.
Graves, N. et al. (1982). Phenytoin dosage predictions using population
        clearances. Drug Intell. Clin. Pharm.,$\underline{16}$,473.
Ludden, T.M. et al. (1976). Optimum phenytoin dosage regimens. Lancet,
        $\underline{1}$,307-8.
Messori, A. et al. (1983 a). A new programmable calculator procedure for
        individualizing phenytoin dosage. Drug Intell.Clin.Pharm.
        (in press).
Messori, A. et al. (1983 b). Comparative analysis of the pharmacokinetic
        techniques available for individualizing phenytoin dosage.
        J. Clin. Hosp. Pharm. (in press).
Mullen, P.W. (1977). Optimal phenytoin therapy: a new technique for
        individualizing dosage. Clin.Pharmacol.Ther.,$\underline{23}$,
        228-32.
Mullen, P.W. & Foster R.W. (1979). Comparative evaluation of six
        techniques for determining the Michaelis-Menten parameters
        relating phenytoin dose and steady-state serum
        concentrations. J.Pharm.Pharmacol.,$\underline{31}$,100-4.
Sheiner, L.B. et al. (1979). Forecasting individual pharmacokinetics.
        Clin. Pharmacol. Ther.,$\underline{26}$,294-305.
Vozeh, S. et al. (1981). Predicting individual phenytoin dosage.
        J. Pharmacokinet. Biopharm.,$\underline{9}$,131-46.
Yuen, G. et al. (1982). Phenytoin dosage predictions using Bayesian
        feedback. Drug Intell. Clin. Pharm.,$\underline{16}$,484.

ANALYSIS OF PHARMACOLOGICAL TREATMENT OF EPILEPSY. RETROS-
PECTIVE STUDY OF 100 CASES

Sala, M.L.; Martí-Vilalta, J.L.; de la Concepción N.; Fernán-
dez, M.P.; Boada, T.; Bonal, J.

Hospital de la Sta. Creu i Sant Pau. Barcelona

The prevalence of epilepsy in developed countries is approximately 6-8 cases per 1,000 habitants according to a study of a WHO study
group (OMS, 1978). Present day technology has brought about a great advance in the diagnosis of the disease as well as in pharmacological and
pharmokinetic knowledge of antiepileptic drugs (Goodman & Gilman, 1980).
This in turn has produced a tendency towards a change from polytherapy
to monotherapy with the reduction of adverse effects and interactions,
and eases therapy compliance on the patient's part (OMS, 1978).

MATERIAL AND METHODS

Due to the lack of quantitative data on epileptic treatment
in our country, we carried out a study of the drugs used in the control
of epilepsy. We analyzed 100 clinical histories of patients with a diagnosis of epilepsy and treated in the Neurology Service of the Hospital
de la Sta. Creu i Sant Pau in 1982. The following data was obtained from
each of the histories studied:

- Sex
- Present age
- Age at first seizure
- Type of seizure according to the International Classifica-
tion of Epileptic Seizures: 1) Elemental partial, 2) Complex partial, 3)
Generalized secondary partial, 4) Generalized convulsive, 5) Generalized
non-convulsive, 6) Non-classified (Gastaut, H 1969).
- Etiology: 1) Primary epilepsy, 2) Secondary epilepsy.
- Number of antiepileptic drugs, type of preparation (simple
and/or compound) and total daily dosis of the drugs used for each patient,
keeping in mind the last prescribed treatment. The drugs studied were:
Phenobarbital (PB), Phenytoin (PHT), Ethosuximide (ESM), Carbamazepine
(CBZ), Valproate Sodium (VPA), Clonazepam (CZP), Diazepam (DZP), Methyl-

phenobarbital (MPB).

RESULTS

The mean age of the 100 patients in the series (51 females and 49 males) was 37 years, the age limits being 8 and 78 years old. The average age at onset of first seizure was 25 (age limits being 2 months and 74 years). The number of patients with late epilepsy (initial age of onset of seizure over 20 years old) was 50%. The type of seizure can be seen in Table I.

TABLE 1

Type of seizure	Nº of patients	
Partial elemental	5	83 %
Complex partial	8	
Generalized secondary partial	13	
Generalized non-convulsive	4	
Generalized convulsive	53	
Mixed crises	15	15 %
Non-classified	2	2 %
	100	

70% of the seizures studied were of primary etiology, and 30% of those remaining corresponded to cases of secondary etiology (alcoholism, cranial trauma,   cerebral tumors, cerebral vascular disease).

The drugs were administered by means of simple preparations (72%), compounds (21%) and mixtures of simple and compound (7%).

The number of antiepileptics drugs used per patient were: 58% with only one drug, 29% with two drugs and 13% with three or more drugs. No patient in the series was treated with more than four drugs.

The data obtained in our series indicates a clear tendency towards monotherapy. Some series published show the following figures of polytherapy: 95.8% in a series of 11720 patients (Guelen & Johannessen, 1977); 48.3% in a series of 94 patients (Hopkins & Scambler, 1977); 41% in 200 patients (Cawthorne & Silas, 1981); 53% in another series of 1104 patients (Beghi et al. 1982).

The percentage of drug use was as follows: PHT 63%, PB 56%, CBZ 22%, VPA 7%, MPB 6%, ESM 1%, PRM 1% and others 2%. The most used drugs (OMS, 1978), (Pht, PB, CBZ) appear to be the most efficient in the treatment of epilepsy.

The associations used in the patients in our series are shown in Table II.

TABLE II

2 DRUGS	Nº PATIENTS	3 DRUGS	Nº PATIENTS	4 DRUGS	Nº PATIENTS
PHT–PB	23	PB–PHT–VPA	3	PB–PHT–MPB–VPA	1
PB–CBZ	4	PB–PHT–CBZ	2	PB–PHT–MPB–CBZ	1
PB–VPA	2	PB–PHT–MPB	4	PB–CBZ–VPA–ESM	1
		PB–PHT–PAC	1		
TOTAL	29		10		3

In nearly all our patients with three or four antiepileptic drugs, the polytherapy was due to the utilization of commercial preparations associated to these drugs.

The majority of patients used daily doses within the therapeutic limits. The use of low doses in some patients was due to suppression of treatment having been begun or to the prescription of compound commercial preparations with low dosage of some antiepileptic drugs.

The doses/day of antiepileptic drugs in the patients of our series can be seen in Table III.

TABLE III

DRUG	DOSES/DAY (mg)	% PATIENTS
PHT	300	34
PB	150	19
	100	14
CBZ	600	11
VPA	250–2000	7
MPB	25–150	6
ESM	750	1
PRM	375	1

CONCLUSIONS

In the 100 patients of our series, <u>antiepileptic monothera-</u><u>phy</u> has been used <u>in 58%</u> of cases. The prescription of two drugs was used in 29% of cases. The mono and bitherapy was therefore established in 87% of our series, as is usual in the correct treatment of epileptic patients. Polytherapy with more than two drugs was used in 13% of cases.

Regarding the prescription of <u>simple</u> or <u>compound prepara-</u><u>tions</u> our figures were <u>72% and 29% respectively</u>. Although these figures are acceptable, we believe the percentage of simple preparations should be 100%. This would be an evident advantage for the clinician, facilitating the regularization of adequate dosage for each patient, and would also be an advantage for the patient by decreasing the adverse effects of some drugs unnecessarily used in compound preparations.

REFERENCES

American Medical Association (1983); Anticonvulsants <u>in AMA</u>; pag. 295-328
         Philadelphia.

Avery, G.S.; (1980) Drug Treatment, pp 1010-27. Adis Press Sidney Chur-
         chill Livingstone. Edimburgh and London.

Beghi, E.; Sasanelli,F. Spagnolli, A. Tognoni, G.; et al. (1982). Quality
         of care epilepsy in Italy: A multi-hospital survey of diagno-
         sis and treatment of 1104 epileptic patients. Epilepsia 23:
         pp. 133-48.

Berciano,J. (1980). "Epilepsia: tratamiento". Inf. Terap. SS. <u>4</u> nº11;
         pp. 205-10.

Fischbacher, E. (1982). Effect of reduction of anticonvulsants on Welle-
         ing. Br. Med. J. <u>285</u> ; nº 6339, p. 423-4.

Guelen PJM & Johannessen SI (1977). Prescription pattern of antiepileptic
         drugs to epileptic patients: A comparison between the Nether-
         lands and Norway In: Antiepileptic drug monitoring. Garden-
         - Thorpe C, Jariz D., Meinardi H, Pippenger CE (Eds), pp.
         345-50. Pitman Medical, umbridge Wells UK.

Goodman L & Gilman A. (1980). Drugs effective in the therapy of the epi-
         lepsies <u>In</u> The Pharmacological Basis of Therapeutics. Macmi-
         llan publishing CO., DNC pp 448-75. New York.

Hopkins A. & Scambler G. (1977). How doctors deal with epilepsy. The Lan-
         cet <u>1</u> nº 8004 pp. 183-6.

OMS (1978). Aplicación de los progresos de las neurociencias en la lucha contra los trastornos neurológicos. Serie de Informes técnicos 629. Ginebra.

Reynolds EH (1978). Drug treatment of epilepsy. The Lancet 2 nº 8092. pp 721-5.

Shorvon S.D. & Reynolds E.H. (1977). Unnecessary polypharmacy for epilepsy. Br. Med. J., 1 6077, pp: 1635-7.

Shorvon S.D. & Reynolds EH. (1979). Reduction in polypharmacy for epilepsy. Br. Med. J., 2 6197, pp: 1023-5.

Sutula, T.,Sackellares,J., Miller, J., Dreiluss,F. (1981). Intensive monitoring in refractory epilepsy. Neurology 31 : 243-7.

THE USE OF ANTIBIOTICS IN SPANISH HOSPITALS

Arrizabalaga MJ, López J, Bachiller MP, Carrasco ME,
Rodriguez-Sasiain JM.
Servicio de Farmacia. R.S. "Ntra. Sra. de Aránzazu"
San Sebastián (Spain)

There is a fair degree of consensus on how antibiotic therapy
should be carried out, what antibiotics should be administered for different diseases and how they should be used (Smith 1981). In many cases the
differences noted in the literature should be attributed to the lack of -
availability of a certain product in a specific country. Nevertheless, -
when the true behaviour of the prescribers is observed, many errors are -
detected in the use of antibiotics, even in hospitals. To try to prevent
this, as well as to try to avoid or delay the development of resistance -
to some products, limiting their use, norms of the use of these antimicro
bian substances have been put into effect in many centres. They consist -
mainly of putting the existing antibiotics on the Formulary at different
restriction levels, thereby allowing the above mentioned objectives to be
complied with.

It can be observed in hospitals as in general medicine, that
a homogeneous behaviour does not exist with regard to the selection of an
tibiotics for specific situations. It is not surprising therefore, that
there are differences between hospitals in the same country, which though
not great, are quite significant. This situation could be motivated by
the existence of a high degree of concern in the respective Pharmacy and
Infections Committees; by the observance of a retrospective review of the
use of antibiotics; by the collaboration between the Pharmacy, Bacterio-
logy and Preventive Medicine Services; by the tendency to accept, with di
ffering degrees of readiness the therapeutic innovations that are conti-
nually appearing in this field, etc. To this effect, no studies have been
carried out that try to detect the differences produced by the use of antibiotics in Spain, not even those that could discover or ascertain the
degree or type of restriction to which these products are subjected when
they are used in hospitals.

METHODS

In order to obtain the information required, an anonymous sur
vey was sent out to 60 General Hospitals in Spain in which the Pharmaceutical Service was questioned on the type of restrictions to which it subjected the antibiotics listed. These products were chosen on the basis of
those commonly used, although, if the case arose, others were also listed.
In the answers, the person filling out the survey classified the products
at different levels; antibiotics that under no circumstances could be used
in the Centre; those that could be freely obtained and finally those that
could only be obtained by some type of medical prescription, signed by the
physician and accompanied or not by the corresponding antibiogram that
would endorse the prescription as far as the Pharmaceutical Service was
concerned.

RESULTS

The number of surveys received was 34, and it could be observed from them that there was a common criteria of restriction for certain
products and of non-admission for others. The total amount of antibiotics
available varies greatly, ranging from a minimum of 17 products to a maxi
mum of 40, although the most frequent number is around 30. The number of
antibiotics that can be obtained without any restriction varies from a mi
nimum of 6 up to a total of 31; the majority of the values are near to 20.
The degree of restriction may vary from a minimum of 25% free (percentage
obtained of the total amount of antibiotics used) up to 100%. The restric
tive behaviour of Spanish hospitals towards antibiotics is shown in the
enclosed Table, where amikacin is at the top, followed by cefoxitin and
cefotaxime.

ANTIBIOTICS SUBJECTED TO MAXIMUM RESTRICTION

Percentage	65%	---------------- AMIKACIN ------------------	65%
of	55%	---------- CEFOXITIN, CEFOTAXIME ----------	55%
hospitals	38%	--------------- AZLOCILLIN ----------------	38%
	36%	------------- CARBENICILLIN -------------	36%
	29%	-------------- MOXALACTAM --------------	29%
	23%	------------- CHLORAMPHENICOL --------------	23%
	19%	--------------- CLINDAMYCIN ---------------	19%
	16%	---------- CEFAMANDOL, VANCOMYCIN ----------	16%

only 22% of the cases the antimicrobial treatment was suspended after having obtained negative cultures; these same authors considered that 19%
of antibiotics were used "irrationally" and 48% "doubtfully". Other authors proved that the use of antibiotics could be reduced by 5% without
increasing the percentage of infections or internments, while at the same
time the total cost of antibiotics would decrease by 20% (Kunin et al.1973)

It is not surprising that in the majority of hospitals restric
tive norms are issued to prevent the liberal use of antibiotics and that
these coincide. This paper will show us that in almost all Spanish hospitals there is an established policy for the use of antibiotics. These
norms establish a different degree of request according to the centres,
products, and probably, the pathology for which they are use. Nevertheless,
certain differences which can be seen from information in this paper may
surprise us. In the first place, the great variability that exists in the
total number of available drugs, which range from 17 to almost all availa
ble in some centres, with an average of 30 products. In its recommendations of 1982, the journal Medical Letter only suggests 20 antibiotics as
selective or alternative drugs, in the same way that in the norms for selecting discs for antibiograms, it uses restrictive criteria that place
the total number of discs near 20. Although it may be that the situation
in Spain is somewhat different from that of other countries, it does not
appear that the ideal number is higher than the aforementioned figure, in
which some hospitals are not included; the majority of hospitals (80%)
permit the use of 26-33 different products. In comparison, marked differences can be observed in the total number of antibiotics of free dispensation or in the highly restricted ones. Some centres restrict almost all,
while others allow more freedom of choice. This attitude could be the result of a very disciplined behaviour by the prescribers, who will faith-
fully comply with the recommendations given by the diverse Committees, or
of a lack of human resources in the pharmaceutical Service to carry out
the restrictive norms.

There is a general tendency, detected from the results of this
paper to restrict more severely those products that are new on the market.
For example, amikacin, latest representative (for the moment) of the amino
glycoside family, is restricted in practically all Spanish hospitals (84%).
This behaviour is a sign of the correct use of the product, since its in-
discriminate use could give rise to the appearance of resistance to the
other components of the group (Apgar 1982).

In the same way, it is interesting to point out that a total number of 16 products are subjected to maximum restriction in only one hospital, followed by 2 hospitals that control 13; the most common behaviour is to control 3 products or even less. If we study separately the groups of antibiotics, among the aminoglycosides only in 58% of the institutions streptomycin is freely obtained; amikacin must be procured by means of some kind of medical prescription in 97% of the hospitals,whereas gentamicin can be freely obtained in 87% of the total amount. Natural peni cillins are subjected to little or no control; the same applies to aminopenicillins: ampicillin is freely obtained in 94% of the centres, amoxicillin in 90% and only 35% admit ampicillin esters. Carbenicillins esters for oral use are proscribed in 2 out of every 3 centres but they can be freely used in 1 out every 3.Ureidopenicillins are heavily restricted; only 12% of hospitals consent the free use of azlocillin. Mezlocillin, like ticarcillin can only be used in very few hospitals.

From the first-generation cephalosporins, the majority of centres prefer cefalexin to cefadroxil for oral administration, using cephradine very seldom. The convenience of substituting cefalotin for cefazolin has been debated for a long time, due to certain advantages of the second product over the first. Nevertheless, in some centres both products coexist, although cefazolin is used more freely in more hospitals than is cefalotin. Among the second-generation cephalosporins, cefuroxime cannot be used in 3 out 4 hospitals and cefamandol is not admitted in 42%; on the other hand cefoxitin is used in almost all hospitals, even though it is higly restricted (to the highest level possible in 55% of institutions). The new third-generation cephalosporins are also greatly restricted in Spain. The majority of centres prefer to use cefotaxime (which has only been rejected in one hospital out of the survey and is free in 16% of the centres) instead of moxalactam which is not used in 58%.

DISCUSSION

For quite some years ago, a higher degree of interest can be detected towards the revision of the use of antibiotics in hospitals (Pien et al. 1979), probably motivated by the many mistakes which, often enough, have been observed in retrospective studies. For example, in 1962, 86.000 cases were revised, of which 29% had received antibiotic treatment, in spi te of the fact that 54% of them did not present infections (Collins & Laza rus 1975). Ten years latter,Gibbs and coworkers (1973) observed that in

(1 out of every 5) restrict gentamicin, which suggests that this product
is the most widely used; probably, the fact that it is more economical ex
plains why this aminoglycoside and not tobramycin is freely used in the majority of hospitals. Among the penicillins, amoxicillin is preferred to ampicillin esters, probably because of economic factors; carbenicillin esters
are also rejected in 65% of hospitals, that prefer parenteral drugs.Ticar-
cillin, recently introduced to Spain is very little used. Ureidopenicillins
are also very limited. Hospitals use cephalosporins very similarly;it appe
ars that as a rule neither cefaclor, cefacetril, cefadroxil,cephaloridine,
cephapirin nor cephradine are used. On the other hand, almost all the hos
pitals allow the free use of cefalexin, one out of every three does not
permit the use of cephalotin and three out of every four permit the free
use of cefazolin. Among the second-generation cephalosporins, cefoxitin is
used almost exclusively. With regard to the third-generation ones, almost
all the centres prefer cefotaxime; moxalactam was not admitted in 58% of
the hospitals surveyed. Without a doubt, the excessive number of products
existing on the market should invite the application of restrictive norms.
Few differences are observed with the attitude towards macrolides and lin-
comycins for example, only 3% use josamycin and 32% spiramycin while only
7% de not use clindamycin and 26% lincomycin. Other products not stated in
the above groups such as tetracycline, doxycycline, rifampicin and fosfo-
mycin are used without restriction in the majority of centres. We can conclude, that in spite of the fact that there are certain differences in the
use of antibiotics, some of which are difficult to justify, the use of the
se products is, on average, quite adequate. Nevertheless, the tendency observed, consisting in the restriction of the newer products should probably be extended to other more venerable ones.

REFERENCES

Anonymous (1982). Antimicrobic drugs selection. Med. Letter. 4,29-36.
Apgar, D.A. (1982). Comment on aminoglycoside evaluation. Drug Intell Clin
       Pharm. 16,956-60.
Collins, G.E. & Lazarus, H.L. (1975). Drug information services handbook.
       Publishing Sciences Group, Acton Mass.
Gibbs, C.N.; Gibson, J.T.; Newton, D.S. (1973). Drug utilisation review
       of actual versus preferred pediatric antibiotic therapy. Am J
       Hosp Pharm. 30,892-7.
Kunin, C.M.; Tupasi, T.; Craig, N.A. (1973). Use of antibiotics. A brief
       exposition of the problem and some tentative solutions. Ann
       Intern Med. 79,555-60.
Pien, F.D. ; Lan, W.K.K.; Sur, N. (1979). Antibiotic use in a small
       community hospital. West J Med. 130,498-502.
Smith, J.K.(1981). Current criteria for selecting an antibiotic. Drug
       Therapy. March, 115-119.

STUDY OF AN ANTI-INTESTINAL INFECTION TREATMENT IN PAEDIATRICS

Antolin Munfort C. and Boquet Jimenez E.

Hospital San Juan de Dios de Manresa (Spain)

In the acute gastrointestinal infections produced by bacteria, the most frequent are <u>Salmonella</u> and <u>Shigella</u>. The majority of children who enter the service - of emergency paediatrics of the Hospital San Juan de Dios - de Manresa for acute gastroenteritis, present with evident signs of dehydration. After obtaining a faecal specimen, we review the method of treating the infection.

We do not want to under-emphasize the importance of the - problem of dehydration for the recuperation of the children, but this problem does not form part of the present study.

The age of the children, the gravity of the illness and the continuous loss of weight means that we do not follow recent ideas of leaving the infection to evolve without administering an antibacterial.

Before the investigation we studied two methods of antibacterial treatment, based on amoxycillin and cotrimoxazole respectively. We rejected them because the Shigellas that we isolated were resistant to both. Moreover - some of the organisms which produced disbacteriosis (an alteration in the bacterial flora of the gut) were also resistant. Our observation was that for amoxycillin the - total resistance was 29%, and for cotrimoxazole 27%.

We rejected the use of the rest of the sulphonamides because the children were very young, many of them nursing, and we rejected neomycin because it produces certain intestinal allergies.

Observing that colistin was effective for all

strains of <u>Salmonella</u> and <u>Shigella</u>, we began to use it as
an initial treatment, without prejudice, but if the cultures and sensitivity studies "in vitro" indicated another
medicine, then we would change the treatment.

The proposal of the present study has been to evaluate the efficacy of the above mentioned treatment,includ-
ing those cases in which it was the only treatment, and to
study the possible existence of resistance.

Material and Methods

We have studied 329 children in the Hospital San -
Juan de Dios de Manresa with symptoms of diarrhoea, during
the period between January 1982 and April 1983. Of all
of them, only 93 showed an acute gastroenteritis and consequently, they were the only ones studied.

The diagnosis was made by the Service of Microbiology, investigating:

a)<u>Rotavirus</u> by techniques of immunofluorescence
(only in cases of acute gastroenteritis.)

b)<u>Intestinal Parasites</u> (<u>Entamoeba histolytica</u> and
<u>Giardia lamblia</u>) observing the faeces in wet preparations
with Lugol for the determination of cysts, and tinting them
with hematoxilina ferrica, for trophozites.

c)<u>Bacterias</u> by growing in selective "mediums",
these were the following:-

Mc. Skirrow and incubation at 43 ^{O}C in microaerophi-
lic atmosphere for <u>Campylobacter</u>.

Mc. Caldo Selenite to enrich <u>Salmonella</u>.

Mc. S.S. to investigate <u>Salmonella</u> and <u>Shigella</u>.

Mc. Saboureaud for <u>Fungus</u> and <u>Yeasts</u>.

Mc. Mannitol Sal for <u>Staphylococcus</u>.

Mc. E M B to observe possible disbacteriosis.

We considered disbacteriosis when the predominant
majority was of one type of micro-organism, which are not
considered pathogenic, with the exeption of <u>E. coli</u>, which
is - always present in abudant proportion. We give path-
ologic significance to a disbacteriosis if the symptom is

acute.

In all cases we made a microscopic study of the - specimen, mixing on a slide a small portion of faeces with a drop of methylene blue, covering it, and observing with an immersion lens, intending to discover leucocytes. Their presence indicates an inflammation of the intestine, which is produced by the Salmonella, Shigella or Escherichia coli.

On the other hand, the gastroenteritis process in faeces without leucocytes, directed our suspicions to a viral - symptom, without reflection in the faeces culture, or toxic bacteria, for example, Vibrio cholerae or - Staphylococcus aureus.

The sensitivity studies were made according to the technique of Kirby-Bauer.

Results

Of the 329 diagnosis of gastroenteritis only 93 presented in an acute form, in consequence, they were the only ones immediately treated after obtaining a specimen, the rest were not given antibacterials.

The micro-organisms which produce acute gastroenteritis were the following:

	Form	Total
Giardia lamblia	2	40
Campylobacter fetus	1	6
Rotavirus	12	-
Salmonella	31	37
Shigella	8	9
Disbacteriosis	10	22
Unknown Aetiology	19	--

The Salmonella strains were identified in the National Center of Microbiology of Majadahonda, and were found to belong to the following serotypes:

S. typhimurium.........10
S. enteritidis......... 6
S. typhi.............. 5

```
        S. heidelberg..........  4
        S. infantis ...........  2
        S. mono ...............  1
        S. agona ..............  1
        S. newport ............  1
        S. kapemba ............  1
```

The <u>Shigella</u> strains all belong to the sp. of -
<u>Shigella sonnei</u>, except one of <u>Shigella boydii</u>.

The species which produce disbacteriosis were the -
following:

```
        Klebsiella pneumoniae ......  2
        Pseudomona aeruginosa ......  2
        Yersinia enterocolitica ....  2
        Aeromonas hydrofila ........  1
        Enterobacter cloacae .......  1
        Staphylococcus aureus ......  1
        Proteus mirabilis ..........  1
```

<u>Discussion</u>

As we found resistant Shigella and other micro-
organisms, which produce acute gastrienteritis, to ampicillin
(29%) and cotrimoxazole (27%). The Committee of Infections
in the Hospital San Juan de Dios de Manresa together with the
Committee of Pharmacy, decided to use colistin orally as a
first choice antibiotic in children with acute gastroenteritis, without prejudice, that once the organism and its
sensitivity is known, the treatment could be changed.

Of the 50 proven bacterial infections, the change
in treatment was made as a result of identifying the organism
in the following cases:

In the 5 infections produced by <u>S. typhi</u>, in which
we changed to a systemic antibiotic.

In the infection produced by <u>Staphylococcus aureus</u>
and <u>Proteus mirabilis</u>, which are by nature resistant to
colistin.

In the infections produced by <u>Campylobacter fetus</u>
the cure was produced spontaneous before changing the

treatment to erythromycin.

In the infection produced by <u>S. enteritidis</u>, we
had to change the treatment by isolating the bacteria by
blood culture.

There were 3 patients who for different reasons we
could not continue in the study, and 6 whose treatment
was varied by the doctor.

In the rest, that is to say, in 32 children, the
treatment with colistin 3,3 - 5mg./kg/daily, divided 3 - 4
times during 4 - 6 days, produced a clinical and
bacteriological cure in all of them.

With the rest of the 19 patients acute gastroenteritis of unknown origin, we practised the same treatment
and observed a cure in 13 of them.

All that has been said, supports the use of
colistin orally as an initial treatment in acute infantile
gastroenteritis.

HOW A PHENYTOIN INTOXICATION CAN LEAD TO AN
ERRONEOUS DIAGNOSIS

LUZ CLARA, M.M.
ARAÚJO PEREIRA, M.E.
MEGA, I.
SILVEIRA MACHADO, F.
Dep. of Pharmacy and Medicine III, University Hospital
Stª. MARIA - LISBON - PORTUGAL

N.L. is a 54 years old male, quite peculiar, who was admitted
in the Emergency Room, because of mental confusion and dehydration,follow
ing a week of intense epigastric pain, nausea, vomiting and diarrhea.

As one would expect, his laboratory parameters had abnor-
malities,such as hypokalemia, hypochloremia and metabolic alkalosis
(Fig. 1). Renal and hepatic function seemed to be normal. Those values
began to be corrected with the administration of parenteral balanced
electrolyte infusions. He had to be admitted for further investigation
of his gastrointestinal tract.

Later on, already in the ward, with an improved mental state,
he told us, he was suffering from epilepsy for the last twenty four years
and that he had been taking 400 mg phenytoin daily, but poorly controlled, as one could guess. This fact impressed the clinical pharmacist
who suggested to the medical team a possible diagnosis of phenytoin intoxication.

The phenytoin plasma concentration was measured at the laboratory of the Hospital Pharmacy, by E.M.I.T. (Enzyme Imuno Assay).

LABORATORY VALUES		
VENOUS		**ARTERIAL**
Na^+ - 138 mEq/l		
K^+ - 2,9 mEq/l ↓	pH - 7.5 ↑	
Cl - 90 mEq/l ↓	pCO_2 - 42 mmHg	

Fig. 1

Its value was 30 μg/ml which was clearly above the therapeutic range. In fact, with plasma concentrations of this anticonvulsant $>$ 20 μg/ml, most patients have central nervous system side effects, mainly of the vestibulo cerebellar type, such as nausea and vomiting.

Nystagmus was not seen in our patient, which was no exception, because in the literature there are many cases reported with plasma concentrations $>$ 30 μg/ml, without presenting this side effect.

Meanwhile, his condition improved just with supportive measures and phenobarbital 100 mg/day. A week later, his phenytoin plasma concentration was measured and the result was $<$ 2.5 μg/ml, which meant that he had already eliminated the drug.

Further investigations on his gastric conditions were negative.

We tried then to use our modest knowledge of non linear pharmacokinetics on our patient, utilizing some key values described for phenytoin, such as apparent volume of distribution (Vd = 0.65 l/Kg), Michaelis-Menten constant (Km = 4.5 mg/l), bioavailability (F = 1) and conversion factor of sodium phenytoin's salt into phenytoin (S = 0.92). Thus, we were able to calculate the maximum metabolic capacity (Vmax) through the following equation, where τ (1 day) is the interval between doses, D is daily dose and Cpss the measured plasma concentration in the steady-state :

$$\ldots Vmax = \frac{S \times F \times (D/\tau) \times (Km + Cpss}{Cpss}$$

$$\ldots Vmax = \frac{(0.92 \times 1 \times 400)(4 + 30)}{30} = 417 \text{ mg/d}$$

With Vmax we also obtained the clearance (Cl), half-life (t 1/2) and desired daily dose (D), to obtain a concentration steady-state level of 15 g/ml of the anticonvulsant.

$$\ldots Cl = \frac{Vmax}{Km + Cpss} = \frac{417}{4.5 + 30} = 12.08 \quad l/d$$

$$\dots \ t\ 1/2\ =\ \frac{0.693\ X\ Vd'}{C1}\ =\ \frac{0.693\ X\ 0.65\ X\ 50}{12.08}\ =\ 1.8\ d$$

$$\dots\ D\ =\ \frac{Vmax\ X\ Cpss\ X\ \mathcal{T}}{(Km\ +\ Cpss)\ (S)\ (F)}\ =\ \frac{417\ X\ 15\ X\ 1}{(4.5\ +\ 15)\ (0.92)\ (1)}\ =\ 350\ mg$$

CONCLUSIONS :

1. The calculated dose which would achieve a plasma concentration of 15   g/ml is very close to that the patient was supposed to take for years. Nevertheless, our patient got intoxicated. This fact confirms the narrow range of security of the drugs, that like phenytoin, may have a non linear pharmacokinetics, even in therapeutic blood concentrations.

2. The reported half-life for phenytoin is approximately 22 hours. Ours, is above this value, which agrees with the clinical state of intoxication . It is also full comprehensive to accept that in a week the drug was eliminated.

3. The calculated values may not be as accurate as we would like because of the patients poor mental state, lack of compliance, use of a large number of reported key parameters.

4. These pharmacokinetic assays were most helpful in the differential diagnosis of this patients condition.

MAGNESIUM DIPYRONE : PRESCRIPTION AND ADMINISTRATION

X.Bonafont Pujol
Clínica Quirón. Pharmacy Department. Barcelona.Spain

Analgesics and anti-inflamatory agents are undoubtedly one of the most often prescribed pharmacological groups inside and outside hospitals. In the Clínica Quirón in Barcelona, it is the second most prescribed group (13%) being somewhat higher than the figure found by DAYER et al. (1977) in Europe and by McKENNEY and WASSERMAN (1979) in North America who quote 10-11%.

On reviewing basic publications (1,6) and articles (8,10) on the treatment of pain, there appear a great many families of drugs and the pyrazolone group is always rejected or ignored.

Many countries have withdrawn dipyrone from the market (U.S.A., Denmark, England, Sweden) and others have made rules to restrict its use (Italy, Japan, Fed. Republic of Germany) (2). But in our centre and in many others in this country (9), it is the analgesic which is most often used.

The aim of this paper is to find out the number of patients in the Clínica Quirón who take magnesium dipyrone, the part played by the doctor and the nurse in its prescription and administration, the length of exposure to the drug, and the dose given.

MATERIAL AND METHODS

We have reviewed 317 medical records belonging to patients who were prescribed or given magnesium dipyrone during April of 1983. The following information was recorded : age, sex, discharge diagnosis, length of stay, allergies reported, type of prescription, length of treatment, maximum daily dose, and total dose.

RESULTS

95 males and 222 females were included in the study, having an average age of 43.15 years and an average stay of 7.76 days.

Prescription

For every 20 patients admitted to our Hospital, 9 were prescribed magnesium dipyrone, which is approximately 45% of the total. According to basic specialities this corresponds to 1 patient out of **every** 10 admitted for general Medicine, 2 patients out of every 5 admitted into the Obstetrics, and 1 patient out of every 2 admitted into Surgery.

The type of prescription was assessed as follows (figure 1):

Value 0 = no prescription (31 cases)

Value 1 = analgesic in case of pain (16 cases)

Figure 1.- Type of prescription

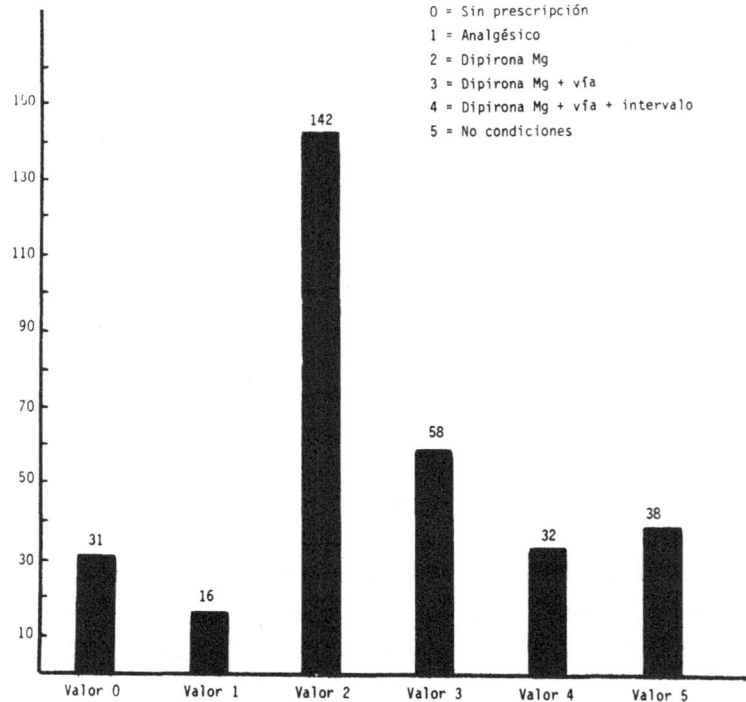

0 = Sin prescripción
1 = Analgésico
2 = Dipirona Mg
3 = Dipirona Mg + vía
4 = Dipirona Mg + vía + intervalo
5 = No condiciones

Value 2 = Magnesium dipyrone in the case of pain(142 cases)
Value 3 = p. r. n. basis, route only (58 cases)
Value 4 = p. r. n. basis, route and interval (32 cases)
Value 5 = Magnesium dipyrone timed basis (38 cases)

      As shown in figure 1, the prescription of the drug is
basically conditional and incomplete and non existent in 31 ca
ses. One of the main principles in the administration of analgesic drugs is to administer the drug at intervals and not in
accordance with the patient's needs as this reduces anxiety
and makes it difficult to remember the painful sensation(10).
Thus, the high values at the right of figure 1 would indicate
a 100% correct prescription of the analgesic, and values on
the left would correspond to 0%. In this case the type of pres
cription is intermediate and mainly indicates the analgesic to
be used.

      The role of nursing staff in the choice of magnesium
dipyrone (value 0 plus value 1) was 14.38% which is a signifi-
Figure 2.- Administration of magnesium dipyrone.

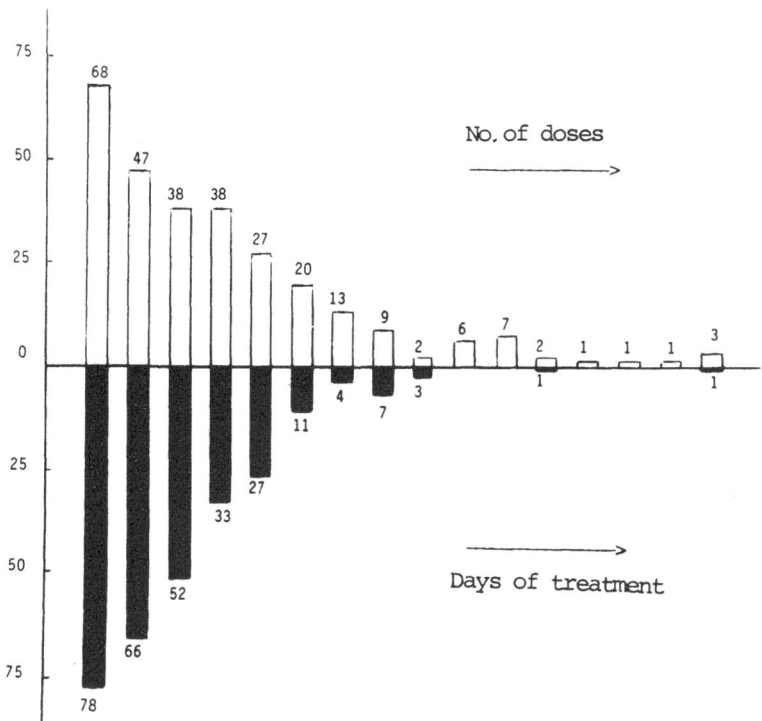

No. of doses

Days of treatment

cant figure.

In cases where the anaesthetist was able to intervene he ordered magnesium dipyrone as a post-operative analgesic in 13.3% of patients.

It should also be pointed out that there were 3 prescriptions for patients who had reported they were allergic to pyrazolone derivates.

Administration
The routes of administration chosen were as follows:

Intramuscular................... 58 %

Oral........................... 37 %

Intravenous.................... 3 %

Rectal......................... 2 %

The results show a clear predominance of the parenteral routes amounting to 61%, making the use of alternative

Figure 3.- Daily dose of magnesium dipyrone.

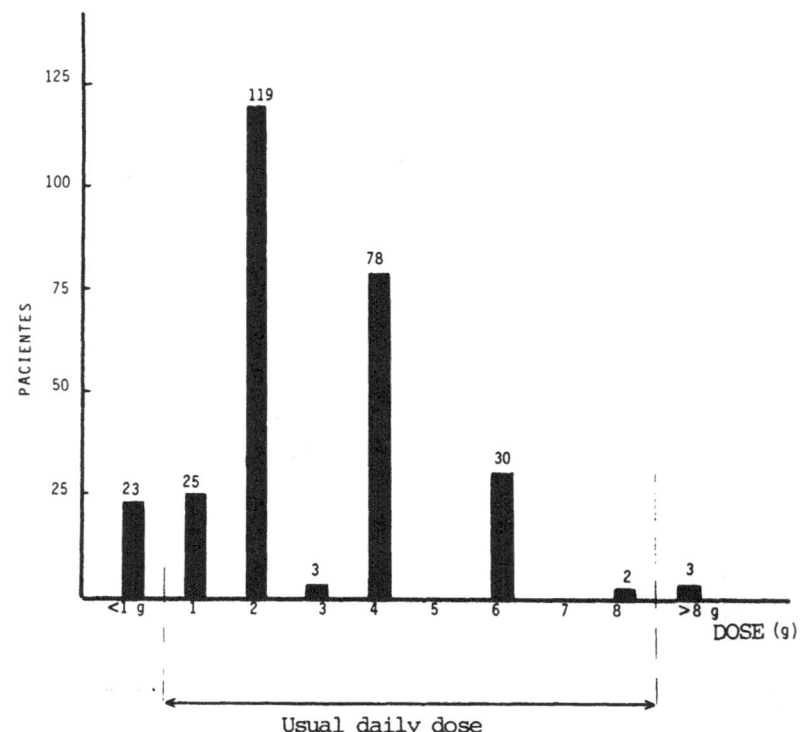

Usual daily dose

analgesics difficult as there are not many available that can
be administered by these routes, if narcotic analgesics are
not taken into account.

On studying the number of doses given and the days'
treatment with magnesium dipyrone (figure 2) we can see that
the majority of patients take from 1-4 doses and carry on the
treatment for 1-3 days (average treatment = 2.96 days).

As shown by figure 3, the maximum daily dose was 2.99
g, being over the usual dose recommended by the manufacturer
(1-8g daily) in only 3 cases. The total average dose received
by patients was 6.74g with oscillations between 0.575g and 56g
(figure 4).

The low number of doses received, short term exposure
to the drug, and slight dosage administered to patients might
suggest the use of narcotic analgesics by way of an alternative, mainly post operatively.

Although the risk of medullar depression by dipyrone
described by some authors(3,4) is low, it is also sufficiently

Figure 4.- Total dose of magnesium dipyrone.

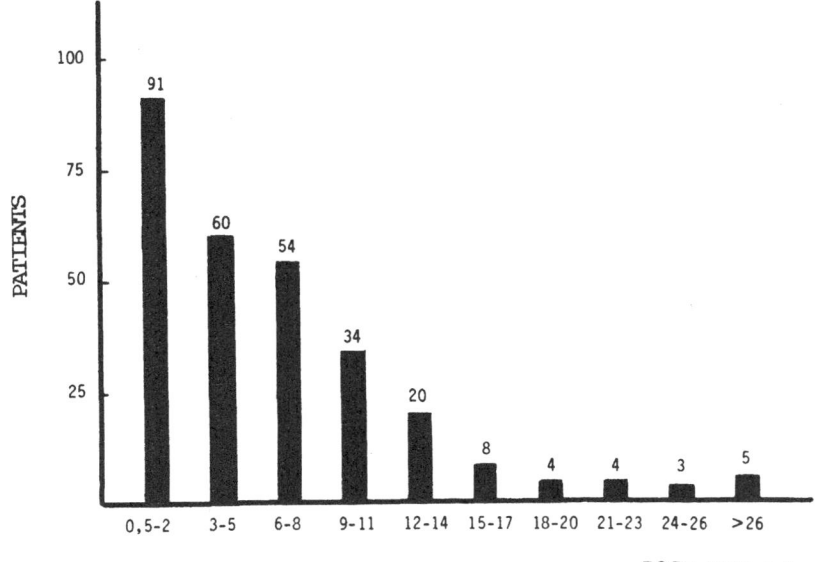

serious to recommend the use of another type of analgesic.

CONCLUSIONS

1. Approximately 1 out of every 3 patients admitted to our Hospital receives magnesium dipyrone as an analgesic.

2. The prescription is fundamentally conditional and incomplete, indicating in the majority of cases only the drug in question from force of habit.

3. The role of the nurse is important in the choice of magnesium dipyrone.

4. In general, the period of exposure and the dose given are both extremely low.

REFERENCES

(1) American Medical Association.(1980). AMA drug evaluations. Chicago. Illinois.
(2) Anonymous.(1982). Medicamentos retirados en otros paises. Inf. Ter. Segur. Soc., 6, 172.
(3) Arneborn, P. and Palmblad, J.(1982). Drug-induced neutropenia: a survey from Stockholm 1973-1978. Acta Med. Scand., 212, 289-92.
(4) Bottiger, L.E., Furhoff, A.R. and Holmberg, L.(1979). Fatal reactions to drugs. A study of 10 year material from the Swedish Adverse Drug Reaction Committee. Acta Med. Scand., 205, 457-61.
(5) Dayer, P., Grossiord, D., Casthelaz, M. et al.(1977). Prescribing patterns in european clinics. J. Clin. Pharm. 2, 205-18.
(6) Goodman, L.S. and Gillman, A.(1981). Bases farmacológicas de la terapéutica. México. Panamericana.
(7) McKenney, J.M. and Wasserman, A.J.(1979). Effect on advanced pharmaceutical services on the incidende of adverse drug reactions. Am. J. Hosp. Pharm.,36, 1691-97.
(8) Nuki, G.(1983). Non-steroidal analgesic and anti-inflamatory agents. Br. Med. J., 287, 39-43.
(9) Triquell, Ll., Mas, M.P. and Pardo, C.(1980). Analgesics in clinical practice: drug use review. In Aulangner,G. Plasse, J.C. and Van der Kleijn, E.Ed. Progress in clinical pharmacy II, 43-53. Elsevier/North-Holland Biomedical Press.
(10) Warfield, C.A. and Stein, J.M.(1982). The use of systemic analgesics. Hospital Practice, july 88 A-88 0.

USE OF PSYCHOTROPIC DRUGS IN A GENERAL HOSPITAL

H. Turakka and J. Johansson
Department of Social Pharmacy, University of Kuopio and
University Central Hospital of Kuopio,
P.O.B. 6, SF-70211 Kuopio, Finland

Consumption statistics on psychotropic drug use have been a special area of interest in recent years (Grimson et al. 1977, Bergman et al. 1979, Westerholm et al. 1979, Hemminki et al. 1981, Cooperstock & Parnell 1982, Idänpään-Heikkilä 1981, Bruun 1983, Cafferata & Kasper 1983). In Scandinavian countries a common comparison on drug use including the most important categories, for instance psychotropics, is published periodically (Nordic Council of Medicines 1982). This Nordic Statistics on Medicines analyses the drug consumption in defined daily dose (DDD) which makes possible the comparison between different countries and institutions. The Scandinavian report includes the total drug consumption, i.e. drug sale from wholesales to the retailers, excluding the hospital sale in Finland. Because of this latter reason and because there are very few reports available on psychotropic drug consumption in hospitals we planned this study. The aims were to analyse the consumption of psycho-tropic drugs and its trends in a general hospital (without psychiatric beds) and to gather information on their prescribing in different specia-lities.

MATERIAL AND METHODS

Hospital. The objective was the University Central Hospital of Kuopio which serves as the area hospital for 250.000 and as special hospital for 1 million inhabitants. All specialities are included, but there were no beds in dermatology, oncology and psychiatry at the time of study. In 1980 there were 786 beds, 204,600 bed days and 139,160 out-patient visits. Since 1977 a Hospital Formulary has been maintained which in 1980 contained 1040 preparations (incl. different dosage forms and strength) and 540 substances (or combination systems).

Material collection. For a trend analysis concerning years 1970-1980 we used the purchase statistics available in the pharmacy codex.

Purchases were counted at two year intervals. Consumption statistics,
i.e. drugs delivered by the pharmacy to the wards were available on computerized form since 1978. Because there are practically no psychostimu-
lants in use and combinations of different psychotropic drug classes
formed less than one per cent we give here the figures for 1) tranquillizers (minor tranquillizers, anxiolytics), 2) hypnotics and sedatives,
3) neuroleptics (major tranquillizers) and 4) antidepressants. As the
measure we used the newest DDD values (Nordic Council of Medicines (1981)
per bed day or 1000 bed days. The figures includes both the bed wards and
out-patient departments.

RESULTS

Total consumption. The total psychotropic drug purchases of
the hospital have decreased by 30 % from 1970 to 1980 and were 0.32 DDD/
bed day in that year (Fig. 1). The real consumption in 1980, counted
from the pharmacy deliveries to the wards was 0.30 DDD. This small difference illustrates the relation between purchase, stocking and supplies and
includes the waste. The waste percentage has been, on average, about 1 %.
The rapid decline in consumption up to 1976 is clearly a result of

Fig. 1. Purchase of psychotropic drugs in 1970-1980 by the
hospital (DDD/bed day)

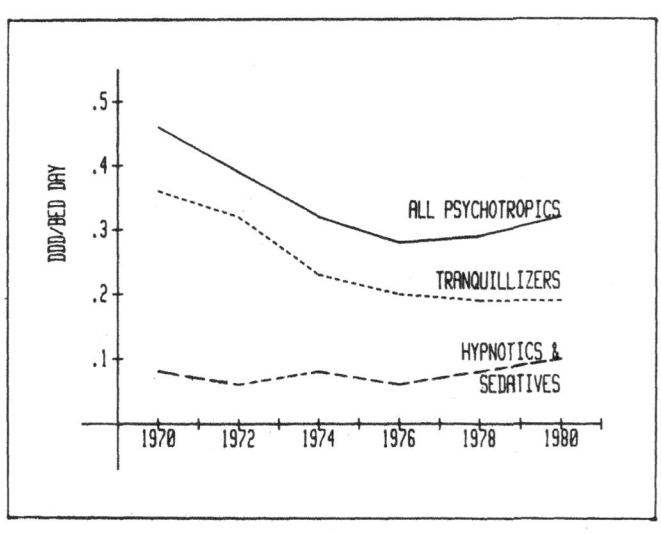

changes in prescribing of tranquillizers. The slight increase during the latter half of the decade is mostly due to an increase of hypnotic and sedative drug use, but also there was an increase in consumption of neuroleptics and antidepressants. The latter was due to establishing the day-time clinic in psychiatry. This decrease in consumption is related to prescribing habits concerning diazepam where the consumption has in ten years decreased from 0.36 to 0.19 DDD per bed day (Fig. 2). The increasing trend in hypnotics is seen in statistics for nitrazepam and oxazepam of which the latter is nowadays preferred by the Formulary Committee as the primary sleeping medication.

Fig. 2. Purchase of some benzodiazepine derivatives by hospital (DDD/1000 bed days)

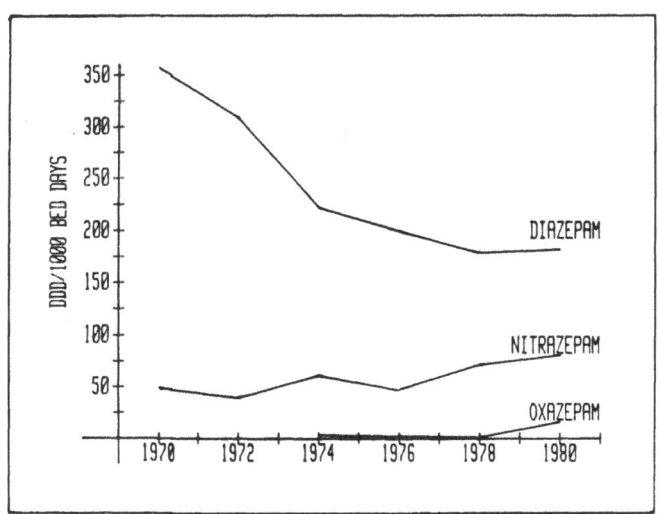

Out-patient departments. Twelve per cent of all consumption (in DDD) in hospital was in out-patient departments. They used 14 % of tranquillizers, 2 % of hypnotics and sedatives, 23 % of neuroleptics and 10 % of antidepressants. These figures should be taken into account when evaluating the figures per bed day in the whole hospital. The distribution of different drug groups in out-patient care was: tranquillizers 74 %, neuroleptics 19 %, sedatives 5 % and antidepressants 2 %. The figures include the day time ward of the psychiatric clinic which accounted for 30 % of the average out-patient use and 95 % of the neuroleptics. Total psychotropic drug consumption was 70 DDD/1000 out-patient visits.

Consumption in different clinics. The highest consumption of
psychotropic drugs was in intensive care (Table 1). There, tranquillizers
were the most commonly used group, more than double that of the average
hospital use, but this was decreasing during the last few years.

Table 1. Psychotropic drug use in intensive care
(DDD/1000 bed days)

	1978	1979	1980
Tranquillizers	663	660	384
Hypnotics & sedatives	66	14	55
Neuroleptics	50	34	31
Antidepressants	3	1	1

The differences in total consumption between the clinics were very small
excluding pediatrics (Fig. 3). However, there were differences between
the specialities in consumption of different drug categories which seemed
to compensate for each other. Between 1978 and 1980 the only significant
changes were a 30 % decrease in tranquillizer and hypnotic & sedative
consumption in gynecology and a 30 % increase in internal medicine and

Fig. 3. Consumption of psychotropic drugs on the patient
wards of different clinics in 1980 (DDD/1000 bed days)

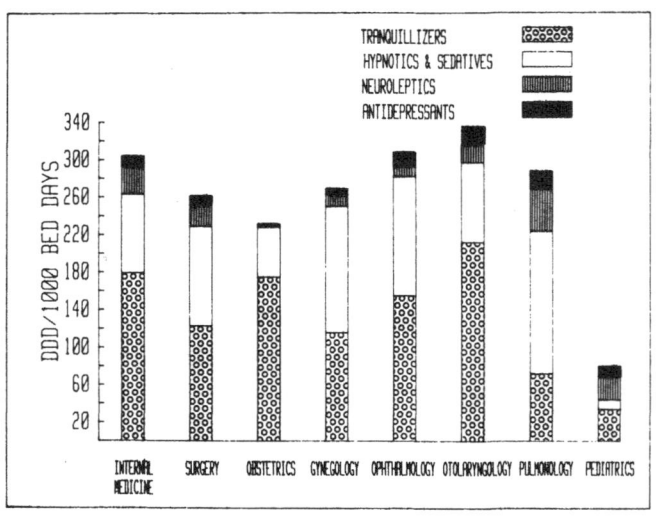

ophthamology as well as 50 % increase in otolaryngology.

Different drug categories. The percentage distribution in consumption of different drug categories is seen in Table 1 and Fig. 1 and the consumption of different drugs in Table 2. Diazepam and nitrazepam but also other drugs with anxiolytic and/or sedative effect were the most consumed substances. Also a part of neuroleptics, for instance haloperidol and levomepromazine often are used for the same indications.

Costs. Total drug costs of hospital in 1978 were about 1 million USD which accounted for 3.3 % of the total hospital costs. The percentage of psychotropic drug costs from all drug costs was 0.8 %. The cost distribution between different drug categories was: neuroleptics 46 %, tranquillizers 40 %, hypnotics & sedatives 9 % and antidepressants 5 %. The difference between the consumption and cost percentages illustrates the price differencies and price competition in some of these groups. In any case, costs is not an important criteria in the control of the consumption of these drugs.

DISCUSSION

The measure DDD/bed day is a useful index in analysing the drug consumption and its trends inside and between hospitals. In the

Table 2. Consumption of different psychotropic drugs in whole hospital in 1980 (DDD)

TRANQUILLIZERS:		SEDATIVES:	
CHLORAZEPATE POTASSIUM	1 165	CHLORALHYDRATE	234
CHLORDIAZEPOXIDE	714	CLOMETHIAZOL	181
DIAZEPAM	31 840	FLUNITRAZEPAM	160
LORAZEPAM	3 528	HYDROXIZINE	817
	37 247	NITRAZEPAM	16 740
	(182 DDD/1000 BED DAYS)	OXAZEPAM	3 871
NEUROLEPTICS:		PENTOBARBITAL	459
CHLORPROMAZINE	427		22 462
CHLORPROTIXENE	697		(110 DDD/1000 BED DAYS)
DIXYRAZINE	478	ANTIDEPRESSANTS:	
FLUPENTIXOLE	33	AMITRIPTYLINE	707
FLUPHENAZINE	-	CLOMIPRAMINE	375
HALOPERIDOL	1 063	DOXEPINE	761
LEVOMEPROMAZINE	602	IMIPRAMINE	163
MELPERONE	307	MIANSERINE	178
PERICIAZINE	233	SULPIRIDE	1 034
PERPHENAZINE	682		3 218
THIORIDAZINE	739		(16 DDD/1000 BED DAYS)
LITHIUM	-		
NON-FORMULARY DRUGS	30	AVERAGE USE: 0.30 DDD/BED DAY	
	5 351		
(26 DDD/1000 BED DAYS)			

long term, prescribing habits (dosing) may vary. Therefore, trend curves
cannot be used, for instance, for drawing conclusions of the percentage
of patients treated with each drug. Also direct comparisons between general and psychiatric hospitals in other than just consumption analyses,
may lead to wrong conclusions because the values of DDD, particularly for
neuroleptics, are defined according to the main use. For instance,
chlorpromazine was mainly used in doses 75-100 mg while the DDD is 300 mg.

The enthusiasm for prescribing benzodiazepine derivatives,
especially diazepam, has significantly decreased during 1970's and
stabilised at the end of the decade. This more critical attitude which
is a reflection of increased concern in the literature (e.g. Marks 1978,
Institute of Medicines 1979, Bratfors 1981, Bruun 1983) can be seen in
consumption statistics, in general (Grimson et al. 1977, Idänpään-Heikkilä 1977, Westerholm et al. 1978, Bratfors 1981, Idänpään-Heikkilä & Khan
1982, Klaukka & Riska 1983).

Prescribing of psychotropic drugs in this general hospital
(0.3 DDD/bed day) is very moderate when compared with some other reports.
In Sweden the average consumption in 1975-1977 has been 0.45-0.66 DDD
(Boethius & Westerholm 1977, Bergman et al. 1980) and in Norway in 1979-
1980 on average 0.67 DDD varying in different hospitals between 0.40 and
0.98 DDD/bed day (Bjørndal et al. 1983, Saugen 1982). Also the differences between the different clinics were in this study surprisingly low
compared with those of other Scandinavian reports. Considering the treatment in non-psychiatric hospitals, one may draw a conclusion that the
differences between different hospitals and even clinics within the same
hospital are more dependent on physicians' attitudes than the patients'
real need for the drug with respect to the prescribing of tranquillizers
and sedatives. Therefore our Formulary Committee emphasizes the necessity
of computerized follow-up of drug consumption and its permanent reporting
to the wards.

REFERENCES

Bergman, U. et al. (1979). Studies in Drug Utilization. Methods and Appli-
    cations. WHO Regional Publications, European Series No. 8,
    Copenhagen.
Bergman, U. et al. (1980). Eur. J. Clin. Pharmacol. 17, 183-187.
Bjørndal, A. et al. (1983). In Drug Utilization in Norway during the
    1970's, eds. S. Sakshaug et al., pp. 203-15. Oslo: Norwegian
    Medical Depot.
Boethius, G. & Westerholm, B. (1977). Svensk Farm. Tidskr. 81, 289-295.

Bratfors, O. (1981). Tidskr. Nor. Laegeforen. 101, 227-231.
Bruun, K. ed. (1983). Controlling Psychotropic Drugs, The Nordic Expe-
          rience. London & Canberra: Croom Helm.
Cafferata, G.L. & Kasper, J.A. (1983). Psychotropic drugs: use expendi-
          tures and sources of payment. National Health Care Expendi-
          tures Study.Data Preview 14. NCHSR/DHSS, Rockville.
Cooperstock, R. & Parnell, P. (1982). Soc. Sci. Med. 16, 1179-1196.
Grimson, A. et al. (1977). Nord. Med. 92, 49-54.
Hemminki, E. et al. (1981). Soc. Sci. Med. 15A, 589-597.
Idänpään-Heikkilä, J. (1977). Suomen Apteekkarilehti 67, 20-31.
Idänpään-Heikkilä, J. & Khan, I. eds. (1981). Psychotropic Substances
          and Public Health Problems. Helsinki: The Government of
          Finland.
Institute of Medicine (1979). Report of Study. Sleeping Pills, Insomnia
          and Medical Practice. National Academy of Sciences.
          Washington D.C.
Klaukka, T. & Riska, E. (1983). Suom. lääk. l. 38, 1595-1597.
Nordic Council of Medicines (1982). Nordic Statistics on Medicines 1978-
          1980. NLN Publications No. 8-10. Parts I-II. Uppsala.
Marks, J. (1978). The benzodiazipines, use, overuse, misuse, abuse.
          Lancaster: MTP Press.
Saugen, N. (1982). Norsk Farm. Tidskr. 90, 380-384.

STUDY OF THE VARIATIONS OF SODIUM AND POTASSIUM
IN PATIENTS ON DIURETICS

SOARES, M.A.
Dep. of Pharmacy, University Hospital Sta Maria,
Lisbon, Portugal

RAMALHINHO, V.M.
Dep. of Medicine I, University Hospital Sta Maria,
Lisbon, Portugal

Diuretics are one of the groups of the drugs that could be
used in a large number of diseases and most of the time for a long therapy.
Certain effects are classically attributed to their action,   like the
depletion of sodium and potassium, glucose intolerance, muscle cramps
and so on. Some of these side effects are assessed by plasma analysis. In
order to try to assess the importance of these changes we developed a
protocol for a retrospective study in wich the variations in plasma concen
trations of sodium and potassium were taken in account.

METHODS
        In the first part of the study we defined the variations of
sodium and potassium that could be considered. So, we recorded any variations of potassium $\geqslant$ 1.5 mEq/l or when ever the serum concentrations of
potassium rose above 5.5 mEq/L . or fell below 3.5 mEq/L.
To serum levels of sodium the limits were 140 mEq/l and 130 mEq/l respectively. We didn't record the alterations of sodium and potassium ever
 if the   initial value was in   the limits that we considered as variation. The patients included in the protocol were into the illness which
need a diuretic regimen, just like heart failure, acute infarction myocardium, hypertension and liver cirrhosis.
        The patients had to have two analyses with, at least, an in-
terval of time of four days. The K^+ and Na^+ levels were determined by
routine clinical laboratory procedures. The diuretics which were considered were the most frequently used in these clinical situations, are those
included in National Hospital Formulary. So, we appreciated the ionic.
variations induced by frusemide and two combinations of diuretics, frusemide and spironolactone and the other with amiloride and hydrochlorothia-
zide. The doses of each diuretic regimen were determined by   analyses.
All of the patients had a diet poor of salt and none of them had taken any

potassium changing resins.

    We chose a group of patients without diuretics but in the same clinical situations, in the same group of ages, to use as a control.

RESULTS

    In this study, the total number of patients that could be included in the protocol was 311; 199 patients were on diuretics and 112 without them. The first group was divided by the three diuretics regimens. The frusemide group, 86 were males and 45 females (table 1), in a total of 131 patients.

GROUP	DIURETIC	MALE	FEMALE	TOTAL Nº PATIENTS
I	WITHOUT DIURETIC	65	47	112
II	FRUSEMIDE	86	45	131
III	FRUSEMIDE SPIRONOLACTONE	39	17	55
IV	AMILORIDE HYDROCHLOROTHIAZIDE	7	6	13
	TOTAL	196	115	311

$\chi^2 \gg 0.05$ D.F.= 3

Table 1

The mean age was 64.5 years old (S.D. $\pm$ 14.4) and the mean dosage was 51.3 mg by day (S.D. $\pm$ 21.2) (table 3). The group on frusemide - spironolactone was constituted by 38 men and 17 women, in a total of 55 patients (table 1). The mean age was 63.4 years old (S.D. $\pm$ 9.5)(table 2), and the mean dosage of each diuretic was 56.4 mg by day (S.D. $\pm$ 22.1) to frusemide and 130.5 mg daily (S.D. $\pm$ 58.2) to spironolactone (table 3). Finally the group on fixed combination of amiloride-hydrochlorothiazide (5 mg-50 mg per tablet), was constituted by 13 patients and 7 of them were men and 6 were women (table 1). The mean age was 61.9 years old (S.D. $\pm$ 15.0)(table 2), ten of the patients were on 2 tablets and 3 of them with just 1 tablet daily.

GROUP	DIURETIC	MEAN (years)	SD	TOTAL Nº PATIENTS
I	WITHOUT DIURETICS	63.9	± 13.7	112
II	FRUSEMIDE	64.5	± 14.4	131
III	FRUSEMIDE SPIRONOLACTONE	63.4	± 9.5	55
IV	AMILORIDE HYDROCHLOROTHIAZIDE	61.9	± 15.0	13

Table 2

GROUP	DIURETIC	MEAN (mg)	S.D.
II	FRUSEMIDE	51.3	21.2
III	FRUSEMIDE SPIRONOLACTONE	130.5-56.4	58.2/22.1
IV	AMILORIDE HYDROCHLOROTHIAZIDE *	10 patients - 5/50 3 patients -10/100	----

* Fixed dose combination 5-50 mg per tablet

Table 3

The control group was constituted by 112 patients, 65 males
and 47 females (table 1). The mean age was 63.9 years old (S.D.±13.7) (table 2).

According to the proposed protocol we observed that in the
group without diuretics 54 patients presented no ionic variations and 58
presented them (table 4). In the groups of diuretics 83 patients presented ionics variations and 116 patients didn't present any alterations of
Na^+ and K^+ (table 4). In the control group the variations of Na^+ were present in 18 patients and 30 showed alterations of K^+. Only 10 patients
suffered variations in both (table 5). In the frusemide group 81 patients
presented no variations and 50 showed alterations in the ionogram (table 4), 30 of them had Na^+ variations, 11 showed K^+ alterations and 9 patients suffered the two possibles variations simultaneously (table 5). In
the frusemide-spironolactone group 27 patients had no modifications of the

plasma levels of Na^+ and K^+ (table 4), 8 had potassium plasma levels altered, 13 patients presented variations of sodium and 7 suffered both (table 5).

GROUP	THERAPY	WITH VARIATON	WITHOUT VARIATION	TOTAL Nº PATIENTS
I	WITHOUT DIURETIC	58	54	112
II	FRUSEMIDE	50	81	131
III	FRUSEMIDE SPIRONOLACTONE	28	27	55
IV	AMILORIDE HYDROCHLOROTHIAZIDE (5 mg/50 mg)	5	8	13
	TOTAL	141	170	311

$\chi^2 = 5.53$ $p = 0.1358$

D.F. = 3 $p \gg 0.05$

Table 4

Finaly, the group on amiloride-hydrochlorothiazide with 13 patients, 5 of them didn't present any plasma level variation (table 4).
This group was too small to be considered by χ^2 analysis to appreciate.
the mean of the variations.

Group	Therapy	FREQUENCY OF CHANGES IN PLASMA LEVELS OF...				Total nº patients
		K^+	Na^+	K^+ and Na^+	without variation	
I	WITHOUT DIURETIC	18	30	10	54	112
II	FRUSEMIDE	11	30	9	81	131
III	FRUSEMIDE SPIRONOLACTONE	8	13	7	27	55
	TOTAL	37	73	26	162	298

$\chi^2 = 7.44$ $p = 0.28$

D.F. = 6 $p \gg 0.05$

Table 5

CONCLUSIONS

In a retrospective study we attempted to analyse the possible role of diuretics in the National Hospital Formulary on the plasma ionogram in the diseases that most frequently use them. The study selected the patients in a ward of internal medicine during an interval of time of 15 months. The diagnoses of the admission of the patients were heart failure, acute infarction myocardium, hypertension and liver cirrhosis.

The choice of the diuretics was made by the physician, according to the National Hospital Formulary.

Using the analysis of χ^2 we didn't note any significant difference in the parameters of the plasma ionogram between the groups on diuretics and the control one. We concluded that there were no significant differences in the plasma concentrations of Na^+ and K^+ determined by all of the diuretics regimens used. Also, the group that used frusemide showed no significant differences comparing with those of the other groups.

We can say that in our patients the sodium and potassium variations in the plasma levels didn't exist.

These plasma levels variations, that are accepted for a long time has been contested by recent works[*], which we can consider to be a support to our conclusions.

REFERENCES

* CDR J. Hamilton Licht, et al.: Diuretic regimens in essential hypertension. A comparison of hypokalemec effects, BP control and cost. Arch. Intern. Med. 1983; 143: 1694-99.

Dargie HJ et al.: Total body potassium in long-term frosemide therapy: Is potassium supplementantion necessary? Br. Med. J. 1974; 4: 316.

Greenblatt DJ et al.: Adverse reactions to spironolactone. JAMA, 1973; 225: 40.

INFLUENCING ANTIBIOTIC USE THROUGH PRESCRIBING
RESTRICTIONS BY HOSPITAL PHARMACY

E. Tendi, G. Donati-Cori, C. Manfriani, A. Messori
Hospital Pharmacy, USL 10/D, Florence, Italy

Since 1979, the Pharmacy Service of the Hospital of
Careggi in Florence (a 2,500-bed hospital) has undertaken a Drug
Utilization Review (DUR) study to survey the use of a number of drugs in
the hospital. The drugs to be included in the study were selected based
on the following criteria: (i) recent arrivals on the market; (ii) most
expensive drugs; (iii) drugs with uncertain therapeutic indications;
(iiii) drugs with low therapeutic index. In the present communication, we
report the data collected from January 1979 to December 1982 regarding
cefuroxime and the data obtained from January 1982 to December 1982
regarding cefotaxime, amikacin, and piperacillin.

For each of the antibiotics included in our analysis, the
following parameters were studied: (i) overall consumption; (ii) patterns
of use; (iii) clinical outcome of therapy. The overall consumption was
estimated from the antibiotic doses that were actually administered to
the patients. The analysis of the patterns of use was focused on the
antibiotic dosage regimens that were employed; furthermore, we assessed
whether the infection to be treated was clinically documented or
microbiologically documented as opposed to prophylactic use.

The clinical outcome of therapy was deduced from the written
comment made by the physicians at the end of treatment. The physicans'
comments were classified into two groups: (i) favourable outcome of
therapy ("improved"); (ii) unfavourable outcome of therapy ("not
improved").

All requests for these antibiotics were handled by using a
form that we developed for this purpose. This form was designed so as to

control the dispensing of these antibiotics via a procedure of requiring justification. When the justification reported by the prescribing physician was accepted by the pharmacist, the drug was provided in the dose amount needed for the first day of therapy; the antibiotic dose required for the subsequent days of therapy could then be obtained through a simple repetition of the physician's signature on the same form used for the initial request. If the physician's justification appeared to be incomplete or inadequate, the physician was usually invited by the pharmacist to discuss by phone his proposed request for the antibiotic. Care was constantly taken to leave to prescribing doctor the last word.

CEFUROXIME

The data for this antibiotic are reported in Table 1. The daily dose and the duration of treatment are in good agreement with the data reported in the literature. It should be noted that the percentage of patients who were treated on the basis of sensitivity information decreases over the period from 1979 to 1982. Since this finding deserves some comment, the following explanations can be offered. First, the initial use of cefuroxime elicited an increase in use of this drug based on the previous own experience of the physicians, as opposed to use supported by microbiological information. Second, a decreased efficiency of the Drug Information Service by the Hospital Pharmacy can be hypothesized. To overcome the lack of information from the Pharmacy Service, in 1983 we undertook a programme of Drug Information for the physicans. For this purpose, we developed a bi-monthly periodical bulletin to report and discuss the results of our DUR studies.

As regards the clinical outcome of therapy, improvement was observed in the highest percentage of cases in the surgical units. At the same time, the lowest percentage of use based on sensitivity information came from the surgical units as well. It therefore appears that cefuroxime was used in these units essentially for prophylaxis.

AMIKACIN, CEFOTAXIME, PIPERACILLIN

The data for these antibiotics are shown in Table 2. It

Table 1. Use of cefuroxime over the period from January 1979 to December 1982.

	1979	1980	1981	1982
Number of patients:	76	137	229	304
Consumption (gr):	2229	3717	6157	8959
Average daily dose (gr):	4.6	3.8	3.4	3.4
Average duration of treatment (days):	6.4	7.0	7.8	8.5
Microbiologically documented infection (%):	25	36	18	8
Favourable clinical outcome (%):	53	38	69	71

Table 2. Use of amikacin, cefotaxime, and piperacillin from January 1982 to December 1982.

	Amikacin	Cefotaxime	Piperacillin
Number of patients:	149	269	382
Consumption (gr):	1434	8609	18735
Average daily dose (gr):	1.2	3.7	7.5
Average duration of treatment (days):	8.0	8.6	6.5
Microbiologically documented infection (%):	37	12.7	8
Favourable clinical outcome (%):	48	45	59

should be stressed that the average daily dose for piperacillin is considerably lower than the one that is usually recommended for this antibiotic. On the other hand, the average daily dose for amikacin and cefotaxime is in agreement with the data available from the literature.

DISCUSSION

Our study has many limitations. For example, all evaluations regarding the clinical outcome of therapy were only made on the basis of subjective criteria; the data collected were incomplete for many patients; the intermediate data that we obtained over the period from 1979 to 1982 were not communicated to the wards nor were they discussed in periodical meetings of pharmacists and physicians. The analysis of the patterns of use of the antibiotics was not, however, the main purpose for which our study was designed. In fact, our restrictive procedure of dispensing antibiotics was mainly aimed at influencing the criteria by which the physician selects an individual antibiotic to treat a given patient. As shown above, we tried different approaches to accomplish this goal, e.g. by restricting the dispensing of antibiotics and by using educational and informative tools such as the afore-mentioned periodical bulletin.

The consumption data resulting from our study deserve to be compared with the data relative to the other Hospital Pharmacies of our hospital. Our hospital is in fact provided with three pharmacies: our pharmacy is a clinically-oriented one, whereas the other two pharmacies have a more traditional approach towards drug distribution. It is worthwhile to analyze comparatively the consumption of the four antibiotics in the three pharmacies. In 1982, in our pharmacy the consumption of these antibiotics was only the 32 per cent of the overall consumption, although the wards serviced by our pharmacy had the 64 per cent of the total patient-days over this period. These data therefore support the view that our procedure of requiring justification may in fact influence the use of antibiotics.

TREATMENT OF POSTOPERATIVE AND CHRONIC PAIN BY THE EPIDURAL ADMINISTRATION OF CRYSTALLIZED MORPHINE

Torres Pons, M.D.; Aguas Compaired, M.; Ribot Roca, A.
Pharmacy Service.
Sanctis Briggs, V.; Mancho Perez, M.T.;
Anesthesia, Reanimation and the Pain Clinic Service
Quinta Salud La Alianza (Hospital Central)
Barcelona. Spain.

For some time morphine sulfate or morphine chlorohydrate, with or without a preservative has been administered epidurally for the treatment of postoperative or chronic pain. The maximum duration of analgesia achieved with this technique is 36 h.(F. Magora 1980)

In order to achieve a longer duration of anesthesia than that obtained with the morphine salts previously mentioned, the Hospital Pharmacy, in cooperation with the Anesthesia Service and the Pain Clinic, studied the results of the epidural administration of morphine base, without the addition of antioxidant or preservative.

The secondary effects of the treatment were also evaluated.

Material and methods:

The study was carried out with a solution prepared from crystallized morphine. Since the solution is not commercially available, it was especially prepared in the pharmacy.

The study was carried out with 63 patients (74% males 26% females) with ages ranging from 16 to 78 years. The patients were divided into two groups: A, corresponding to surgical patients in good general health (56 cases) and B, corresponding to patients in average or poor gene-

TABLE 1. TIPE OF SURGERY

TYPE OF SURGERY	DOSE			
	5 mg	%	10 mg	%
Colorectal	16	40	4	25
Herniorraphy	17	42,5	6	37,5
Angiography	2	5	1	6,25
Urology	2	5	5	31,25
Traumatology	1	2,5	—	—
Vascular	1	2,5	—	—
Plastic	1	2,5	—	—
Total cases	40	100	16	100

ral health because of terminal cancer (7 cases).

In order to better evaluate the results, no preoperative medication was administered to the surgical patients. The same technique was used in all the patients. The patient was placed in the left lateral decubitus position with the lumbar puncture done between L_3 and L_4. Mepivacaine 0,5% was used for infiltration of the skin; then, using a polyvinyl intravenous catheter and No. 17 Tuohy needle, the epidural space was identified with the Dogliotti technique.

The degree of muscular relaxation necessary for the surgical procedure determined the anesthesia used, either 60-66 mg of 0,37% bupivacaine without epinephrine or 200 mg of 1% etidocaine with epinephrine. The dose was decreased in the patients with chronic pain because no surgical procedure was performed. In all cases a solution 5 or 10 mg of crystallized morphine without preservative or antioxidant was added to the bupivacaine or étidocaine. The anesthesia was potentiated in some cases with atropine 0,6 mg, diazepam 10 mg, and fentanyl.-dehydrobenzoperidol 3 ml and in others with atropine 0,6 mg, diazepam 10 mg, and flunitrazepam 1,5 ml.

All patients in group A and those who required hydration in group B received a polyionic dextrose intravenous solution at the rate of 15 ml per kilo per hour.

All the information was noted in individual protocols: patient identification, vital signs, latency of anesthesia, duration of the surgical procedure, time of analgesia and any possible complication.

GRAPH 1. DURATION ANALGESIC (Doses: 5 mg)

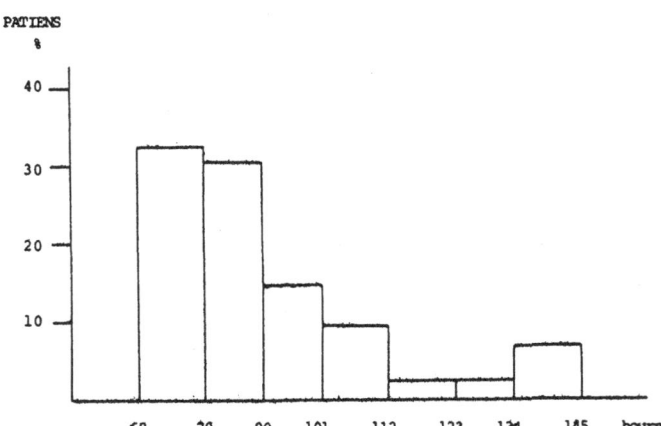

There was no significant variation in the vital signs, nor were there any autonomic reactions with the manual dilatation of the anal
sphincter in colo-rectal surgery or in the postoperative period while re-
moving the hemostatic tampon.

The patient evaluated the duration of the analgesia.

Results:

The average age of the patients was 45 years. The average surgical procedure lasted 49 minutes. The type of surgical procedure and
number of cases in the group A are tabulated in Table 1. Seven patients
were treated for chronic pain; each received 10 mg of crystallized morphine.

The latency of the anesthesia varied according to the agent
used, bupivacaine, or etidocaine. The average latency of bupivacaine was
$\bar{X}$ = 12,93 $\pm$ 3,33 minutes; and of etidocaine $\bar{X}$ = 10,67 $\pm$ 1,22 minutes. Because 1% etidocaine caused greater relaxation compared to 0,37% bupivacai-
ne, the former was used in general surgery and the latter administered in
colo-rectal surgery and Pain Clinic patients. The duration of the analgesia in the patients in group A is expressed in graphs 1 and 2 . The patients (graph 1) who were administered 5 mg of crystallized morphine presented analgesia for a average of $\bar{X}$ = 90,55 $\pm$ 20,28 hours; and those who
received 10 mg (graph 2), for a average of $\bar{X}$ = 98,12 $\pm$ 13,03 hours. All
patients in group B (graph 3) were administered 10 mg of crystallized
morphine; the analgesia was effective for a average of $\bar{X}$ = 143,71$\pm$ 30,66
hours.

GRAPH 2. DURATION ANALGESIC (Doses : 5 mg)

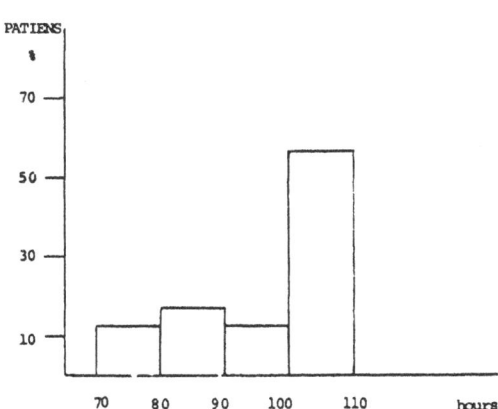

No secondary effects of the crystallized morphine were observed except nausea and vomiting four hours after surgery in one casethe
symptoms were controlled with 10 mg of metoclopramide intravenously. With
respect to the secondary effects of the anesthesia, urinary retention
occurred with both bupivacaine and etidocaine. This effect was decreased
by reducing the dose of bupivacaine from 66 to 60 mg

Conclusions:

Use of epidural morphine base without a preservative or antioxidant, achieves analgesia superior to that obtained with the use of morphine sulfate or hydrochloride with, or without preservative.

The average duration of the analgesia in surgical patients administered a solution of 5 mg of crystalized morphine was $\bar{X} = 90,55 \pm$
20,28 hours. With the same dose, 10 mg of crystallized morphine, a longer
duration of analgesia ($\bar{X} = 143,71 \pm 30,66$ hours) is achieved in the Pain
Clinic patients than in the surgical patients ($\bar{X} = 98,12 \pm 13,03$ hours)

With these doses the secondary effects of morphine are practically indetectable

The duration of the analgesia is independent of the anesthetic
agent and the dose used.

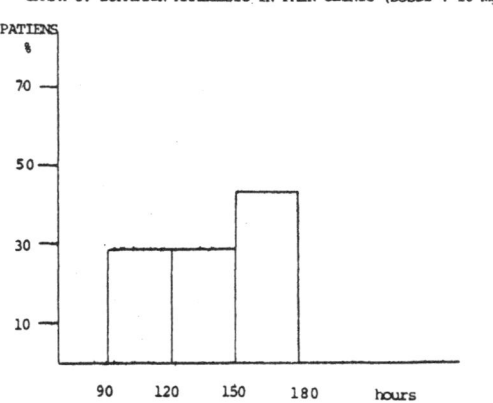

GRAPH 3. DURATION ANALGESIC IN PAIN CLINIC (Doses : 10 mg)

References:

Behar, M; et al. (1979). Epidural morphine in treatment of pain. The Lancet. 527-528

Coombs, Dennis W; et al. (1981) Continuous epidural analgesia via implanted morphine reservoir. The Lancet. 425-426.

Chambers, W.A.; et al. (1981). Extradural morphine for pain after surgery Br. J. Anaesth. 53 , 921-925

De Castro, J; et al. (1980) Perspectives d'utilisation de morphinoides en anesthesie loco-regionale. Anesth. Analg. Reanin. 37, 17-24

Coombs, Dennis W; et al. (1982). Epidural Narcotic Infusion Reservoir: Impantation Technique and Efficacy. Anesthesiology. 56, 469-473

Engquist, A; et al. (1980). Epidural morphine-induced catatonia. The Lancet. 984,

Galindo, A; et al. (1979). Local anesthetics and pain. Anesthesiology. 213

Gustafsson, L.L; et al. (1982). Disposition of morphine in cerebrospinal fluid after epidural administration. The Lancet. 796

Havdala, H.S; et al. (1979). Chronic naltrexone anhancement of morphine action. Anesthesiology. 235.

Mc Clure, J.H; et al. (1980). Epidural morphine for postoperative pain. The Lancet. 975-976

Magora, F; et al. (1980). Observations on extradural morphine analgesia in various pain conditions. Br. J. Anaesth. 52, 247-252.

Reitz, Sebastian and Mats Westberg. (1980) Side-effects of epidural morphine. The Lancet 203-204

Rutter, D.V; et al (1981). Extradural opioids for postoperative analgesia. Br. J. Anaesth. 53, 915-920

Willian A. Woods; et al. (1982) High-Dose Epidural Morphine in a Terminally III Patient. Anesthesiology. 56, 311-312

Zenz, M; et al. (1981) Long-Term peridural morphine analgesia in cancer pain. The Lancet. 91

THE HOSPITAL PHARMACIST IN THE CONTROL OF PHARMACO-LOGICAL TREATMENT

Borrego,A.M., Rafart,MªA., Fábrega,C.
Hospital San Juan de Dios. Barcelona. Spain.
Pharmacy Service

In this paper we are concerned with an area that we believe fundamaental within the context of the functions of a Hospital Pharmacy Service, namely the control of pharmacological treatments, and more precisely, the role played by the pharmacist in our Centre within this control.

This control should extend from the day the patient enters the Hospital till he is discharged. The process is shown diagrammatically in figure nº I; it begins, as we may see, with the preparation or, when applicable, with the review of the Drug History, continues with its practical utilization during the course of the stay, as well as being supplemented with new data, and finally concludes with the possible immediate application of everything that has been compiled in the information that is supplied to the patient.

To achieve the control, it is necessary for the Drug History,(drawn up beforehand) to have a dynamic nature, as it would not fulfil the function indicated if it were to remain filed in the Pharmacy Service and were only consulted to draw overall conclusions or to carry out statistical studies; we have to see to it that it reaches the medical staff committed to the daily care of the patient and, above all, the doctor responsible for him.

Sending the doctor the Drug History just as it is will most probably not be of much use, since he will either not have specific knowledge of such subjects as incompatibilities, exact composition of the drugs, etc. or he will not have time to spend on the analysis of this History.

We believe that the most effective way of ensuring maximum utilization of the information contained in the Drug

History is to draw up a written report (figure nº 2), of the incidences that this History may have on the final Medical Orders. This report is attached to the patient's chart board and may be consulted at any time by any doctor, although he may not be directly responsible for the patient.

The Pharmacy Service attaches to this report the list of the drugs included in the Hospital Pharmacological Guide that contain any of the additives or excipients that may produce allergy or intolerance in the patient. These components are generally not known by the doctor and it is common knowledge that they may produce disagreeable reactions to an equal or greater extent than the actual active principles.

In the light of this report the doctor is in optimum condition to make a definite decision on what the active principles are and on the most suitable pharmaceutical forms and ways of administration for the patient in question.

A control of pharmacological treatment like the one we describe cannot be established if there is no rational system of drug distribution in the Hospital, such as distribution by unitary doses. Using this system, a copy of the Medical Orders (figure nº 3) reaches the Pharmacy Service every day and the patient's pharmacotherapeutic record card is compiled from it.

The information regarding the most suitable form of administration of the medicaments and the progress of the treatment are covered partly by the individual pharmacotherapeutic record as well as by internal notes nurses-pharmacy, doctor-pharmacy, proper labelling of the infusion bottles, remarks in the Hospital Pharmacological Guide...

The section referring to Adverse Drug Reaction Monitoring A.D.R.M. deserves special attention. In this sense we act on two levels, on the one hand collecting daily the reports of adverse reactions observed both by the medical and nursing staff, and on the other, keeping a check on the foreseeable adverse reactions.

In the light of the different A.D.R.M. programmes currently established, we have reached the conclusion that

the best way of keeping a check on adverse reactions at in-
trahospital level is by carrying out an organized and systematic daily collection of data, whether adverse reactions e-
xist or not, in order to prevent possible errors or omissions
that may be put down to lack of practice in taking part in
programmes of this type. Bearing in mind that the information comes from two different sources (Medical Staff and Nursing Department) the forms used to gather it should be different, as the signs and symptoms that may be detected by both
groups are different.

The information provided by the Medical Staff reaches us together with the Medical Orders document (figure
nº 3) with the result that, as we explained before, it involves a daily communication of the presence or not of adverse
reactions in a given patient.

For the Nursing Department the form is according to
the model attached (figure nº 4). It contains the identification of the patient, the existence or not of adverse reactions and, if so, their description. An informative list of
possible adverse reactions that may be detected by the nurse
is given on the back. It is completed every day by each nursing shift.

Lastly, the Pharmacy Service completes the final
A.D.R.M. record with the data received from the medical staff,
the nurses and in the light of the patient's file and Therapeutic History (figure nº 5).

If we achieved a type of standardized final record
cards, identical for all hospitals and prepared by a commission of hospital pharmacists, it would assist the interhos-
pital task of A.D.R.M.

On reaching the last stage of the patient's stay in
the Hospital and prior to his discharge, a final report is
prepared on the progress of the treatment in which any incidences that may have arisen are commented upon. This report
has two purposes:

- To complete the Drug History, which will be filed
in the Pharmacy Service.

- To provide the information that should be given
to the patient about the use of medicaments.

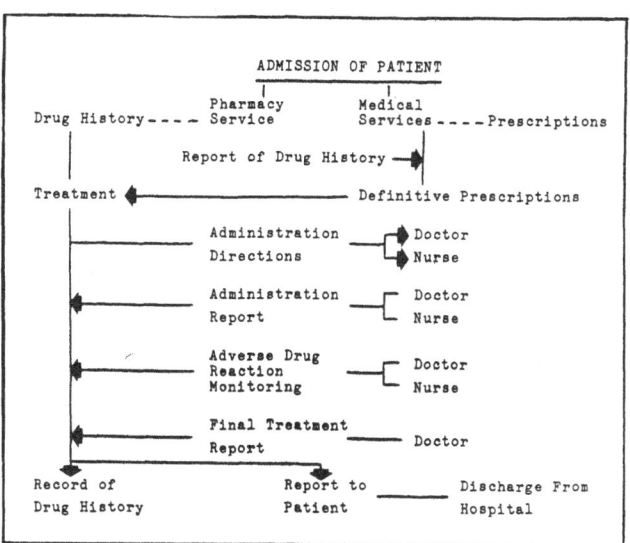

figure nº I

ADMISSION OF PATIENT

Pharmacy Service — Drug History

Medical Services — Prescriptions

Report of Drug History

Treatment — Definitive Prescriptions

Administration Directions — Doctor / Nurse

Administration Report — Doctor / Nurse

Adverse Drug Reaction Monitoring — Doctor / Nurse

Final Treatment Report — Doctor

Record of Drug History   Report to Patient   Discharge From Hospital

figure nº 4

HOSPITAL SAN JUAN DE DIOS
BARCELONA
Pharmacy Service

ADVERSE DRUG REACTION MONITORING SHEET
(TO BE COMPLETED BY NURSE)

Ward or Department......... Date......
Has any patient shown signs of any adverse reaction to drugs:

    yes ☐   no ☐

If Affirmative:

Patient	Drug(s)	Type of Reaction	Diet
....	....	....	.....
....	....	....	.....
....	....	....	.....

Name and Signature of Nurse:

figure nº 3

HOSPITAL SAN JUAN DE DIOS
BARCELONA
Pharmacy Department

PRESCRIPTION

PATIENT	Hospital San Juan de Dios PRESCRIPTION	Date	Time
ADVERSE DRUG REACTION MONITORING			
Adverse Drug Reaction			
yes ☐ no ☐			
If Affirmative: Drug Involved:			
Type of Reaction:	Signature of Doctor		

figure nº 2

HOSPITAL SAN JUAN DE DIOS
BARCELONA
Pharmacy Service   PATIENT

DRUG HISTORY
REPORT OF PHARMACY DEPARTMENT

- Possible allergies to drugs:...............
- Possible allegies to food:................
- Other allegies:................
- Drugs currently taken:................
    Preventative:................
    Diagnostic:................
    Therapeutic:................
- Interactions:................
    Drugs:................
    Food:................
    Laboratory Test:................
- Remarks:
    Habits: Tobacco:....Alcohol:... Others:....
- Others Remarks:................

                    Signature of Pharmacist

figure nº 5

HOSPITAL SAN JUAN DE DIOS
BARCELONA
Pharmacy Service   PATIENT

ADVERSE DRUG REACTION MONITORING

- Diagnostic: ....
- Associated diseases: ....
- Description of supposed adverse reaction
  and its development: ....
- Drugs associated with adverse reaction:

Drug	Dose	Mode of Admin.	Admin. Route	Duration of Treatment
....	....	....	......	....
....	....	....	......	....
....	....	....	......	....

- Diet: ....
- Allergies of patient: ....
- Allegies in family: ....
- Remarks: ....
- Laboratory data, X-Rays, etc.: ....

REFERENCES

Alberola,C.(I976). Bases para la iniciación de un programa de
      farmacovigilancia intensiva. pp. I75-I8I.XXI Asam-
      blea Nacional de Fârmacéuticos de Hospitales.Cuenca

Allwood,M.C.; Fell,J.T.(I980). Textbook of Hospital Pharmacy.
      Blackwell Scientific Publications.

Bonal,J.(I973). Información de Medicamentos entre el farma-
      céutico de Hospital y el enfermo. pp.97-III. XVIII
      Asamblea Nacional de Farmacéuticos de Hospitales.
      Canarias.

Gerbino,Ph.P. et al. (I975). Patient Communication. Reming-
      ton's Pharmaceutical Sciences. Fifteenth edition.
      pp. I702-I709. Pennsylvania: Mack Publishing Com-
      pany.

Mitchell, A.A. et al. (I980). Adverse Drug Effects and Drug
      Surveillance. Pediatric Pharmacology Therapeutic
      Principles in Practice. S.J. Yaffe ed. pp. 65-77.
      Grune and straton,Inc.

Triquell,Ll.(I980). Distribución y control de medicamentos en
      Hospitales. Puesta en marcha de sistemas en dosis
      unitarias. Asociación Española de Fârmacéuticos de
      Hospitales ed.

Van der Kleijn,E.; Jonkers,J.R. (I977). Clinical Pharmacy.
      Proceeding of the International Symposium on Clini-
      cal Pharmacy held in the Hague. The Netherlands:
      Elsevier/North Holland Biomedical Press.

PHENYTOIN AND PHENOBARBITAL DRUGS WITH INVARIABLE DOSES

N.V.Jiménez Torres
Pharmacy Service.General Sanjurjo Hospital.Valencia.SPAIN
A.Sánchez Alcaraz
Pharmacy Service.General Sanjurjo Hospital.Valencia.SPAIN

ABSTRACT.- The ponderal ratio between the doses of Phenytoin/
Phenobarbital (PHT/PB) in the different medicaments of PHT and
PB commercialized in Spain, varies from 0.5 to 6. Now, in a-
greement with the theoretical pharmacokinetic expositions, it
becomes impossible to obtain therapeutic plasma levels of both
active principles outside the interval of 1 to 4.
The aim of the present work is to confirm the fact that the
therapeutic plasma levels are specifically reached with medicaments having a PHT/PB ratio of 2. This thesis has been established after analyzing the experimental plasma PHT and PB levels
of 72 patients, treated with different commercial drugs composed of PHT and PB with invariable doses.

I INTRODUCTION

Of the different medicaments with antiepileptic drugs currently
on the market in Spain, there are 16 which consist of fixed doses of Phenytoin (PHT) and Phenobarbital (PB). This number represents more than 36% of
the total of these medicaments (1). This percentage is closely related to
the consumption of these medicaments, both at a national and provincial levels, as in 1981 they formed 33.3% and 34.7% respectively of the group of
antiepileptic drugs (2).

The abundance of this kind of drug in Spain bears no relation
to what happens in France (3), Great Britain (4) or the USA (5), where there are respectively 1, 2 and 2 commercial medicaments of the above mentioned characteristics.

On the other hand, the ponderal ratio between doses of PHT/PB
in the 16 drugs ranges from 0.5 to 6. The justification of this fact has
not been dealt with sufficiently in the bibliography, as only Gastaut (6)
in 1966 advises, without arguing his criterion, that for the treatment of
generalized tonic-clonic seizures, the dose of PB should be 50% of that of
PHT. More recently, Muller et al (7) have indicated that fixed dose PB and
PHT combinations with a ratio of 1:2 are acceptable for obtaining therapeu-

tic plasma levels (PL) of each drug.

'Along these lines, and in 1981 (8), after applying Wagner's equation for calculating dosage regimes to each drug, the hypothesis was established that, of all those medicaments formulated with fixed dose PHT and PB, those with a ponderal PHT/PB ratio of 2 would be the most suitable for achieving, simultaneously, therapeutic PL of both drugs.

Thus, the aim of the present work is to corroborate this hypothesis, by studying the experimental PL of PHT and PB presented by a group of 72 patients, under continuous treatment, with one of the following drugs Comital L; Disfil; Epilantin; Episindrome; Redutona and Trinuride H Forte.

The present study covers a period of over two years.

II MATERIALS AND METHODS

II.1 Patients and Medicaments

We have studied a group of 72 adult patients, diagnosed with generalized seizures (40.7%), partial complex seizures (22.0%) and others.

The last column of table 1 shows the number of patients who took each of the specified durgs. All the patients, in personal interviews, confirmed that they carried out the treatment. Also, in table 1 we show the ponderal ratio of PHT/PB and the daily dosages advised by the manufacturer and calculated for a patient of 60 kg and plasma clearance for PHT and PB of 0.02 and 0.005 l Kg^{-1} h^{-1} respectively were considered.

TABLE 1. Medicaments with PHT and PB and daily doses

Registered Name	Ratio PHT/PB	Daily Dose Manufacturer	Calculated[*]	Number Patients
Comital L	1	1.5 - 8	6	11
Epilantin	2	3 - 6	3 - 6	26
Redutona	2.3	4	5 - 9	13
Trinuride H Forte	2.7	3 - 6	10 - 15	5
Disfil	3	3 - 10	8 - 10	9
Episindrome	3.3	3	5 - 6	8

II.2   Assay Method

Blood samples were taken coinciding with the minimal concentration in steady-state (C_{min}^{ss}). The drug monitoring was carried out following the technique of homogeneous enzyme immunoassay (EMIT).

III   RESULTS AND DISCUSSION

Figure 1 shows the C_{min}^{ss} of PHT (square) and PB (triangle) corresponding to the 72 patients. Each segment corresponds to one patient.For each drug, the patients have been ordered from lowest to highest dose/day.

In view of the experimental PL at normal doses of PHT and PB, with the drugs whose PHT/PB ratio is well below 2, the PL of PHT will always be subtherapeutic. With drugs whose PHT/PB ratio is much greater than 2, the PL of PB will be subtherapeutic. This generalization is corroborated by the excellent lineal correlation found between the ratios of C_{min}^{ss} (y) and the ponderal ratios of PHT/PB doses (x) which are presented by the drugs given to the patients (figure 2).

Table 2 intends to show, through the analysis of frequencies, the grade of the PL obtained (therapeutic and non-therapeutic) with drugs which have a ratio PHT/PB different from 2, as opposed to those obtained with drugs of the ratio PHT/PB 2.

FIGURE 1. Plasma levels of PHT and PB in differents patients

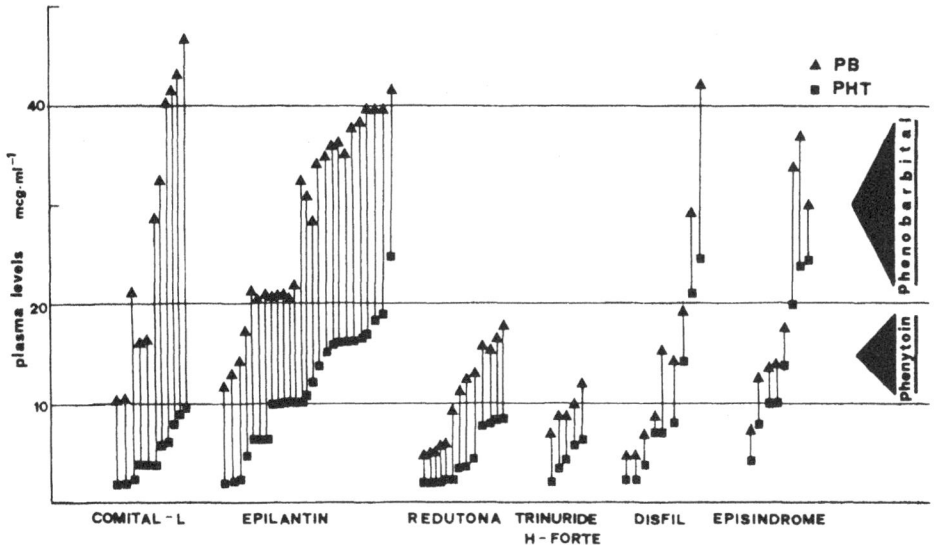

The important statistical significance obtained does not only explain the fact that there were 20 changes of treatment in the 72 patients of whom more than 90% were patients undergoing treatment with drugs whose PHT/PB ratio was different from two. The reasons for the modification of the treatments were in 25% to pass to drugs with a ratio of 2; in 30% one single drug (PHT or PB) was used; and in 45% there was a change to Carbamazepine. This situation also explains the abandoning of these drugs, a fact

FIGURE 2. Correlation between ratios C_{min}^{ss} and doses of PHT/PB

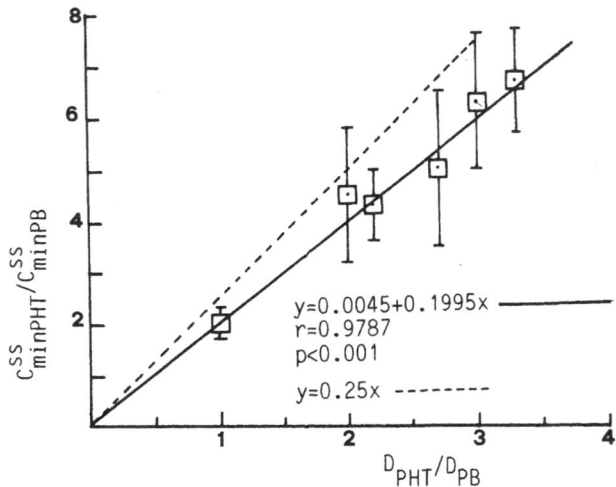

$$y = 0.0045 + 0.1995x$$
$$r = 0.9787$$
$$p < 0.001$$
$$y = 0.25x$$

TABLE 2. Distribution of the plasma levels (therapeutic and not) calculation of chi squared and value of P

| Medicament (NR) | Patients | Plasma levels of PHT and PB | | x^2 | P |
		Therapeutic	Non-Therapeutic		
Epilantin	26	18	8	-	-
Redutona	13	0	13	16.7	4×10^{-5}
Comital L	11	0	11	14.8	1×10^{-4}
Disfil	9	0	9	12.8	3×10^{-4}
Episindrome	8	1	7	7.9	5×10^{-3}
Trinuride H forte	5	0	5	8.3	4×10^{-3}

which is clearly reflected in the percentage of prescriptions.Thus, at the beginning of this study (1980) they constituted 41.1% and two years later, they represent only 16.8% of the total consumption of these medicaments(2).

IV CONCLUSION

The present work firmly supports the fact that drugs formulated with PHT and PB at fixed doses, with a ponderal ratio of 2, are the most suitable for obtaining plasma concentrations in the steady-state which achieve the therapeutic ranges currently established for both drugs. Therefore, the use of other commercial preparations should be avoided according to their distance from that value.

V REFERENCES

1 Câtalogo Especialidades Farmaceuticas. (1983). Madrid:Consejo General de Colegios Oficiales de Farmaceuticos.
2 SANCHEZ A. & JIMENEZ N.V. (1983) Medicamentos Antiepilépticos:(I) Análisis de su consumo. XXVIII Congreso Nacional de la AEFH. Barcelona
3 Dictionaire Vidal. (1978). Paris:O.V.P.
4 British National Formulary. (1981). London: British Medical Association and the Pharmaceutical Society of Great Britain.
5 Physician's Desk Reference. (1982). Oradell N.J.: Medical Economics Company.
6 LITTER M. (1975) Farmacologia Experimental y Clínica.Buenos Aires: El Ateneo. pag.347.
7 MULLER F.O. et al.(1974). Diphenylhydantoin-Phenobarbitone combination therapy:Analysys of serum level findings. S A Medical Journal (Sept.),1894-1895.
8 SANCHEZ A. & JIMENEZ N.V. (1981) Antiepilépticos: Determinación de niveles plasmáticos. Revista AEFH V(3), 253-260.

TREATMENT OF ARTERIAL HYPERTENSION IN THE OLD PATIENT

M.I.Genua
Servicio de Farmacia

F. Almagro
Medicina Interna

A. Cabarcos
Director Médico. Hospital General Geriátrico "José Matía Calvo"
San Sebastián. Spain

INTRODUCTION

In the aged patient the quantity of documents on the treatment of Arterial Hypertension (A.H.T.) is clearly smaller than in the young and the guidelines to be followed have not been set out definitely.This is due to the fact that amongst other causes there exist greater difficulties in defining the concept of hypertension itself, greater diagnostic difficulties and above all a greater complexity in the use of hypertension medicines for such patients.

The common use of beta-blocking drugs with intrinsical, (ASI) mimetic sympathetic activity and previewed fewer side effects, as well as the better knowledge of the bio-disposing of medicines in the organism of the aged patient causes us to consider the possible application of staged therapeutics used in middle aged patients for older patients.

An exhaustive study of drugs usually used for the treatment of A.H.T. has led us to the conclusion that beta-blockers, even considering exclusively those with ASI, present in determined doses a depressive action on the myocardic function of the senile heart. Consequently, these drugs have been excluded from our study, apart from in very concrete cases.

Diuretics play an important part in the case of the aged patient. A single doses per day when dealing with chlorthalidone (thiazide family) is enough to control A.H.T. in a high number of patients, which is something to be specially considered for those out patients where the amount of medicine administered daily will determine in many cases the accomplishing of the treatment. The difficulties described are diverse, amongst others , postural hypertension and dehydration. In order to control these adverse effects it is necessary to calculate the dosage with regard to the patient constants.

We should not forget the calcium vasodilators and antagonists which, although they represent the inconvenience of a short half life with the result that the dosage must be increased (2 or 3 times per day), their efficiency and the surprisingly few number of adverse side effects noted, make them a group of drugs essential in this type of treatment.

Methyldopa, a drug used extensively for its good anti-hypertensive performance, has not been chosen for consideration within this study due to the large number of side effects described and observed in our hospital.

Once we had selected the drugs to be used, 222 patients were chosen who had shown a high level of arterial pressure on their admission to the Medical Centre.

Only 96 of these 222 maintained this high level of arterial pressure on 2 occasions with an interval of 24 hours and in 2 positions, either orthostatic or supine decubitus. We considered high arterial pressure to be present in all those whose systolic rate remained above 160 mm Hg and whose diastolic rate was above 95 mm.

RESULTS

We intended to normalise the pressure,applying measures as non-aggressive as possible in the 96 patients.

33% of the patients (32) normalised their pressure only by regulation of their diet. Of the remaining 64 patients, 52 only needed to be treated with a single drug, chlorthalidone in 40 of these cases and nifedipine or prazosin in the other 12, due to the fact that they also presented cardiac problems which required the use of these drugs.

Only 10 patients had to be treated with 2 associated drugs, and 2 with 3. In the latter case, beta-blockers and methyldopa were used on 2 occasions.

Making use of the drugs described above, we noticed that some of those patients treated with chlorthalidone on a dose of 50 mg per day showed signs of slight dehydration over a long period of time and when already at the out-patient stage, which was resolved by giving a dose of 25 mg chlorthalidone per day, maintaining the efficiency of the treatment as described in a case in the extensive bibliography.

No adverse effects were observed with any of the drugs used.

CONCLUSIONS

1) We showed the high number of patients who appear to be hypertensive if the mistake is made of evaluating exclusively the arterial tension when taken on admission to the hospital.

2) Once again it was shown that control is absolute in the majority of patients, only with hygienic-dietetic measures alone or including a mild diuretic.

3) We should nor forget that lower doses than those usual in young adult may, for the aged patient, reduce to a minimum the collateral effects, maintaining their effectiveness.

REFERENCES

Because the bibliography about this matter is so plentiful, if you are interested on it,please,ask Dra. Genua.

ADDRESS: Servicio de Farmacia. Hospital General Geriátrico "José Matía Calvo". Avda. de Zarauz, 123. San Sebastián. SPAIN.

PASSIVE/ACTIVE IMMUNIZATION AND FOLLOW-UP OF NEWBORN
BABIES OF MOTHERS WHO ARE CARRIERS OF THE HEPATITIS
B VIRUS. THE ROLE OF THE PHARMACIST IN THE CLINICAL
TEAM

Fábrega,C.[1], Calvet,E.[2], Mainou,C.[3]
Hospital San Juan de Dios. Barcelona. Spain
1 Pharmacy Service
2 Biochemistry Service
3 Department of Pediatrics

The vertical transmission of Hepatitis B Virus(HBV)
from a mother to her infant is a major mechanism of spread
and persistency of the virus B in the environment.

Vertical transmission can be achieved intrauterus,
during the labour or in the perinatal period, either the mother had acute hepatitis B during pregnancy, specially in the
third trimester, or when she was a chronic carrier. The frequency of transmission depends on the rate of chronic carriers in the environment and on the ethnic origin. There is considerable geographic variation in the pattern of transmission and the risk of the newborn to be infected (Papaevangelou
Hoofnagle 1979; Polakoff 1982.).

The resolution of the disease in the chronic carrier state is related inversely with the age at which the infection is attained. Thus, the perinatal infection increases the
risk of chronic liver diseases, cirrhosis and/or primary liver carcinoma, because the association between these pathologi-
es and chronic antigenemia (Zuckerman 1982,a; Chin 1983).

During a two years period we determined the serological markers of HBV in blood donors and pregnant women in
our hospital, (N=3,000), finding a 1.7% rate of asymptomatic
chronic carriers. That fact place our country in a middle endemic situation, between those with a low persistence (0.1-
0.5%) and those with a high persistence (10-20%). These results are similar to other data observed in our country (Caba-
llería & Bruquera 1981; Pujals i Ferrús 1983).

The possibility to use specific measures for the
prophylaxis of newborns of chronic carrier mothers, gave rise
to a study conducted by clinicians of Pharmacy, Biochemistry,

Gynaecology, Neonatology Pediatric and Gastroenterology Services, in order to establish the selection and treatment criteria.

A specific hyperimmune immunoglobulin, with an antibody titer of near I:I000.000, is available for passive immunization. It will give a quick but brief protection. Although
the available data are limited, no reaction due to immunocom-
plex formation has been reported when the immunoglobulin was
administered to positive HB_SAg patients (Palmer et al. I98I;
Working party on the Clinical use of specific immunoglobulin
in hepatitis B. I982; Centers for disease control, Department
of health and human Services; Atlanta, Georgia. I982).

Recently has been marketed a vaccine whose special
characteristics makes it of limited supply and very expensive.
This vaccine is a suspension of purified surface antigen particles, obtained from plasma of healthy chronic carriers, i-
nactivated by biophysical and biochemical procedures (Maupas
et al. I98I,a; Hilleman et al. I982). The vaccine proved to
be safe and highly immunogenic in children, inducing protective antibody titers with only two doses, smaller. than those u-
sed in adults, in 97% of all healthy children tested (Krugman
I982; U.S. Department of Health and Human Services. I982). Recent studies seem to prove the immunogenicity of the vaccine
at birth. Regarding the efficacy of the vaccine, the induced
antibody protect from the acute and the asymptomatic infection as well as from the chronic carrier state, regardless the
subtype of virus B involved. The efficacy is total in those
individuals vaccinated prior to the infection. The use of the
vaccine   post-exposure to the virus could be effective due to
the long incubation period of type B hepatitis (Krugman I982;
U.S. Department of Health and Human Services.I982).

·The passively acquired antibody, either from the mother or by means of the administration of the immunoglobulin,
do not interfere the active immunologic response to the vaccine. Therefore, it is possible passive/active immunization to
obtain an immediate and permanent protection. The accumulated
data about the active immunization at birth, are limited and
the optimum timing for vaccination in conjunction with immuno-

globulin administration has not been established (U.S. Department of Health and Human Services. 1982).

Until more data are available we propose, the selection and treatment of newborns of asymptomatic chronic carrier mothers, as follows:

Within the usual control of pregnant women we shall include at sixth-month control the HB_SAg and HB_cAc determination. This should be repeated in all cases at the 9th month control or if it is impossible, during labour. If one or both of them were positive, the complete serological markers must be detemined as well as the study of liver function, that should be repeated at the 9th month control or if it is impossible, during labour.

All newborns of those mothers who were positive to HB_SAg or HB_cAc (without HB_SAc) or both in any of the controls, will receive prophylactic treatment. Newborns of mothers either positive or negative to HB_eAg are also included, assuming that the available data are not enough to make therapeutic differences based on the presence or absence of this antigen (Zuckerman 1982; Delaplane et al. 1983; Rosendahl et al. 1983).

All newborns described above will receive a course of 3 doses of specific immunoglobulin (0.5 ml. within the first 24 hours of life, 0.5 ml. I month later and 0.5 ml. 3 months after the first dose) and a course of 3 doses of vaccine given intramuscularly (IO mcg in conjunction with the third dose of immunoglobulin, IO mcg. I month later and IO mcg. 6 months after the first dose of vaccine). They will receive a single booster dose of vaccine at 5 years of age. Follow-up blood samples, to test serological markers, will be taken before the first dose of immunoglobulin and at 3,9,I2 months ant 2,3,4 and 5 years. If there is some positive HB_SAg result, the liver function will be studied. If there is clinical or laboratory evidence of active liver disease, the established schedules will be followed.

We hope that collaboration between Pharmacists, Biochemists, Obstetricians and Paediatricians will contribute, with the results obtained with this group of children, to the

studies underway in order to attain the optimal use of the a-
vailable therapeutic measures.

REFERENCES

Barin, F. et al. (1983). Immune response in neonates to hepa-
        titis B vaccine. Lancet I, 251-253.
Cabellería,J.(1981). Hepatitis vírica. Medicine 2,3ª serie,
        116,123.
Centers for disease control. Department of health and human
        Services; Atlanta,Georgia.(1982). Immune globulins
        for protection against viral hepatitis. Recommen-
        dations of the immunization practices advisory co-
        mmitee. Ann. Inter. Med. 96, 193-197.
Chin,J. (1983). Prevención de la transmisión de la infección
        crónica por el virus de la hepatitis B de madres a
        hijos en los E.E.U.U. Pediatrics ed.esp.2,79-82.
Delaplane,D. et al. (1983). Hepatitis B mortal en la fase pre-
        coz de la infancia. Importancia de la identificaci-
        ón de las gestantes con HB_SAg positivo y de la in-
        munoprofilaxis de sus hijos. Pediatrics(ed.esp.)
        Vol. 16, Nº 2, 107-111.
Hilleman,M.R. et al. (1982). The preparation and safety of
        hepatitis B vaccine. Symposium: Worlwide control of
        hepatitis B. Athens. Greece.
Krugman,S.(1982). The newly licensed hepatitis B vaccine.Jama.
        Vol. 247 ,Nº 14, 2012-2015.
Maupas,P. et al. (1981)a. Hepatitis B vaccine; rationals,
        principles and application. Elsevier/North Holland
        Biomedical Press. Nº 18.
Maupas,P. et al. (1981)b. Efficacy of hepatitis B vaccine in
        prevention of early HB_SAg carrier state in children.
        Lancet.I.289-292.
Palmer Beasley,R. et al. (1981). Hepatitis B immune globulin.
        Efficacy in the interruption of perinatal transmi-
        ssion of hepatitis B virus carrier state. Lancet,
        388-393.
Papaevangelou,G. & Hoofnagle,J.H. (1979). Transmisión de la
        infección por el virus de la hepatitis B a través

de madres asintomáticas portadoras crónicas del an-
tígeno de superficie de dicho virus. Pediatrics (ed.
esp.) Vol. 7,Nº 4, 317-320.

Polakoff,S. (1982). Immunization of infants at high risk of
hepatitis B. British Medical Journal. Vol. 285,
I294-I295.

Pujals i Ferrús,J.Mª. (1983). Prevenció de l'hepatitis B. But
Soc. Cat. Pediatr. 43, I6I-I69.

Rosendahl,C. et al. (1983). Avoidance of perinatal transmission of hepatitis B virus; Is passive immunization
always necessary. Lancet. II27-II29.

Szamuness,W. et al.(I98I). Passive-Active immunization against hepatitis B: Immunogenicity studies in adult
americans. Lancet. 575-577.

U.S. Department of Health and Human Services.(1982). Inacti-
vatede hepatitis B virus vaccine. Recommendation of
the immunization practices advisory commitee (ACIP).
M.M.W.R. Vol. 3I,24, 3I7-328.

Working party on the Clinical use of specific immunoglobulin
in hepatitis B. (1982). Use of immunoglobulin with
high content of antibody to hepatitis B surface antigen (anti-HB$_S$). British Medical Journal. Vol. 285.
951-954.

Zuckerman,A.J.(1982)a.The Association of Hepatitis B with Primary Hepatocellular Carcinoma. Symposium: Worldwide
Control of hepatitis B. Athens. Greece.

Zuckerman,A.J.(1982)b.Priorities for immunisation against hepatitis B. Br.Med.J. Vol. 284. 686-688.

INTRATHECAL INJECTION OF MORPHINE FOR ANALGESIC TREATMENT OF
TERMINAL CANCER

A. Idoipe, Mª P. Pardo, M. Mendaza, Mª A. Sagredo, P. Palomo
Servicio de Farmacia. Ciudad Sanitaria de Zaragoza (Spain)

L. Carcavilla
Servicio de Neurocirugía. Ciudad Sanitaria de Zaragoza (Spain)

The present work presents the manufacture, control and use of
intrathecal morphine injection in the treatment of patients in
pain due to untreatable terminal cancer. We have prepared a
hypertonic solution of 3.33 mg ml^{-1} morphine hydrochloride in
6.66% glucose. The manufacture of these injections takes place
under sterile conditions where the solution for injection is
submitted to sterilizing filtration and is dosified in 1 ml
ampoules. Control of sealing, contents, sterility and pH of
the ampoules also takes place. The therapeutic response
obtained in the treatment of four patients has been
satisfactory. The absence of side effects, so common after
injection via systemic, shows evidence of the direct medullar
action of the morphine. The implantation of a morphine
reservoir in two patients allowed constant administration,
carried out even in outpatient conditions and thus
considerably increasing the perspectives that this new
analgesic technique offers.

The administration of intrathecal morphine in analgesic
therapeutics is a technique that is being investigated at present with
different types of pain: preoperative, postoperative, obstetrics and
terminal cancer (Babcock et al. 1981; Besson 1977; Besson et al 1978;
Tung et al. 1980; Wang et al. 1979; Yaksh & Rudy 1977). The Department of
Pharmacy has started the preparation of intrathecal morphine injections
for its routine application to patients controlled by Department of
Neurosurgery who suffered from irreducible pains caused by terminal
cancer, what constitutes the object of this paper.

MATERIAL AND METHODS

Manufacture of morphine injection: morphine hydrochloride (1%)
90 ml, glucose (10%) 200 ml, and water for injections 10 ml are added to
a 300 ml sterile flask in laminar flow hood. The morphine solution is
submitted to sterilizing filtration and is dosified in 1 ml ampoules.
Control of sealing, contents, sterility (Farmacopea Europea 1981) and pH

are carried out,

In relation to the use of the **prepared** intrathecal morphine
injections, they have been actually administered to four patients, three
male (A,B and C) and one female (D). The patients A,B,C and D were 46, 67
73 and 42 years old, respectively, All of them suffering from irreducible
pain caused by terminal cancer, Intrathecal morphine has been injected in
all the cases by lumbar puncture and subarachnoid injection according
to the method described by Lazorthes et al. (1980). The dosage is
dependent on each patient and reservoir is introduced in cases C and D.

RESULTS AND DISCUSSION.

An injectable solution of 3.33 mg ml^{-1} morphine hydrochloride
in 6.66% glucose, hypertonic enough, has been prepared, as Lazorthes el
al. (1980) claim, to limit the narcotic diffusion to supraspinal
arachnoid regions by means of which the side effects commonly observed
after systemic injection are noticed (Glynn et al. 1979; Liolios &
Hartman-Andersen 1979; Miralles et al. 1980). Oca (1963) shows that the
oxidative decomposition of morphine into pseudomorphine is helped by
heating, **lighting** and alkaline medium. In order to favour stability,
the whole **preparation** process has been realized under sterile conditions
where the injectable solution is submitted to sterilizing filtration.
This solution presents a pH lower than 6, **threshold value from which**
morphine may precipitate (Del Pozo 1977). The sterility assay has been
satisfactory,

The therapeutic response obtained by intrathecal morphine
administration for irreducible pain treatment in terminal cancer has been
satisfactory, achieving the analgesic effects to lower doses than
required when administering morphine by via systemic (Baraka et al. 1981).

Analgesia induced in patient A has been partial, He has been
injected with two ampoules of intrathecal morphine at an interval of
five days. Patient B: The pain reappears progresively and with different
characteristics than his habitual ones. He has injected two intrathecal
morphine ampoules within an interval of four days, Patient C: The
analgesia has been almost total and up to 80-90%. Positive response to
the four injections firstly administered within an interval of five days,
encouraged the reservoir implantation for chronic dosage. Patient D
showed pain regression 6 minutes after the first injection. After 15

minutes it had decreased 75% and after 30 minutes it had almost
disappeared; the analgesia lasting for about 30 hours. The pain
reappearing progresively in the same location but with different features
than was habitual. This positive response encouraged the posterior
reservoir insertion.

Analgesic response features relating to intensity and
duration are the same as the ones assesed by Baraka et al. (1981) and
Lazorthes et al. (1980). All the cases have presented a significant
relief on pain within 30-45 minutes following the injection. Analgesia
has been intense and its effects remained for periods of time range from
5 hours in patient A to 72 hours in patient C.

As Lazorthes et al. (1980) claim morphine analgesia after
intrathecal injection is certainly a result of the narcotic fixing and
selective medulla opiate receptors of the gelatinose substance in the
spinal cord and it **mimics** and reinforces a physiological mechanism
commonly assured by **enkephalins** .

Patient	A	B	C	D
Clinic	Gastric neoplasia possible metastasis	Adeno- carcinoma in pancreas	Rectal tumor renal surgery	Rectal tumor abdomino- perineal amputation
Pain	Abdominal	Abdominal & dorsolumbar	Perineal region	Intergluteal & left gluteal
Analgesia start	45 minutes	40 minutes	30 minutes	6 minutes
Analgesia duration	5 hours	10 hours	48-72 hours	30 hours
Side effects		Nauseas Vomiting	Vomiting itching drowsiness	Drowsiness

The period of time analgesia remains latent varies from one patients to another and it does not seem to depend on morphine dose, it corresponds to the time morphine takes to diffuse in cerebrospinal fluid to receptors of the dorsal horn of the spinal cord. Its slow posterior redistribution due to the hydrophilic feature of molecule, thus accounts for its prolonged effect.

Side effects such as drowsiness, nausea   vomiting and itching disappear without naloxone administration. The lack of significant side effects, which normally appear after systemic injection states again morphine medullar direct action, its diffusion being confined to supraspinal arachnoid spaces mainly due to hypertonicity of the administered solution.

Morphine reservoir has been implanted in two patients, which has enable intrathecal administration repeated easily even in outpatients conditions. As Onofrio et al. (1981) and Lazorthes et al. (1980) state the employment of morphine reservoir inserted through the spinal subarachnoid space permits chronic administration avoiding repeated lumbar puncture, because of which injection risk decreases, the possibilities offered by this new analgesic technique greatly increase.

REFERENCES.

Babcock, N.K. et al. (1981). Respiratory arrest after intrathecal morphine. J.A.M.A., 245, 1528.

Baraka, A. et al. (1981). Intrathecal injection of morphine for obstetric analgesia. Anesthesiology, 54, 136-140.

Besson, J.M. (1977). Effects de la morphine sur la transmission des messages nociceptifs au niveau médullaire. Actualités Pharmacol. Paris, 119-141.

Besson, J.M. et al. (1978). L'analgésie morphinique: données neurobiologiques. Ann. Anesth. Franc., 19, 343-369.

Del Pozo, A. (1977). Farmacia Galénica Especial, 2 edition. Barcelona: Romargraf.

Farmacopea Europea (1981). Madrid: Consejo General de Colegios Oficiales de Farmacéuticos.

Glynn, C.J. et al. (1979). Spinal narcotics and respiratory depression. Lancet, 2, 356-357.

Lazorthes, Y. et al. (1980). Aanlgésie par injection intrathécale de morphine. Neurochirurgie, 26, 159-164.

Liolios, A. & Hartman-Andersen, F. (1979). Selective spinal analgesia. Lancet, 2, 357-358.

Miralles, F. et al. (1980). Analgesia con morfina intratecal y depresión del S.N.C. Caso clínico. Rev. Española Anest. Rean., 27, 511-513.

Oca, J. (1963). Manual de Farmacotecnia. I. Inyecciones. Zaragoza: edited by author.

Onofrio, B.M. et al. (1981). Continous low-dose intrathecal morphine
        administration in the treatment of chronic pain of malignant
        origin. Mayo Clin. Proc., 56, 516-520.
Tung, A.S. et al. (1980). Opiate withdrawal following intrathecal
        administration of morphine. Anesthesiology, 53, 340.
Wang, J.K. et al. (1979). Pain relief by intrathecally applied morphine
        in man. Anesthesiology, 50, 149-151.
Yaksh, T.L. & Rudy, T.A. (1977). Studies on the direct spinal action of
        narcotics in the production of analgesia. J. Pharmacol.
        Exp. Ther., 202, 411-428.

ACUTE DERMATITIS DUE TO ZINC DEFICIENCY ASSOCIATED TO LONG TERM TPN WITH ZINC SUPPLEMENT: A CASE REPORT

Cardona, D.*, Llistosella, E.**, Coma, I.*, Navarro, S.***, Queraltó, J.M.****, Sanz, M.* and Bonal, J.*
Hospital de la Santa Creu i Sant Pau. Services of: *Pharmacy, **Dermatology, ***Surgery and ****Biochemistry

In this report we are presenting the case of a patient who was taken into our hospital and received treatment of TPN zinc supplementation and who showed a deficit of this oligoelement.

CASE REPORT

A 28-year-old woman was hospitalized with an acute digestive hemorrhage, gastric neoplasia was diagnosed, and a total gastrectomy of the Henley type was performed.

After 20 days, it underwent volvulation, became necrotic and was resected. Later, an esophagus-jejunal plastia of the colon was tried, but it also became partially necrotic.

After the second intervention, TPN was initiated with the mean composition values as follows: 1 l of crystalline aminoacids, 1 l of glucose 50% and 250 ml of Intralipid 20%. 2.1-2.4 g proteins/Kg/day were administered; 9-10 g glucose/Kg/day; 0.55-1.1 g lipids/Kg/day and 50-55 Kcal/Kg/day. The solution also contained electrolytes. On alternate days a multivitamin complex and a solution of trace elements (Zn:3 mg; Cu: 1 mg; Cr: 2.25 ug was added. Once a week, via IM, the patient received 3 mg of folic acid, 10 mg Vit. K and 1 mg Vit B_{12}. The iron supplement was calculated according to the haemoglobin level.

The patient was administered this parenteral diet for one month, initiating a continuing enteral elemental diet (Elemental Diet[R]) by the duodenostomy (5 g of Nitrogen, 1665 Kcal and 8 mg Zn/day).

After the third intervention, a mixed diet was maintained with TPN and EN, after having withdrawn the parenteral diet. However, there was an intolerance of the EN wich produced a clinical picture of diarrhea and abdominal pain that caused an increase of the TPN again and a withdrawal of the EN. (Fig.1)

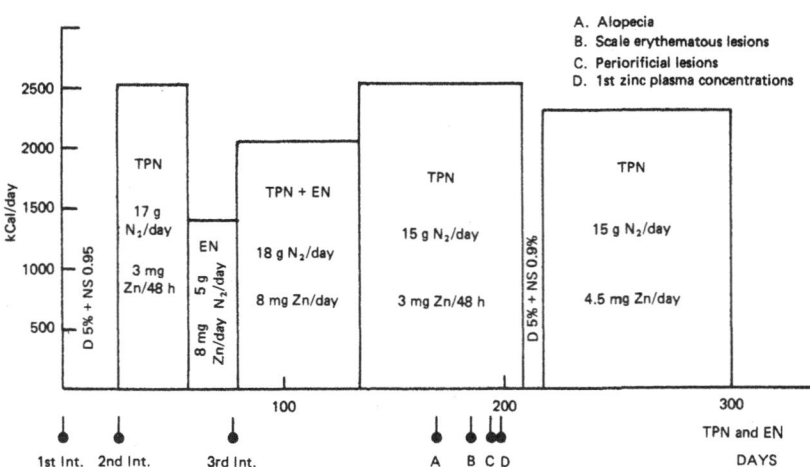

Following the two months of the initiation of the TPN, the
patient showed a clinical picture of depression. During the third month,
a diffuse hairloss had already been observed. In the first dermatological
consultation the alopecia was attributed to either a hyposideremy or a
deficit of essential fatty acids. The laboratory test showed normal iron
values. As far as the essential fatty acids were concerned, those were
perfectly covered by the lipids administered with the TPN.

        After one month, the patient developed a generalized pruritus
and painful cutaneous lesions in periophtalmic, perinasal and perimouth
areas as well as in axial, inguinal and perianal areas, producing greyish-
blue spots with scales and scabs evolving in about 15 days.

        The clinical pharmacist that was responsible for the follow
up and control of the parenteral nutrition suggested that a zinc deficiency should not be ruled out, even though the TPN was **being** supplemented
and therefore, a plasma   level was ordered.

        Serum zinc concentration was determined by Atomic Absorption
Spectroscopy. The first values obtained were of 3 umol/1. (Reference values: 10-23 umol/1).

        In the Galenic section of the pharmaceutical services,ampou-
les containing 15, 10 and 3 mg zinc, respectively, were prepared.

        The treatment continued, administering for 3 days 15 mg of
zinc IV, followed by 10 mg of zinc IV for 3 more days and maintaining
3 mg of zinc daily, above and beyond the 1.5 mg/day that were administered
through the TPN. (Fig.2)

        The cutaneous lesions were healing spectacularly and had dis-
appeared within a short time. The alopecia also improved, although not as

quickly as the cutaneous lesions.

DISCUSSION

Kay described the zinc deficiency syndrome in adults after surgery of the digestive tract of patients receiving TPN (Kay,1975). Until then, the sources of aminoacids had been solutions of hydrolyzed proteins rich in zinc, which were substituted by solutions of crystalline aminoacids, containing less of this oligoelement, and then started to appear zinc deficiency syndromes in patients on total parenteral nutrition. (Walravens,1976).

During recent years, some cases have been observed of zinc deficiency in patients on TPN supplemented with this oligoelement. (Latimer,1977), (Mozzillo,1982), (Moran,1982), (Holbrook,1980), (Hayat,1983).

Zinc deficiency may manifest itself already prior to TPN due to:

A diminished absorption of the cation (Crohn´s disease, cancer of colon, pancreatitis. (Haver,1978), (Regan,1979).

Gastrointestinal losses. (Postoperative patients with short bowel syndrome, drainages or severe diarrhea). (McClain,1980).

Whenever TPN is administered:

There is an increase of urinary losses of zinc, primarily in patients with catabolism. (Ladefroged,1982). In hypoalbumineous patients the free zinc plasma increases, if it is found in great proportion aligned with the albumin. (Freeman,1975). Some aminoacids contained in the TPN (cysteine and histidine) are able to combine with the zinc, forming complexes which are then easily eliminated by the urinary tract. (Mozzillo, 1982).

There is an increase of zinc requirements in patients on TPN with positive nitrogen balances, that is, in phases of anabolism or protein synthesis. (Prasad,1979), (Kay,1976 b).

In our case report, the nitrogen balances of the controlled TPN were always positive. (Fig.3).

What then is the quantity of zinc that should be given to patients on total parenteral nutrition?.

According to Wolman, the patient maintains positive balances of this element with 2.5 mg Zn/day, whenever there are no diarrhea or gastrointestinal losses present. (Wolman,1979).

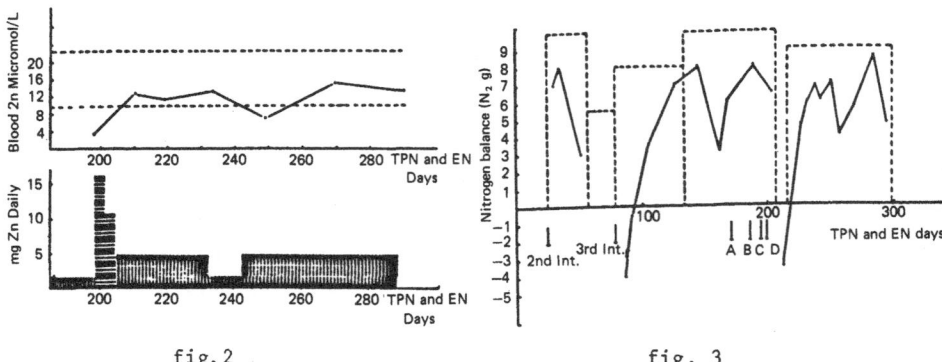

fig. 2   fig. 3

The American Medical Association (AMA) recommends 2.5–4.0 mg of Zn/day, wich may be increased by 2.0 mg more in patients with severe gastrointestinal fluid losses.

In our case 1.5 mg of Zn/day was administered, a lower dose than recommended by the two authors mentioned above.

However, there should be kept in mind the contamination of the TPN solutions (due to aminoacids and the Intralipid), which has already been studied in various reports (Wolman,1979), (Chevranky,1982), and which may reach values of 1.0–1.2 mg of Zn/day.

In this report, the plasma zinc values are 3 umol/l (r.v. 10–23 umol/l) confirmed the deficit of this oligoelement and explained the symptoms wich the patient showed: alopecia, depression and cutaneous lesions. The administering for 3 days of 15 mg of zinc IV, followed by 3 days of 10 mg normalized the low levels of zinc in the blood. The plasma values were maintained within refernce interval by administering 4.5 mg Zn/day IV.

Alkaline phosphatase enzyme contains zinc. Some authors (Mozzillo,1982), (Jiménez Torres,1980), (Kasarkis,1980), encountered low levels of alkaline phosphatase in patients with zinc deficiency. In our case, the alkaline phosphatase values were always higher than reference limit. (Fig.4)

CONCLUSION

From this case report it can be concluded that it is necessary to control the zinc plasma levels of all patients who are on total parenteral nutrition for more than one month and to adjust the dose

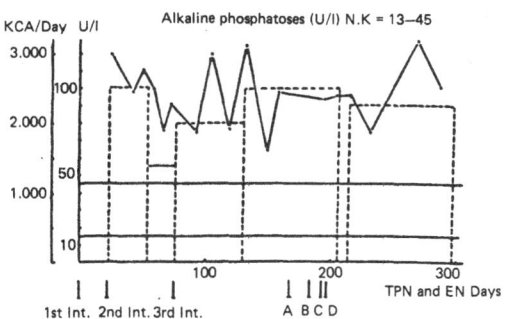

fig. 4

administered according to the clinical evolution of the patient.

REFERENCES

CHERURANKY, T. EFFECT OF GROWTH HORMONE ON HAISERUM AND URINE ZINC IN GROWTH HORMONE-DEFICIENT CHILDREN. AM.J.CLIN.NUTR. 35: 668-670. 1982.

FREEMAN,J.B. EXCESSIVE URINARY LOSSES DURING PARENTERAL ALIMENTA. J.SURG.RES.18:463-468.1975.

HAUER,E.C. TRACE ELEMENT PROFILE OF T.P.N. AM.J.CLIN.NUTR. 31: 264-268. 1978.

HAYAT,D. R.CLINI.ZN DEFICIENCY IN T.P.N.: ZN SUPPLEMENTA. J.P.E.N. 72-74,1983.

HOLBROOK,I.B. LOW SERUM ZN AND LONG-TERM T.P.N.. AM.J.CLIN.NUTR. 33: 1891-1982.

JIMENEZ TORRES,V. PRESENCIA ELEMENT. TRAZA EN SOL. COMERC. N.P. A.E.F.H. IV.2.87-90.1980.

KASARKIS,E.J. SERUM ALKALINE PHOSPHATASE AFTER TREATMENT OF ZINC DEFICIENCY IN HUMANS. AM.J. CLIN.NUTR. 33: 2609-2612. 1980.

KAY,R.G. ACUTE ZN DEFICIENDY IN MAN DURING T.P.N. AUST.N.Z.J.SURG. 45:325-330. 1975.

KAY R.G. A SYNDROME OF ACUTE ZN DEFICIENCY DURING T.P.N. IN MAN.ANN.SURG.183:331-340.1976.

LADEFOGET,K.INTESTINAL AND RENAL LOSS OF INFUSED MINERALS IN PATIENTS WITH SEVERE SHORT BOWEL SYNDROME.AM.J.CLIN.NUTR. 36: 59-67. 1982.

LATIMER,J.S. CLINI.ZN DEFICIENCY DURING ZN-SUPPLEMENTED T.P.N. J.OF PEDIA. 97:434-437.1980.

M$_C$CLAIR.C. ZN DEFICIENCY: A COMPLICATION OF CROHNS DISEASE. GASTROENTER. 2: 272-279.1980.

MORAN,D.M. ZN DEFICIENCY DERMATITIS ACCOMPANYING T.P.N. SUPPLEMENTED WITH TRACE ELEMENTS. CLINICAL PHARMACY.1: 169-176.1982.

MOZZILLO,N. ZN DEFICIENCY SYNDROME IN PATIENT ON LONG-TERM T.P.N. LANCET 1.744.1982.

PRASAD,A.S. ZN IN HUMAN NUTRITION.PP1-80: BOCA RATON FLORIDA: CRC.PRESS.1979.

REGAN,P.T. THE MEDICAL MANAGEMENT OF MALAPSORTION.MAYO CLIN.PROC.4: 267-274.1979.

WALRAVENS,P.A. GROWTH OF INFANTS FED A ZN SUPPLEMENT FORMULA.AM.J.CLIN.NUTR.29:1114.1979.

WEISSMANN,K. SERUM ALKALINE PHOSPHATASE ACTIVITY IN ACRODERMATITIS ENTEROPATHICA: AN INDEX OF THE SERUM ZN LEVEL. ACTA DERMATOVENER 59: 89-90.1978.

WOLMAN,S.L. ZN IN T.P.N.: REQUIREMENTS AND METABOLIC EFFECTS. GASTROENTEROLOGY 76:458-467.1979.

INFORMATION FOR PATIENTS WITH PARENTERAL HYPERALIMENTATION

Torres Pons, M.D., Argemí Fuentes, M.T., Aguas Compaired, M.,
Ribot Roca, A.
Quinta de Salud La Alianza. Pharmacy Service . Hospital Central
Barcelona, Spain

There are many services which the Hospital Pharmacy can perform within the institution. One activity in development is informing the
patients and/or their families about their medication. To initiate this
service in our hospital we selected patients receiving parenteral hyperalimentation for various medical indications because there appears to be
little information generally available for the patients and their families.

Material and methods:

A hospital pharmacist informed the patients directly about parenteral hyperalimentation, regardless of age or sex.

The following data were collected according to a protocol to
evaluate the effectiveness of the program: patient identification, diagnosis, physician responsible for the parenteral hyperalimentation, date of
initiation and termination, education and social-economic level of the patient, dates of visits and notes of interviews with the patient.

TABLE 1. PERCENTAGE THE EDUCATIONAL AND SOCIAL-ECONOMIC LEVELS

LEVELS	Educational		Social-economic	
	Nª cases	%	Nª cases	%
Upper	0	0	0	0
Upper middle	4	16	3	12
Middle	4	16	5	20
Lower middle	8	32	9	36
Lower	9	36	8	32
Total	25	100	25	100

Because the patients come from a wide variety of educational and social-economic levels, this section was subdivided into upper, upper middle, middle, lower middle and lower levels.

A few days after beginning the hyperalimentation, we interviewed the patient to avaluate the following areas of information:

- comprehension (very good, good, average, poor, doesn't know/ no answer)
- breadth of coverage: (Very complete, average, incomplete)
- and patient and family acceptance: (yes, no, indifferent)

These data were noted in the file along with any questions of the patient. (All notes were made after completion of the interview to avoid any misunderstanding by susceptible patients.)

The physician responsible for the parenteral hyperalimentation, together with the pharmacist, decided the composition of the parenteral fluid for individual cases. After receiving the prescription, and before the administration of the hyperalimentation, began, the pharmacist visited the patient to inform him or her clearly and concisely using vocabulary appropriate for the patient. During the interview, according to the social and educational level manifested the process was explained in more or less detail.

FIGURE 1. PAMPHLET OF INFORMATION

QUINTA DE SALUD LA ALIANZA

WHAT YOU OUGHT TO KNOW ON:

PARENTERAL NUTRITION

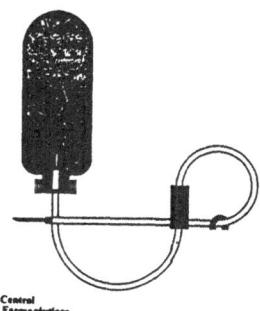

Hospital Central
Servicios Farmacéuticos
C/ San Ant. M.ª Claret, 135
BARCELONA-25

·WHAT CARE MUST BE TAKEN?

·To avoid infection, the conection points of the intravenous infusion set and the paper tape on the injection site should not de ma-mipulated. If any anomaly in the machine or the infusion set is detected, call immediately a member of the nursing staff.

WHAT COMPLICATIONS CAN OCCUR?

Normally, Parenteral Nutrition, does not produce complications but one should be aware of the following: fever, diaorrhea, displacement of the catheter, intolerance to the components of Parenteral Nutrition and vein inflamation

* * * * * *

For futher information, please contact the Pharmacy Department.

Before terminating the interview the patient was asked if he had understood the explanation and if he desired more information. At the same time the patient received a pamphlet (figures, 1, 2) which served to remind the patient of the explanation given.

The points mentioned in the pamphlet are:
- the objective of parenteral hyperalimentation
- its composition
- cases in which it is administered
- the preparation by the pharmacist
- the administration by the physician
- the duration of the treatment
- precautions necessary with the treatment
- possible complications which may occur

The information on puncture catheter technique is carried out by the medical service.

Results:

The study was carried out with 25 patients (52% male, 48% female) with an average of 63 years. The distribution of diagnosis among the patients was 58% neoplasia and 42% various.

FIGURE 2. PAMPHLET OF INFORMATION

WHAT IS THE AIM OF PARENTERAL NUTRITION?

To feed a patient by intravenous route (central o perypheral), in order to administer him the adequate feeding for his state

WHAT IS THE COMPOSITION?

The same basic or elemental components of a normal nutrition but adequately prepared: sugars, fats, proteins (meat, fish, eggs, milk...) vitamins, ect. The doctor, through a series of tests, knows the daily needs of the patient and prescribes the diet with the right proportion of each of its components.

IN WHICH CASES SHOULD BE USED?

When the patient cannot eat, should not eat or does nor want to eat. Also, sometimes, before surgical operations to increase the defenses and/or improve the nutritional state.

WHO, WHERE AND HOW IS PREPARED?

A specialized pharmacist from the Pharmacy Department prepares it in a sterile room and in conditions of maximum cleanness.

WHO AND HOW IS IT ADMINISTERED?

A specialized doctor localizes a vein. Through this vein the Parenteral Nutrition is administered. The nursing staff will place and control it. A machine called "Nutribomb" controls the Parenteral Nutrition rate. Its function is to meassure in a precise form the rate flow, drop by drop.

HOW LONG IS THE TREATMENT?

The contents of a bag of Parenteral Nutrition should be given in 24 hours. The total length of the treatment will depend on the state of the patient and is decided by the specialized doctor.

The average duration of treatment was 21,6 days

The educational and social-economic level of the patients is expressed in Table 1. Because of the predominance of a lower middle and lower level education + social-economic state, the original explanations were modified accordingly

The acceptance of the information by the patient and family is indicated in Table 2 . More than 50% of the cases (68% of the patients and 75% of the families) accepted the information favorably.

The majority of cases of refusal correspond to the very sick patients. We think this is due not to the patient's lack of interest but to state of his illness. A later acceptance of the information when he improves is the rule.

In the cases where the acceptance was indifferent, although the percentage is the same, the patient and families did not correspond to each other.

The grade of comprehension and evaluation of the information is expressed in Table   3   . In 72% of the cases the comprehension was good or very good. In 48% more verbal information was requested.

More ample information was especially requested regarding:
- skin testing with various antigens
- participation of the digestive system in hyperalimentation
- secondary effects
- clarification of the label of the parenteral liquid.

TABLE 2. ACCEPTATION OF INFORMATION

	Patients		Families	
	Nª cases	%	Nª cases	%
Yes	17	68	15	75
No	4	16	1	5
Indifferent	4	16	4	20
Total	25	100	20	100

Conclusions:

- We conclude that the patient is not familiar with the concept of hyperalimentation.

- The patient accepts and appreciates all the information received.

- Contrary to the original idea, the information, although given in terms comprehended by the patient, should be more extensive.

- We consider the patient information about hyperalimentation to be necessary and affective.

- Having observed the results of the pilot study in our hospital, informing the patient about hyperalimentation is now a routine procedure.

References:

Charles, M. Karnack; and col. (1981). Pharmacist involvement in home parenteral nutrition programs. American Journal of Hospital Pharmacy. 38, (2) 215-217

TABLE 3. COMPREHENSION (C) AND VALORATION (V) OF INFORMATION

LEVELS	Nº CASES		%	
	(C)	(V)	(C)	(V)
Very good	9	5	36	20
Good	9	15	36	60
Average	4	4	16	16
Poor	0	1	0	4
Doesn't know/ no answer	3	—	12	—
Total	25	25	100	100

THE USE OF COMPUTER PROGRAMS IN CLINICAL NUTRITION

Elizabeth M Zola, PharmD
Ross Laboratories
and
Assistant Clinical Professor
The Ohio State University of Pharmacy
Columbus, Ohio 43210

Introduction

The role of microcomputers in the health care system is
constantly expanding and includes applications in the areas of
patient care and medical education. This paper will describe
examples of microcomputer programs designed to increase the clinical
knowledge base of members of the nutritional support team composed
of the physician, clinical pharmacist, dietitian and nurse.

Applications in Patient Care

Microcomputers have applications in the daily clinical
activities of nutrition support team members. A large amount of
clinical and laboratory data must be analyzed daily by team members
to assess the nutritional status of a patient. Calculation of some
of the more complex anthropometric indices frequently requires
time-consuming mathematical and statistical analyses and the use of
nonograms which may produce inaccurate results. Computer programs
have been developed that can greatly decrease the time between
collection of laboratory and anthropometric measurements and documentation of the nutritional status of a patient. These programs
are designed to be operated by any member of the nutrition support
team and prior computer training is not a prerequisite for computer
users. The computer operator inputs anthropometric measurements

including weight, height, mid-arm circumference, and skinfold
thickness. Laboratory data are input including white blood cell
count with percent lymphocytes and monocytes, serum electrolyte
values, serum albumin, and 24-hour urine creatinine. The computer
output is in the form of a graphic printout with the patient's data
expressed as the number of standard deviations from the mean for
each measurement. This is represented as a bar graph with the
patient's measurements lying above or below a horizontal line. Any
measurement more than +2 or less than -2 standard deviations from
the mean is automatically considered abnormal. The patient's
nutritional status can easily be read from a graph which is attached
to the patient's chart for documentation.

Microcomputer programs can also be used by the pharmacist
monitoring nutritional formula preparation. Simple programs can be
written to perform routine calculations and print out copies of
worksheets and labels for the preparation of total parenteral
nutrition solutions. These programs may be particularly time-saving
in the calculation of caloric intake and fluid requirements for low-
birth-weight infants in the neonatal intensive care unit who must
receive their daily nutrient requirements in small volumes of
intravenous solutions. A controlled study conducted by Giacoia
et al using a parenteral nutrition formula program for 15 low-birth-
weight infants showed a reduced incidence of hyperglycemia,
decreased serum sodium fluctuations, and a reduction in weight loss
in the first days of life.[1] In addition, total parenteral
nutrition profiles may be stored and generated for each patient for
monitoring purposes.

Companies in the United States are presently marketing
microcomputer software for use on a rental basis for which the user
must pay a monthly fee for each patient profile generated.

Applications in Education

In addition to applications in daily practice, micro-

computers are easily adaptable to medical educational needs. Ross
Laboratories and Hospital Products Divisions of Abbott Laboratories
have developed an ongoing series of self-paced, interactive educational programs on nutrition-related topics using computer-assisted
instruction for use by practicing physicians, medical students, and
members of the nutrition support team. The programs are designed to
increase the awareness of the importance of nutrition and to integrate knowledge of clinical nutrition into daily practice.
Physicians, clinical pharmacists and dietitians are consulted in the
preparation of these programs to ensure the clinical applicability
of the material. The programs may be reviewed by all nutrition
support team members as well as students, residents, or interns
participating in nutrition support rotations. Currently available
topics include "Protein-Calorie Malnutrition: A Preventable Complication of Hospitalization", "Protein Malnutrition: Clinical Expression and Assessment", "Nutrition Intervention Techniques", and "Case
Study in Crohn's Disease". Additional programs specifically
designed for instruction of the clinical and hospital pharmacist and
clinical dietitian are under development. The programs operate on
Apple microcomputers, with each diskette containing both a short (15
minutes) and a long (60 minutes) version of each program. A monograph containing the text of each program is provided. The program
is "user friendly" and can be operated by individuals unfamiliar
with computer programming by following a simple set of instructions. Each program consists of an introductory didactic section on
a specific area of nutrition with the user asked to respond to
questions that test understanding of the material. The concluding
section consists of an in-depth case presentation which requires the
user to make a clinical assessment and determine the proper nutritional management of the patient.

Conclusion

        Microcomputer applications in clinical nutrition include
both the areas of daily practice and education. Programs can be

developed that perform routine calculations, store patient data, and instruct health professionals in nutritional management.

Bibliography

1. Giacoia G.P. Chopra R. (1981) The use of a computer in parenteral alimentation of low-birth-weight infants. JPEN, $\underline{5}$, no. 4. 328-31.

INSULIN DELIVERY FROM DIFFERENT TOTAL PARENTERAL NUTRITION SOLUTIONS

Bassons,T*, Cardona,D*, Bassas,L.**, Ordóñez,J.***, Sánchez,J#, Bonal,J*
Hospital de la Sta Creu i S. Pau. Services: * Pharmacy, ** Endocrinology,
*** Biochemistry and # Intensive care

It is well established that insulin (I) has affinity for plastic or glass. Thus when (I) is mixed with solutions contained in plastic or glass containers it may adhere to these materials with decrease in its delivery from these solutions.

In present study we have assayed the degree of adherence of(I) to different plastic containers when mixed with five types of Total Parenteral Nutrition (TPN) solutions. Adherence has been evaluated as percentage of (I) delivered from these containers and solutions.

MATERIAL

1. Total Parenteral Nutrition Solutions:

The study was carried out in five different TPN solutions whose compositions, the same that we utilize in clinical use, are detailed in Table 1.

TABLE I.   Composition (in ml) of TPN solution in the study

Content of solution	A	B	C	D	E
Glucose 5% in water	2000	–	–	–	–
Glucose 50% in water	–	1000	875	1000	875
Aminoacids (15gN$_2$/l)	–	1000	875	1000	875
Intralipid^R 20%	–	–	250	–	250
Multiple Vitamin complex	–	–	–	3	3
Electrolytes*	–	–	–	50	50
Distilled water	53	53	53	–	–

* mEq electrolytes contents are: Chloride 80, Potassium 70, Sodium 20, Phosphate 10, Calcium 9 and Magnesium 8.

2. Plastic Supports

(I) delivery was tested for two different types of plastic bags: Polyvinylchloride (PVC)-Mixiflo^R- and Ethylvinylacetate (EVA)-Nutri-bolsa^R-.

The same administration set was attached to both type of bags. Regular flow rate from administration set was obtained by means of percusion device (Dial-a-flo^R).

3. Insulin Preparations

Two different type of (I) preparations were utilized in the study: 40 units of regular insulin - Velosulin^R-

40 units of regular insulin and sufficient amount of ^{125}I-labelled insulin to provide 3500 dpm/ml of TPN solution.

METHODS

1. Insulin preparations were added to TPN solutions by direct injection to the bags. Solutions containing TPN and (I) were well mixed by shaking 1 minute. Aliquots for (I) assay were collected from the end of ad ministration sets.

2. The amount of (I) recovered was determined from(I) delivered from bags by two methods: Radioimmunoassay(RIA)-Insulin Bioria^R- of aliquots of TPN containing added(I), or radioactivity counting of aliquots of TPN containing the mixture of(I)and labelled (I).

3. All TPN solutions were assayed by two methods, but only PVC bags were used in radioactivity count experiment.

4. Constant flow rate was adjusted to 85.8 ml/h and 2-ml aliquots were collected at 0, half, 2.6, 12 and 24 hours. Aliquots were diluted to 1/500 prior to RIA determinations, but no dilution was done for radioactivity count.

5. Purity of labelled(I) was assayed by gel-filtration chromatography in Sephadex G-25, PD-10 colums. When recovery of(I)was calculated from recuperation of ^{125}-I labelled(I), the percentage of impurity found was substracted from the results.

6. Percentage of(I) recovery was compared between PVC and EVA bags with RIA results. In PVC bags recovery results from radioactivity count were compared to those obtained by RIA methods. All comparisons were made for each of the time-collections studied. Statistical comparison between recoveries was done by percentage-comparison test.

RESULTS

Results obtained in recovery study are shown in Table II and Figures. Gel filtration chromatography of labelled(I)showed less than 10% of unbound iodine for the product utilized.

TABLE II. Insulin recovered in TPN solutions at the end of delivery.

Solution	Radioimmunoassay		125-I counting
	EVA(%)	PVC(%)	PVC(%)
A	46'3	43'3	67'9
B	56'8	40'1	78'8
C	93'7	86'8	86'9
D	97'7	95'7	79'1
E	94'1	89'5	85'1

AMOUNT OF INSULIN (%) RECOVERED FROM DIFFERENT TOTAL PARENTERAL NUTRITION.

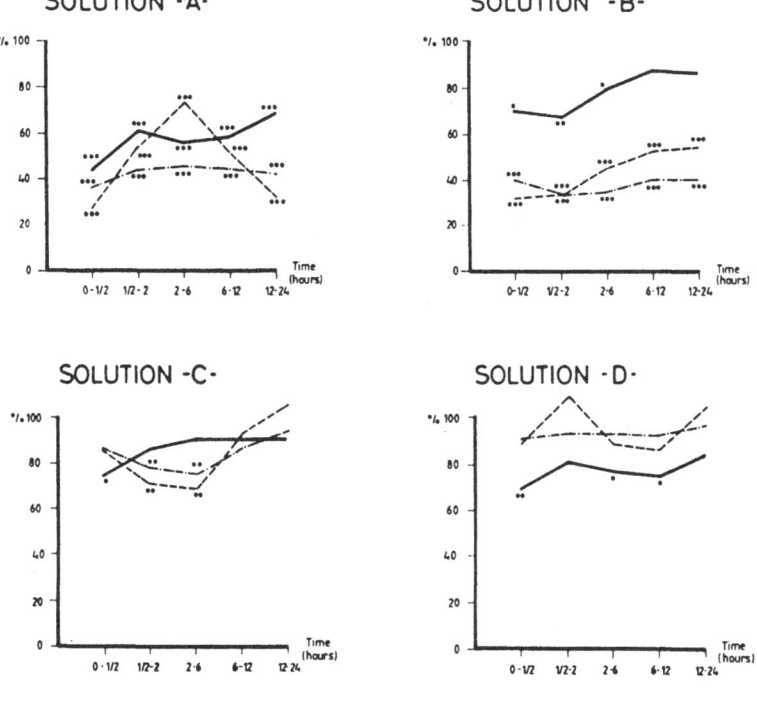

SOLUTION ·E·

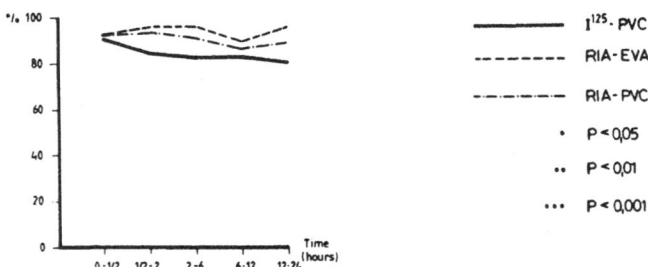

CONCLUSIONS

1. No significant   differences in recovery of (I)between PVC
and EVA bags were found, except for solutions A and B. From the slope of
recovery curves it seems that PVC(I)delivery is more regular than EVA(I)
delivery.

2. No identical results for all studied recoveries were obtained by RIA or radioactivity count methods. RIA results for solutions A
and B gave lower recovery values than radioactivity count results.

3. Intralipid[R], electrolytes and vitamins addition decreased
the(I)loss.

4. TPN solution E (mixture of Glucose 50%, Aminoacids, Intralipid[R], Electrolytes and Multiple Vitamin complex) showed the best behaviour in (I)delivery. Solution E had the highest recovery among all TPN
solutions tested and the most regular slope in recovery curves.

5. The present study suggests that clinical trial must be done to assess the "in vivo" reproductiveness of present "in vitro" results.

A ddress reference requests to the authors at the Department of Pharmacy
Service.
Hospital de la Sta. Creu i S. Pau. Avda. S. Antoni Mª Claret, 167.
Barcelona-25. Spain.

PARENTERAL NUTRITION MIXTURES - STABILITY AND TRI-
GLYCERIDES ELIMINATION RATE IN LIVER PATIENTS

M.O.Rodrigues[*], M.L.Valdeira[***], J.A.Morais[***],
M.E.Camilo[**], J.Pinto Correia[**]. Departments of
Pharmacy[*], and Medicine II[**], University Hospital
of Santa Maria; Faculty of Pharmacy[***] Lisbon -
Portugal

Introduction
    Significant Malnutrition is often found in patients
with chronic liver disease. However, the utilization of paren
teral nutrition (PN) is still controversial, specially when -
ever standard aminoacid solutions and lipid emulsions are con
sidered. The present study was carried out in order to evalua
te: the stability of PN mixtures of aminoacids solution plus
lipid emulsion , its clinical tolerance and plasma levels of
exogenous triglycerides in patients with cirrhosis submitted to
such treatment.

Material and Methods
    We studied six cirrhotic patients (age range 35-70
yrs), admitted to an Intensive Care Unit of Gastroenterology
after an episode of upper gastrointestinal bleeding. None presented any evidence of encephalopathy, 4 had moderate ascites,
4 hypoalbuminaemia and one severe malnutrition. One control
study was performed in a patient with no liver disease.   The
following protocol was observed: 1) patients were included in
the study at least 12 hours after settlement of haemorrhage ;
2) mixtures' composition was calculated daily on an individual
basis: 0.1 g nitrogen/kg body weight (as Vamin 7%); non-pro -
tein energy: 20-25 kcal/kg b.w. provided by Intralipid 10%
(500 ml=50 g) and the remaining as glucose; 60-80 mEq of po -
tassium; 60-90 mEq of sodium; phosphorus 310-610 mg;   trace
elements (one vial of Addamel); total volume 1500-2000 ml. Dai
ly adjustments of electrolytes were made according to needs ;
3) the nutrient mixtures were prepared within plastic bags of

ethyl vinyl acetate (E.V.A.) under a laminar air flow and ri-
gorous aseptic technique; 4) the mixture osmolality was de -
termined by routine laboratory technique and ranged from 840
to 1100 mOsm/kg; 5) samples of mixtures were stored at 4°C for
examination of lipid particles at 24, 48, 72 hours and one week
after preparation: evaluation of coalescence, morphology and
diameter of lipid particles on electron microscopy (Yeol 100 C
at 80 Kv) according to Pamperl technique; 6) PN was adminis -
tered continuously over 72 hours through peripheral vein; 7)
plasma levels of exogenous triglycerides were determined   by
nephelometry, and 24 hours urine collection for urea nitrogen
determined   by routine technique.

Results

In the study of stability control the following re
sults were obtained. Standard Intralipid 10% emulsion (control):
particle's surface layer thin and linear; some particles atta
ched, no coalescence; mean diameter: 0.6 μ. Mixture at 24 hrs:
surface layer electron-dense coarse rim sometimes thick; rare
protusions and impressions; no coalescence; mean diameter   :
0.4 μ. Mixture at 48 hrs: similar morphological appearance ,
yet rare globules with a bright core were observed; mean diameter; 0.5 μ. Mixture at 72 hrs: similar features; mean diame
ter: 0.5 μ. After one week, one mixture presented coalescen
ce with rare osmiophilic inclusion bodies, not found in the re
maining three mixtures observed, where the mean diameter was
0.6 μ. This particular result could be due to its higher glu
cose and electrolytes concentration.

There was good clinical tolerance with no systemic
side effects, but local phlebitis in 4 patients.This reaction
could be due to the high osmolality of the mixture or a mecha
nic reaction to the catheter. So we consider either to modify
the mixture in order to get a lower osmolality or to administer the same mixture in a central vein. The nitrogen
balance shifted in all patients studied towards an equilibrium
state (Fig. 1).

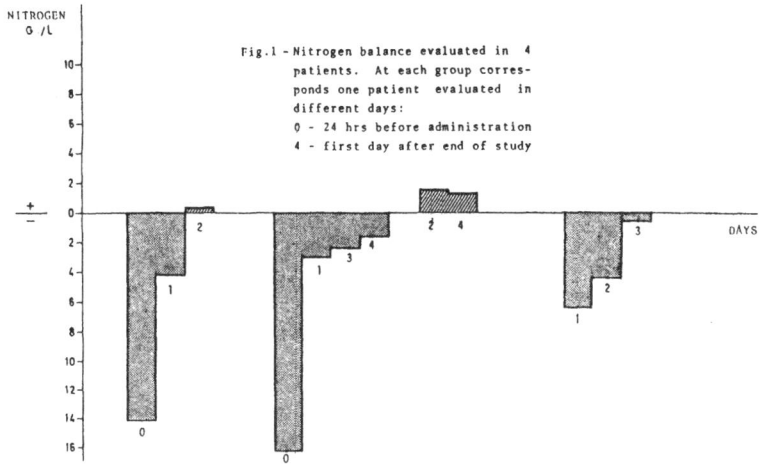

Fig.1 - Nitrogen balance evaluated in 4 patients. At each group corresponds one patient evaluated in different days:
0 - 24 hrs before administration
4 - first day after end of study

Plasma levels of exogenous triglycerides were determined in only one patient (table 1). A striking increase was observed at 24 hours with a posterior rapid progressive decrease.

TABLE 1

Plasma levels of exogenous triglycerides in one hepatic and one non-hepatic patient

Triglycerides (T.G.)
(mg/l)

Hours	Hepatic patient	Non-hepatic patient
0	0	0
24	465	26.0
48	152	24.9
72	72.6	28.1
96	2.70	7.60

Non hepatic patient: $K_2 = 0.732$ min.$^{-1}$ where:

$$K_2 = \frac{Ko}{V.C^{\infty}}$$

Ko: infusion rate (mg/min.)
V: plasma volume (l)
C^{∞}: "steady-state" TG (mg/ml)

At 96 hours values obtained were similar to those
verified in a control subject where a k_2 value was calculated.
Since patients with liver disease don't reach a steady-state,
it is necessary to perform serial determinations in order to
obtain an elimination curve and k_2 calculation. A study is in
progress to clarify this problem.

Conclusions

1. In 3 out of 4 mixtures there was good stability
with a stable profile size distribution of lipid particles un
til 72 hours.

2. There was good clinical tolerance, except for the
phlebitis in the peripheral vein.

3. The i.v. lipid administration must be monitor -
ed in cirrhotic patients since the triglyceride elimination
rate suggests a delayed clearance.

References

Black, C.D. and Popovich, N.G. (1981). A study of intravenous
       emulsion compatibility: effects of dextrose, amino-
       acids and selected electrolytes. Drug Intell.Clin.
       Pharm., 15: 184-193
Pamperl,H. and Kleinberger,G. (1982). Morphologic changes of
       Intralipid 20% liposomes in all-in-one solutions du
       ring prolonged storage. Infusionstherapie 9:86-91
Pamperl,H. and Kleinberger,G. (1983). Compatibility of two
       different fat emulsions with aminoacids, carbohydra
       tes and electrolytes in parenteral nutrition mixtu-
       re. Concept and Practice of Therapeutic Teams, ed.
       H.Clercq, J.W.Poston, J.Bonal, p.p. 61-67. Cambrid-
       ge University Press.

DRUG INDUCED AGRANULOCYTOSIS: THIRTY-THREE OBSERVATIONS

Ga Díez, J.; Sanz M.A.; Colomina P., Cuenca A.;
Gallego C., Ramírez I. and Ruiz C.
Ciudad Sanitaria "La Fe". Pharmacy and Hematology
Services. Valencia. Spain

In the present study, thirty-three episodes of agranulocytosis are evaluated restrospectively in 30 patients admitted to the Hematology Service over a 12-year period (1970-82). The distribution by sex was very similar (14 males 16 females), and the average age was 49 (range 18-77). In 30 episodes of agranulocytosis (91%) the relation to exposure to 1 or several potentially toxic drugs could be established, pyrazolone derivatives being the most frequently implicated (Palva & Mustala 1970 and Goudemand et al 1976). The rest of the drugs constitute a mixture of which the tetracyclines and chloramphenicol were of greater incidence. The minimum duration of the neutropenic period (PMN $<$ 1000/mm^3) was of 8.5 days, without appreciable differences as to age or sex. Occasionally alteration of other hematopoietic lines could be confirmed (thrombopenia $<$ 100.000/mm^3 in 18% and anemia below 30% of hematocrit value in 12%). A rise in temperature of a probable infectious etiology was observed in 32 episodes (97%), at least one localization being discovered in 28 (84.8%). Five patients developed a septic shock with fatal evolution in all of them. The mortality observed was specially important in the group of patients older 60 (4 out of 8; 50%), while only 12% of the 25 patients under 60 evolved fatally (p $<$ 0.05).

After tracing the clinical hematological profile of agranulocytosis induced by drugs in our medium, and in the light of the progress made in the last few years in the field of antibiotic therapy and support measures, a strategy of control adapted to the different prognostic group is being designed.

INTRODUCTION

Drug-induced agranulocytosis is characterized by a
selective and severe reduction in the circulating neutrophiles
usually to levels lower than 200/mm^3, due to an idiosyncratic
reaction after the administration of a drug(Young & Vincent
1980). Incidence varies between 2.6 and 100 cases/10^6
inhabitants/year, and represents 40% of the hematological
toxicity resulting from the use of drugs. Incidence is
slightly higher in women and increases with age.

Diagnostic criteria are based on the existence of less
than 200 granulocytes/mm^3 in peripheral blood, together with a
history of recent exposure to a drug, exclusion of other
causes of severe neutropenia, and recuperation in a period of
less than three weeks after withdrawal of the drug.

MATERIALS AND METHODS

Of the 30 patients studied, 14 are men (46.7%) and 15 are
women (53.3%). The men's ages range from 33 to 77 years
($\bar{X} \pm SD = 51.2 \pm 13.6$) and the women's from 18 to 77
($\bar{X} \pm SD = 46.7 \pm 18.7$).

Thirty-three cases were evaluated. In 16 of them (48.4%)
dyscrasia was caused by a single drug, and in 14 several
drugs were potentially responsible. In one case (3.1%)
responsibility could not be imputed to any known drug, and in
two cases (6.1%) anamnesis was impossible. The participation
of pyrazolone derivatives in the toxic phenomena is presented
in Tables 1 and 2.

TABLE 1. ETIOLOGY DRUGS RESPONSIBLE A SINGLE DRUG
POTENTIALLY RESPONSIBLE (16 CASES)

PYRAZOLONES = 12   PENICILLAMINE = 1
PENICILLIN = 1   QUINIDINE   = 1
          CHLORAMPHENICOL = 1

To establish the duration of the neutropenic period, we
evaluated the latency from the time of detection of the lowest
number of granulocytes in peripheral blood to the time of
detection of the lowest number of granulocytes in peripheral
blood to the time of recuperation to the level of 500 and

TABLE 2.   ETIOLOGY. DRUGS RESPONSIBLE SEVERAL DRUGS
           POTENTIALLY RESPONSIBLE (14 CASES)

PYRAZOLONES = 11   TETRACYCLINE = 6
CHLORAMPHENICOL=5   SULFAMIDES = 2
LYNCOMYCIN = 1   AMPICILLIN = 1
CYPROHEPTADINE=1   METOCLOPRAMIDE= 1
STREPTOMYCIN = 1   ATENOLOL= 1

$1000/mm^3$. It was impossible to demonstrate latency in all 33
cases of agranulocytosis studied because several patients
died before reaching these levels (27 cases could be evaluated
see Table 3).

TABLE 3.   DRUG-INDUCED AGRANULOCYTOSIS DURATION OF NEUTROPENIA
           PERIOD (IN DAYS).

		>500 GRANULOCYTES MEAN ± SD	(RANK)	> 1000GRANULOCYTES
MEN	(13)	7.8 ± 3.5	(2 -16)	8.8 ± 3.1
WOMAN	(14)	7.4 ± 3.8	(2 -15) N.S.	8.2 ± 4.0
<45 YEARS	(14)	7.6 ± 3.2	(2 -12) N.S.	7.9 ± 3.2
>45 YEARS	(13)	7.5 ± 4.1	(2 -16)	9.1 ± 3.9
TOTAL		7.5		8.5

It was sometimes demonstrated that other hematopoietic
lines were affected, giving rise to myelemia, indirect
leucocytosis, anemia, thrombopenia and thrombocytosis.

TABLE 4.   DRUG-INDUCED AGRANULOCYTOSIS

- MYELEMIA 18/27 (66.66%)
- INDIRECT LEUCOCYTOSIS 10/23 (43%)
- ANEMIA (HEMATOCRIT< 36%) IN THE BEGINNING 14/33
                             (42.4%)
   (HEMATOCRIT< 30% WHEN DX WAS REACHED
                  4/33 (12.1%)
- THROMBOPENIA (< 100.000/mm3) WHEN DX WAS REACHED
                  4/33 (12.1%)
   (< 40.000/mm3) WHEN DX WAS REACHED
                  2/33 (6.1%)
- THROMBOCYTOSIS(> 400.000/mm3)WHEN DX WAS REACHED
                  1/33 (3.0%)

In 32 of the 33 cases of agranulocytosis, fever was involved
The patient's temperature exceeded 38.5°C in 23 cases(69.7%)
and slight fevers (37°C-38.5°C) were detected in nine cases
(27.3%). In only one case of agranulocytosis was there no
fever at all (Apyrexia).

With regard to the clinical focus point of the infection, the following distribution was found: in 5 cases(15.2%)there was no focus point; 10 cases (30.3%) showed a single focal point; and in 18 (54.5%) there was more than one focal point In Table 5 we show the location of the lesions.

TABLE 5.   INFECTIONS IN DRUG-INDUCED AGRANULOCYTOSIS.CLINICAL FOCAL POINT OF INFECTION IN 33 CASES.

ORAL-PHARYNGEAL = 18	UPPER RESPIRATORY TRACT = 3
PULMONARY = 6	ABDOMINAL = 6
GENITAL-URINARY	CUTANEOUS =10
TRACT = 2	ABSCESSES IN SOFT PARTS = 5

Five cases of probable septic shock were also found and there were two cases of acute renal breakdown (see Table 6)

TABLE 6. DRUG-INDUCED AGRANULOCYTOSIS: 33 CASES

MORTALITY   7(21.2%)
  $<$60 YEARS: 3/25 (12%) $P < 0.05$
  $>$60 YEARS: 4/8   (50%)
CAUSES OF DEATH:5 RESULTING FROM SEPTIC SHOCK
                1 ACUTE PULMONARY EDEMA
                1 ACUTE RENAL FAILURE. COMPLICATIONS

TREATMENT

Antibiotics were widely used, alone or in combination, in 28 cases. In 15 of these a parenteral combination of a beta lactamic antibiotic + an amino glycoside antibiotic was used. Only three of the patients who died received this combination.

Other therapeutic recourses and instruments used were: Isolation=7; Corticosteroids=6; Androgens=6; Lithium salts=4; Granulocyte transfusions=1.

CONCLUSIONS

1. Drug-induced agranulocytosis is not frequently found in young people. We have not been able to demonstrate an increase in the incidence of the disorder among the elderly(24% $>$ 60 years).
2. In two thirds of all the cases it was demonstrated that pyrazolone derivates had been taken prior to the onset of agranulocytosis. In 36.3% of all the cases it was demonstrated

that these derivatives were solely responsible for the disorder.

3. No relationship could be demonstrated between agranulocytopenia and the age or sex of the patients.

4. In a large percentage of the cases studied there was a clinical focal point. The most frequent focal points were: oral pharyngeal, lung, abdomen and skin.

5. Shock, probably caused by infection, was fatal in all cases in which it appeared.

6. Our research showed a significant mortality rate.

7. The use of an adequate antibiotic therapy could reduce in the future the morbidity and mortality rates that go along with this serious hematological disorder.

REFERENCES

Goudeman,J.; Plouvier, F.; Bauters,F.; et al.(1976). Les agranulocytoses aigues induites par le Pyramidon or les Phenothiazines. A propos de 31 observations. Sem.Hop.Paris, 52: 1513-20.

Palva,I.; Mustala,O.(1970). Drug induced Agranulocytosis with special reference to Aminophenazone I.Adults. Acta Med.Scand. 187: 109-15.

Young,G.; Vincent,P. (1980). Drug-induced Agranulocytosis. Clin.Haemat. 9: 483-504.

TWO-COMPARTMENT TIME-SHARED COMPUTER PROGRAMS FOR PLANNING, MONITORING, AND ADJUSTING DIGITOXIN AND DIGOXIN THERAPY

R.W. Jelliffe, M.D., A. Schumitzky, Ph.D., D.Z. D'Argenio, Ph.D., D. Katz, Ph.D., and J.H. Rodman, Pharm. D.
Laboratory of Applied Pharmacokinetics, Section of Clinical Pharmacology, University of Southern California School of Medicine, Los Angeles, CA, USA

The clinical effects of cardiac glycosides correlate poorly with serum level data until at least eight hours after a dose, when distribution from the central (serum) compartment into the peripheral (effect) compartment is complete. Because of this, physicians have traditionally avoided obtaining serum glycoside levels for therapeutic drug monitoring prior to 8 hours after a dose. Usually serum levels are not obtained until just before the daily dose is given. Such management of digitalis therapy is logically equivalent to managing aminoglycoside therapy by obtaining only trough levels and omitting the peaks. Much dynamic information about the patient's pharmacokinetic model is lost. The only reason for waiting 8 hours before getting a serum glycoside level is that only 1-compartment models of the drug were being used.

Two-comparetment models of digitoxin (1) and digoxin (2) have recently been made. In these models, the rise and fall of drug in the peripheral compartment correlate well with changes in ejection-time indices and with the other known clinical effects of the drugs.

THE 2-COMPARTMENT PROGRAMS

Our laboratory has developed time-shared computer programs for planning, monitoring, and adjusting digitoxin and digoxin therapy which employ these 2-compartment models. The initial oral dosage regimen is developed to achieve and maintain a chosen peak total body glycoside concentration in the peripheral, rather than the central, compartment. Using the chosen tablet size, the regimen is then apportioned into the appropriate number of tablets for each day of a typical week of therapy.

MONITORING THERAPY WITH SERUM LEVELS.

These programs permit a serum level to be obtained at any time. There is no need to wait 8 hours after a dose, nor is it desirable. Indeed, considerations of optimal monitoring strategies for a 2-compartment pharmacokinetic model show that an optimal pair of serum levels is one that is obtained at the peak serum level after the first dose (1.5 to 2.0 hours) and then at the latest trough before some subsequent maintenance dose that one is willing to wait for on clinical grounds, depending upon the urgency to know. Such a strategy will best characterize the volume of distribution and the elimination rate constant from the central (serum) compartment. For characterization of the rate constants to and from the peripheral compartment, preliminary computations also suggest that levels at 0.5 and 7.0 hours after the first dose should optimally monitor the distribution phase of the drugs.

THE FITTING PROCEDURE

When serum level data, obtainable at any time, become availab-le, the models are fitted to such data using a maximum a posteriori Bayesian procedure. The fitted model can then be used to reconstruct the time course of both serum and peripheral compartment data over any de-sired period of his past therapy. This can then be compared with the patient's clinical behavior at all times, and in this way one can choose a therapeutic goal in the form of a desired peripheral compartment total body glycoside concentration. As with initial therapy, the regimen is again apportioned into so many of the chosen tablets for so many days of a typical week.

CLINICAL APPLICATIONS - ATRIAL FIBRILLATION

In addition to providing more information for monitoring of patients under routine circumstances, these programs have improved the ability to acheive and maintain proper rate control for patients with atrial fibrillation, greatly reducing or eliminating loss of control from trying to choose such a regimen intuitively, and may well shorten a patient's hospital stay by 2 to 3 days with respect to this aspect of his care.

CLINICAL APPLICATIONS - DIGOXIN AND QUINIDINE

The programs also have provided valuable insights into pa-tients receiving both digoxin and quinidine. They quantify the magnitude of the digoxin-quinidine interaction in each patient, and show not only the degree to which each patient's serum levels are elevated, but also suggest the degree to which his tissue uptake is impaired, resulting in diminished inotropic effect. Such data improves the assessment of risk and benefit easily and rapidly in each patient as part of their ongoing care.

These programs are currently in use by hospitals over an international time-sharing facility (3) with local telephone numbers for access in the USA, UK, France, Germany, Holland and Belgium. They can also be accessed via the TELENET network in Spain, Italy, and other countries, including the Far East.

1. Jelliffe RW, Bechtol LD, and Crabtree R: The Bioavailability of Digi-toxin. Clin Pharmacol Ther., 27(2): p 261, 1980.

2. Reuning RH, Sams RA, and Notari RE: Role of Pharmacokinetics in Drug Dosage Adjustment. 1. Pharmacologic Effects, Kinetics, and Apparent Volume of Distribution of Digoxin. J. Clin. Pharmacol., 13:127-141, 1973.

3. Comshare, Inc. (Mr. Suda), 3325 Wilshire Boulevard, Suite 500, Los Angeles, California, 90033. (213) 387-1177.

LUMBAR CEREBROSPINAL FLUID CONCENTRATIONS OF METHOTREXATE FOLLOWING HIGH-
DOSE INFUSION THERAPY

Cubells, J*; Mangues, M.A.** and Bonal, J.**
* Pediatric Service. ** Pharmacy Service. Hospital de la Santa Creu i Sant
Pau. Barcelona. Spain

The principal complication of the Acute Lymphocytic Leukemia
(ALL) and some Lymphomas is the location of leukemic cells within the
central nervous system (CNS). High dose infusion therapy of Methotrexate
(MTX) tries to reach CNS cytotoxic concentrations of the drug for long
enough to remove the potential leukemic or lymphocytic meningosis. Likewise,
it seems that high dose MTX therapy has good possibilities in the treatment
of CNS tumors.

The purpose of the present study is to analyze the maximum
concentrations of MTX reached in lumbar cerebrospinal fluid (CSF) as well
as the time that cytotoxic concentrations of the drug are maintained after
high dose infusion therapy.

Twelve patients (4 males and 8 females) from the Pediatric
Service of our Hospital, receiving high dose MTX therapy, participate in
the study. Their clinical diagnosis were ALL, non-Hodgkin Lymphoma, Burkitt
Lymphoma, CNS tumor and osteosarcoma. Their ages ranged between 3 and 11
years and the doses administered between 15 and 400 mg/kg. The MTX was
infused i.v. over 4 hours. Hydration (3000 $ml/m^2/24$ h) and urinary alkali
nization (pH 7-8) with $NaCO_3H$, started 12 hours before the MTX administration.
Two (for doses $>$ 200 mg/kg) or six hours (for doses $\leqslant$ 200 mg/kg) after the
end of drug infusion, leucovorin administration was initiated and continued
at 6 hours intervals until MTX serum concentrations below 10^{-7} M. All
patients were followed with MTX serum determinations for 3 days following
the administration of high dose MTX in order to minimize systemic toxicity
(Mangues et al 1983). The total number of infusions studied was 78. 2 and
24 hours after the completion of the infusion, CSF samples were collected
and analyzed by enzyme immunoassay for determination of the MTX concentration.

Cytotoxic levels of MTX ($\geqslant 5.10^{-7}$M) in CSF were achieved 2 hours
after the administration of all, except 3, infusions. The exceptions were
3 infusions at doses of 30 mg/kg. According to the Rosen results (Rosen 1977),

the CSF MTX concentration 2 hours postinfusion is, in effect, the maximum
MTX concentration obtained in CSF after the administration of this therapeutic protocol.

Three patients kept the CSF MTX concentrations over 5.10^{-7} M,
24 hours after the completion of the infusion, at doses of 300 mg/kg.

Figure 1 shows the maximum CSF MTX concentrations obtained in
two different groups of patients: those with intact CNS and those with CNS
tumors. We found that the maximum CSF MTX concentrations achieved, after
high dose therapy, increase when the MTX doses are augmented and they are
always higher for the group of patients with CNS tumors than for those with
intact CNS.

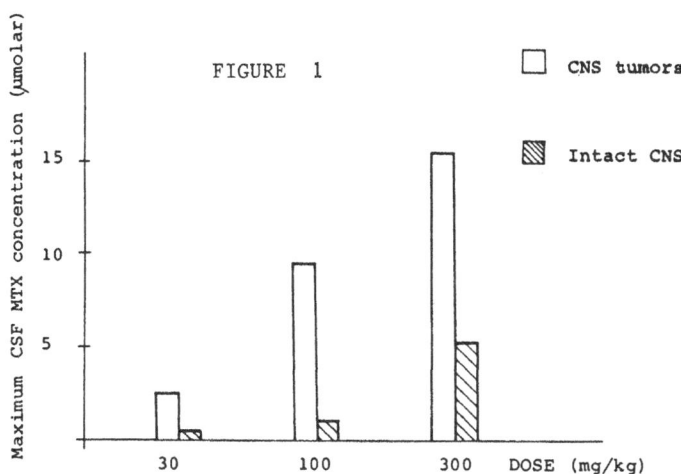

The clinical results were as follows:

Overt CNS leukemia: The patients were kept free of disease when the high
dose of MTX was administered at intervals shorter than 3 months.

Rabdomiosarcoma: A total reduction of the tumor was obtained and the patient
is free of disease, 16 months after the MTX therapy.

Burkitt lymphoma: The patient has not developed meningosis and she is free
of disease, 1 year after the treatment.

CNS tumors: The results were quite poor although the cytotoxic action of
the MTX after high dose therapy was proved as some of the patients had
objective evidence of tumor regression.

Osteosarcoma: The efficacy of HDMTX in this diagnostic has been previously
reported by some authors (Rosen et al 1974). We obtained very good results.

REFERENCES

Mangues M.A. et al. (1983). In Progress in Clinical Pharmacy: VI (in press).
Rosen G et al. (1974). Cancer, 33, 1151-1162.
Rosen G et al. (1977). Cancer Treat Rep, 61, 681-690.

MANAGEMENT OF EXTRAVASATION OF ANTINEOPLASTIC DRUGS: A CASE
REPORT OF THE TREATMENT OF A MITOMYCIN C EXTRAVASATION

R.H. BURR
6808 16th N.E.
SEATTLE, WASHINGTON 98115
U.S.A.

Highline Community Hospital in Seattle is a small community
hospital (104 beds) with an active outpatient and inpatient chemotherapy
program. We administer approximately 250 doses of antineoplatic drugs
per month.

Early in 1981 when the oncology program began, an attempt was
made to prepare for the possibility of extravasation. The literature was
searched for approaches to the treatment of these problems. Approaches
varied from the treatment of an area with only ice packs to aggressive
treatment with theoretical "antidotes".(Ignoffo & Friedman 1980; Larson
1982; Dorr1980) Only vincristine, vinblastine, and mechlorethamine
carried manufacturers' recommendations for the treatment of extravasation.
These being local injection of hyaluronidase and heat application for
vincristine and vinblastine, and local injection of 1/6 molar solution of
sodium thiosulfate for mechlorethamine.(Eli Lilly 1982 a,b; Merck 1979)
Unfortunately there was virtually no scientific evidence to support the
value of the various approaches.

When the program began it was decided to adopt the recommendations of Ignoffo and Friedman (1980) with certain modifications. These
modifications were that ice packing was chosen over the application of
heat and that dexamethasone 4 mgm ml^{-1} was chosen over hydrocortisone.
The specific "antidotes were packaged and labeled for each particular
chemotherapeutic drug. Packages were made for 6 vessicant drugs commonly
used in our program. These packages are kept together in a box and are
at hand when chemotherapeutic drugs are being administered. This is the
extravasation protocol under which the following case report was treated.

Subsequent to the development of our extravasation protocol
a limited amount of additional information has become available. The vast
majority of information concerns the treatment of doxorubicin extravasations. The results cast doubt on the value of local injection of

of sodium bicarbonate, the antidote incorporated in our protocol. Other
proposed doxorubicin antidotes, based on a variety of rationales, which
showed little or no benefit in animal testing include cimetidine, heparin,
diphenhydramine, lidocaine, N-acetylcysteine, hyaluronidase, and alpha-
tocopherol.(Dorr 1981 a,b,c; Cohen 1979) Apparently beneficial results
have been reported by Dorr(1981 c) and Cohen(1979)in the treatment of
doxorubicin extravasation in animals using low dose steroids locally
injected as well as isoproterenol and propranolol.

References to the treatment of extravasations of other chemotherapy drugs in the literature consist mostly of isolated case reports.
Recent case reports describe mitomycin C extravasations which were said
to have healed after treatment with locally injected hydrocortisone
(Johnston-Early 1981) and local soaks with Burow's solution (Fuller 1981).
However, there is still little solid information available regarding the
treatment of extravasation of chemotherapy drugs other than doxorubicin.

The extravasation protocol at Highline Community Hospital is
currently being reviewed for the purposes of updating and revision.

A CASE REPORT OF THE TREATMENT OF A MITOMYCIN C EXTRAVASATION

On October 25, 1982 a man being treated for advanced carcinoma
of the colon with hepatic metastases experienced an extravasation of 2-3
ml of mitomycin C (0.5mgm ml^{-1} at the site of injection on the dorsum of
the right hand. The needle was immediately removed contrary to protocol
recommendations. The area surrounding the injection site was locally
injected with 8 ml of a solution of sodium thiosulfate made by mixing 4 ml
of sodium thiosulfate 10% with 6 ml of sterile water for injection. This
was followed by the local injection of dexamethasone 4mgm (1ml). After
completion of these injections the area was packed with ice.

On November 1, 1982 the patient returned to the clinic reporting severe pain of 24 hours duration. At this time a discolored blistered
area was evident. The remainder of the hand demonstrated swelling but
was without evidence of extravasation. The lesion evolved to become two
separated areas of involvement. These two areas were separated by a seem-
ingly uninvolved area which was the region treated at the time of extravasation.

During the following several weeks the lesion showed only
moderate improvement. On January 25, 1983 the dorsum of the right hand
was surgically grafted. Immediately prior to the grafting the hand

demonstrated full range of motion and showed no tenderness. The patient did describe some numbness in the dorsum of the right hand.

Conclusion: This may represent a partially successful treatment of a mitomycin C extravasation.

REFERENCES

Cohen, M.H. (1979). Amelioration of adriamycin skin necrosis: An experimental study. Cancer Treat. Rep.,63, 1003-4.

Dorr, R.T., Alberts, D.S., Chen, H.S.G. (1980). The limited role of corticosteroids in ameliorating experimental doxorubicin skin toxicity in the mouse. Cancer Cheother. Pharmacol.,5, 17-20.

Dorr, R.T. (1981). Extravasation of vessicant antineoplastics:Clinical and experimental findings. Ariz. Med.,38, 271-5.

Dorr, R.T. & Alberts, D.S. (1981). Modulation of experimental doxorubicin skin toxicity by beta-adrenergic compounds. Cancer Res.,41, 2428-32.

Dorr, R.T. & Alberts, D.S. (1981). Pharmacologic antidotes to experimental doxorubicin skin toxicity:A suggested role for beta-adrenergic compounds. Cancer Treat. Rep.,65, 1001-6.

Eli Lilly and Company (1982). Oncovin package insert. Indianapolis, IN.

Eli Lilly and Company (1982). Velban package insert. Indianapolis, IN.

Fuller, B., Lind, M., Bonomi, P. (1981). Mitomycin C extravasation exacerbated by sunlight. Ann. Int. Med.,94,542.

Ignoffo, R.J. & Friedman, M.A. (1980). Therapy of local toxicities caused by extravasation of cancer chemotherapeutic drugs. Cancer Treat. Rev.,7,17-27.

Johnston-Early, A. & Cohen, M.H. (1981). Mitomycin C induced skin ulceration remote from infusion site. Cancer Treat Rep.,65,529.

Larson, D.L. (1982). Treatment of tissue extravasation by antitumor agents. Cancer, 49,1796-9.

Merck, Sharpe and Dome. (1979). Mustargen package insert. West Point, PA.

HIGH- DOSE METHOTREXATE: PHARMACOKINETIC MONITORING AND TOXICITY

Mangues, M.A.*, Cubells, J.**; Queraltó, J.M.*** and Bonal, J.*
Hospital de la Santa Creu i Sant Pau. * Pharmacy Service. ** Pediatric
Service. *** Biochemistry Service. Barcelona. Spain

The purpose of the present study is to analyze retrospectively
the complications associated with high-dose Methotrexate (HDMTX) as well
as the criteria for identification of patients at high risk for toxicity,
described by some authors (Tatterall 1975; Isacoff 1976, 1977; Niremberg
1977; Stoller 1977 and Evans 1979).

Thirteen patients (5 males and 8 females) from the Pediatric
Service of our Hospital, receiving HDMTX therapy, participate in the study.
Their clinical diagnosis were Acute Lymphocytic Leukemia, non-Hodgkin
lymphoma, Burkitt lymphoma, CNS tumors and osteosarcoma. Their ages ranged
between 3 and 11 years and the doses administered between 15 and 400 mg/kg.
The MTX was infused i.v. over 4 hours. Hydration (3000 $ml/m^2/24$ h) and
urinary alkalinization (pH 7-8) with $NaCO_3H$, started 12 hours before the
MTX administration. Two (for doses > 200 mg/kg) or six hours (for doses $\leq$
200 mg/kg) after the completion of the infusion, Leucovorin administration
was initiated and continued at 6 hours intervals until MTX serum concentra
tion below 10^{-7}M. The total number of infusions were 97. 0, 2, 12, 24, 48
and 72 hours postinfusion, blood samples were collected and analyzed by
enzyme immunoassay for determination of the MTX concentration.

After infusion, biphasic elimination curves were obtained. The
half-life of the first and the second phases were 2.4 ± 0.5 and 15.6 ± 2.3
hours, respectively, for patients that did not developed toxicity.

Four out of the thirteen patients developed clinical toxicity.
Two infusions were followed by moderate symptoms: one patient presented a
erythemapapulo   rash after the first infusion of 350 mg/kg and another
one showed very high hepatic enzymes values after the infusion of three
doses of 300 mg/kg of MTX, administered weekly. None of these patients
fulfil any criteria of high-risk for toxicity and the symptoms did not
require treatment.

Two patients developed severe toxicity. The first one had
bleeding stomatitis, exanthema, renal failure, thrombocytopenia, severe

leukopenia and cardiorespiratory arrest that could not be solved, after
one dose of 100 mg/kg. The second patient developed stomatitis, oliguria,
pancytopenia and renal failure, after one dose of 100 mg/kg. The renal
failure was treated and the toxic picture was solved without consequences.

When the 97 infusions were administered, Niremberg's criteria
of toxicity were applied (Niremberg 1977). None of the patients met the
parameters of high-risk for toxicity at 24 hours postinfusion. They were
not identified as high risk patients, and conventional low-dose Leucovorin
rescue was continued. Applying "a posteriori" the Evans' criteria (Evans
1979) we can observe that the infusions causing severe toxicity fulfil
such criteria (24 MTX plasma concentration$>$5.0 mcM and t 1/2 of the first
phase of elimination$>$3.5 h). The t 1/2 values were available retrospecti
vely (3.7 h for the first patient and 3.6 h for the second patient). The
24 h MTX concentration was only available for the second patient (10.0 mcM).
This values would have prospectively identified these patients as being at
high risk for toxicity and would have allowed to start a superrescue thera
py with Leucovorin in order to avoid toxicity. The most important advantage
of the Evans' criteria is to allow an earlier identification of high risk
patients.

Another patient did not meet the criteria of high risk but he
had a 48 h MTX serum concentration too high (1.42 mcM). Rescue with Leuco
vorin was continued until MTX serum concentrations below below 0.1 mcM and
no signs of toxicity were developed.

In relation to toxicity, due to the above mentioned, and line
with our administration protocol, we have established 3 groups of patients:

RISK OF TOXICITY	T 1/2 FIRST PHASE OF ELIMINATION	mcMOLAR MTX PLASMA CONCENTRATION AFTER THE END OF THE INFUSION		
		24 H	48 H	72 H
LOW	$<$3.5 H	$\leq$5	$\leq$1	$\leq$0.1
MEDIUM	$<$3.5 H	$\leq$5	$>$1	$>$0.1
HIGH	$>$3.5 H	$>$5		

PATIENTS WITH LOW RISK OF TOXICITY REQUIRE
RESCUE WITH LEUCOVORIN AT CONVENTIONAL DOSES.
IN PATIENTS WITH MEDIUM RISK, THERAPY RESCUE
HAS TO BE CONTINUED WITH THE CONVENTIONAL
DOSES UNTIL MTX PLASMA CONCENTRATIONS BELOW
0.1 mcM. IN PATIENTS AT HIGH RISK, A SUPER
RESCUE THERAPY WITH LEUCOVORIN HAS TO BE
ESTABLISHED AS SOON AS POSSIBLE, WITH THE
DOSE DEPENDING ON THE MTX LEVELS (SIROTNAK 1978).

Application of these criteria in a large number of patients will determine
whether they retain their validity as an early indicator of impending toxicity.   REFERENCES

Evans WE et al. (1979). Cancer Chemother Pharmacol, 3, 161-166.
Isacoff WH et al. (1976). Med Pediatr Oncol, 2, 319-325.
Isacoff WH et al. (1977). Cancer Treat Rep, 61, 1665-1674.
Niremberg A et al. (1977). Cancer Treat Rep, 61, 779-783.
Sirotnak et al. (1978). Cancer Res, 38, 345-353.
Stoller RC et al. (1977). N Engl J Med, 297, 630-634.
Tattersall MHN et al. (1975). Cancer Chemother Rep, 6, 25-29.

INDIVIDUALIZATION OF FACTOR VIII DOSAGE

M. Matucci, G. Longo, M. Morfini, S. Vannini
Haemophilia Centre, USL 10/D, Florence, Italy

A. Messori, G. Donati-Cori, C. Manfriani, E. Tendi
Hospital Pharmacy, USL 10/D, Florence, Italy

S. Ruffo
Department of Physics, University of Pisa, Italy

Abstract. We assessed the extent of the intraindividual variability of Factor VIII kinetics in patients with classic haemophilia. Eight patients were included in our study. On two different occasions, each of these patients received a single dose of Factor VIII after which the time-curve of plasma Factor VIII levels was measured. Good agreement between the two measured curves of plasma levels was found. Our data show that the kinetics of Factor VIII do not demonstrate considerable intraindividual variability.

The kinetics of Factor VIII concentrates in haemophiliacs have a considerable intersubject variability (Biggs, 1978). In light of this variability, recent studies (Matucci et al., 1983; Longo et al., 1984) have addressed the need to individualize the dosage of Factor VIII, pointing out that individualization of Factor VIII dosage involves both clinical and economical aspects.

In fact, over the past decade several reports have demonstrated that the use of appropriate dosage regimens of Factor VIII has a beneficial effect upon the clinical outcome of the haemophilia patients who are being treated for a bleeding episode. Furthermore, it has also been shown that the choice of a proper dosage is also an important issue from a cost-effectiveness point of view, since Factor VIII concentrates are very expensive.

The most recent technique for individualizing the dosage of Factor VIII (Longo et al., 1984) is based on complete characterization of Factor VIII kinetics in each patient who is treated with Factor VIII. The Longo method, which is a modified version of the Sawchuk and Zaske

(1977) method, is designed to calculate the dosage of Factor VIII when repeated doses are necessary. According to this technique, individual kinetic variables of the one-compartment open model are estimated in each patient from the concentration-time data obtained after a test-dose of Factor VIII. Then, the calculated kinetic variables are used to predict the dosage regimen that will elicit the desired plasma level of Factor VIII activity. All mathematical calculations required for determining dosages have been incorporated into a program for a hand-held calculator. In this way, the Longo method becomes easily applicable in the clinical setting.

The Longo method is based on the following assumptions: (i) The pharmacokinetics of Factor VIII are linear and obey the superposition principle; (ii) Factor VIII kinetics can be appropriately described by using the one-compartment open model with constant rate i.v. administration; (iii) Factor VIII kinetics have a low intraindividual variability.

The first two assumptions are supported by numerous data available from the literature (Biggs, 1978; Matucci et al., 1983). Conversely, further studies are needed to assess the extent of the intraindividual variability of Factor VIII kinetics. In this report, the data of eight patients with haemophilia-A were analyzed to gain insight into the intraindividual variability of Factor VIII kinetics.

PATIENTS AND METHODS

Eight patients with haemophilia-A were included in the study (mean age 23.8 yrs; range 9-39 yrs). None of the patients had demonstrable inhibitors to Factor VIII. Six patients were treated with Factor VIII for minor bleeding episodes; the other two patients received Factor VIII for prophylaxis. After inclusion in the study, each of these patients received a single dose of Factor VIII by constant-rate i.v. infusion on two separate occasions. The clinical condition of each patient when the second single-dose treatment was given was similar to that of the first treatment. Although three different Factor VIII prepa-

rations were used (Kryobulin-Immuno; Koate-Cutter; Hemofil-Travenol),
each patient was treated with the same product on both occasions. Each
patient received the first dose of Factor VIII by i.v. infusion over
approximately 15 minutes (range of doses: 8.2 to 20.8 units/kg). Seven
blood samples were drawn before infusion and at 0.5, 1, 3, 6, 12, and 24
hrs after the end of the infusion. The baseline Factor VIII:C plasma
level was measured from the blood sample taken before the start of the
infusion. The concentration-time data were fitted to the two-compartment open model with constant rate infusion by using a nonlinear
least-squares program (Messori et al., 1983). The kinetic correction for
endogenous synthesis of Factor VIII (Matucci et al., 1983) was employed.
The variables of the kinetic model were estimated for each patient.

After a time interval of at least a week since the first
dose, each patient was given a second dose of Factor VIII. For practical
reasons, only one blood sample was taken following the second dose at a
time ranging from 8 to 24 hrs after the dose. For each patient, the
theoretical time-curve of plasma levels of Factor VIII following the
second dose was predicted based on the two-compartment kinetic variables
estimated after the first dose. (The two-compartment open model with
constant rate infusion was used for carrying out these predictions).
Then, the plasma concentration of Factor VIII (mC) that was measured
after the second dose was compared with the corresponding value (pC) of
the theoretical time-curve of predicted levels.

Plasma VIII:C activity (units/dl) was measured by a one-stage
assay (Ingram, 1965).

The intraindividual variability between the two administered
doses was assessed by comparing the values of mC and pC. The mC-versus-pC
data pairs obtained from the patients were analyzed by linear regression.
The correlation coefficient was also calculated.

RESULTS

The correlation coefficient between the measured and

predicted values of Factor VIII concentration was 0.925. The equation of the regression line was: mC = 0.855 pC + 2.315.

DISCUSSION

The problem of individualizing Factor VIII dosage deserves to be studied because on the one hand the availability of Factor VIII concentrates has increased in recent years and on the other the high cost of Factor VIII therapy makes the choice of a proper dosage an important issue from a cost-effectiveness point of view.

The Longo method appears to be a useful tool for use in clinical practice. This method was developed by assuming that the intraindividual variability of Factor VIII kinetics is not relevant from a clinical point of view. Specific data concerning the intraindividual variability of Factor VIII kinetics are useful to assess the potential use of the Longo method in clinical practice. Indeed, the findings resulting from our study support the above assumption. Therefore, in our view further, prospective studies are warranted to evaluate the usefulness and the reliability of the Longo method in clinical practice.

REFERENCES

Biggs, R. (1978). Plasma concentrations of Factor VIII and Factor IX and treatment of patients who do not have antibodies against these Factors. In The treatment of haemophilia A and B and von Willebrand's disease, ed. R.Biggs. Oxford: Blackwell Scientific Publications.

Ingram, G.I.C. (1965). Blood coagulation Factor VIII: genetics, physiological control and bioassay. Adv.Clin.Chem.,21:189-99.

Longo, G. et al. (1984). A calculator program for individualizing Factor VIII dosage. Drug Intell. Clin. Pharm. In press.

Matucci, M. et al. (1983). Pharmacokinetics of Factor VIII: appropriateness of the one-compartment model for estimating clearance. Farmaco Prat.,38,306-11.

Messori, A. et al. (1983). Iterative least-squares fitting programs in pharmacokinetics for a programmable hand-held calculator. Am. J. Hosp. Pharm.,40,1673-84.

Sawchuk, R.J. et al. (1977). Kinetic model for gentamicin dosing with the use of individual patient parameters. Clin. Pharmacol. Ther. 21,362-69.

DIFFICULTIES IN EPILEPTIC PATIENT MONITORING IN WHICH THE
PHENYTOIN LOT HAD INADVERTENTLY BEEN CHANGED

CHINITA, I.M.

MEGA, I.M.
Quality Control Laboratory, Dep. of Pharmacy
Stª. MARIA - LISBON - PORTUGAL

In this study we intend to show the difficulty with an epileptic out patient monitoring, using several lots of tablets from the same
manufacturer, which showed on being tested great differences in dissolution values (Fig. 1).

All these lots were analysed in quality control laboratory,
Department of Pharmacy, Hospital Santa Maria.

DISSOLUTION   DATA :

LOT Nº	% OF THE LABELED AMOUNT
H.C.	40,6
1568	70
1282	42
482	18,4
M	-
LOT M = different lots	

FIG. 1

The apparatus used for dissolution test was apparatus I of
USP XX and the procedure was the same of Prompt Phenytoin Sodium Capsules
USP XX page 622. The method employed to determine the serum concentration
was enzyme imunoassay - EMIT[r] and the apparatus was a SP GILFORD STASARIII

E. A. C. is a 56 years old white male with 64 Kg, whose past
medical history was a A. V. C. onset age 54 years old. At the present the
patient has epilepsy.

He is taken Phenytoin Sodium Tablets 100 mg and Ibuprofen Tablets 400 mg - S. O. S.

The Laboratory parameters were normal.

The patient has been monitored for six months.

The changing of lots was due to the patient who has got medicines in different departments and Community Pharmacies.

The review of the different data (Fig. 2) allow us to be sure
about the influence of different dissolution values on the serum levels.

DATA	DAILY DOSE	LOT Nº	SERUM CONCENTRATION
2.3.83	300 mg	H.C.	4,6 ug/ml
16.3.83	300 mg	1568	5,2 ug/ml
23.3.83	300 mg	1568	5,6 ug/ml
30.3.83	350 mg	1568	10,5 ug/ml
6.4.83	350 mg	1568	10,5 ug/ml
11.5.83	350 mg	482	8,5 ug/ml
18.5.83	350 mg	1282	8,25ug/ml
22.6.83	350 mg	1282	8,25ug/ml
1.7.83	350 mg	1282	Ibuprofen crisis
6.7.83	350 mg	1568	Phenobarbital,inj. 7 ug/ml
13.7.83	350 mg	1568	7,5 ug/ml
20.7.83	350 mg	1568	10 ug/ml
27.7.83	350 mg	M	9,5 ug/ml
3.8.83	350 mg	M	8,2 ug/ml
9.8.83	350 mg	1568	9 ug/ml
THERAPEUTIC RANGE :		10 - 20 ug/ml	

FIG. 2

Conclusion:

It seems we can conclude that the different changes presented on the values of blood levels are due to the different dissolution values in several lots of Phenytoin. These lots were able to put the patient out of the therapeutic range, normally admitted for Phenytoin, causing a crisis of difficult medical interpretation.

It is of the greatest importance the lots from the same manufacturer have always an homogeneous dissolution (GMP),particularly when used in patients on chronic therapy.

ANALGESIC CONSUMPTION, RATIONALIZATION AND MODIFICATION OF PRESCRIBING

M.C. Antolin, P.M. Vidal
Hospital Sant Joan de Deu. Manresa

F.MD. Berna, T.MQ. Gorgas, J.C.Codina, P.E. Homs, V.J. Miralles, A.M. Tosa, J.A. Perello, V.M. Riva, S.J. Ribas
Five general hospitals. Barcelona

Introduction

The consumption of pyrazolone analgesics in the hospital circle is high,partly due to the great number of conditional analgesic norms that are resolved by the medical department with the use of this type of medicine, often in high doses, underrating the appearance of adverse effects which are sometimes very serious. In this paper we show the combined effort of a group of six general hospitals to make   the pyrazolone analgesics   only   by medical prescription and so reduce their consumption.

Material and methods

The information on the consumption of analgesics for the first six months of 1982 was collected.

A common standard of analgesia was established in which the use of paracetamol and diclofenac was recommended as an alternative to the salicylates, and the dipyrones were left as the last choice,and always under medical prescription.

The standards were presented to the district Pharmacy and Theraputic Commissions, and each hospital was adapted accordingly, dissemination being carried out through the Information Bulletins and through meetings with the different Services and medical departaments. A month was given for its introduction.

Periodic follow-up meetings were held and the collection of the results was done over a period equivalent to the first six months (March-August 1983) .

Results and discussion

On comparing the results obtained during the two periods, a lowering of the consumption of pyrazolone analgesics by 50% was shown favouring the recommendations made by us in the standards.

A stabilizing of the consumption of salicylates and opiates was noted.

Although we haven't been able to eliminate the dipyrones,their prescription being firmly established, it has been possible to achieve that they are only available through medical prescription.

Conclusions

A rationalization of the prescription and use of analgesics has been obtained.

As a result a reduction of 50% in the consumption of dipyrones has been observed.

We have obtained a better information about analgesia from the medical centre personal.

It has been possible to know the use pattern of analgesics for each hospital and compare it with others of similar characteristics.

It shows that collaboration between hospitals is an adequate way to establish standards for rationalising therapeutics.

TREATMENT OF HYPERTENSION ARTERIAL IN NEPHROLOGY

García,L.[I], Iñiesta,M.[2], Gimenez,A.[I], Borrego,A.M.[2],
Camacho,J.A.[I], Rafart,A.[2]
Hospital San Juan de Dios. Barcelona. Spain
I Nephrology Service
2 Pharmacy Service

The lack of specific therapeutic guidelines in the treatment of abnormally high renovascular pressure, which are at the same time suitable in pediatrics, urged us to carry out a study with the aim of establishing suitable standards for the treatment of this symptom which is caused by different types of nephropathies.

The Pharmacy Service carried out an inspection of drugs already used in treating such cases of high blood pressure, and the conclusion was reached that the most effective were those such as captopril,which had an inhibitory effect upon the angiotensin converting **enzyme** (I.A.C.E.). The guidelines we are proposing were formed in conjunction with the Nephrology Service, and the patients treated were continously studied during a period of two years.

MATERIAL AND METHODS

I Renal artery stenosis..................... 3 cases
2 Adult type renal polycistic disease...... I case
3 Segmental hypoplasia (Ask-up mark kidney) I case
4 Idiopathic pulmonary fibrosis............ I case
5 Following the administration of ACTH..... I case
6 Hereditary haemolytic-uremic syndrome.... I case
7 Oligomeganephronia....................... I case

Age varied from 5 months to I0 years old.($\overline{X}$=5,7 years). Before treatment with captopril was begun blood pressure ranged from I90/I30 to I45/90 mmHg.

The recommended children dosage. is of I mg /kg per day. Which may, if necessary, be increased by I mg /kg per day up to a maximum of 6 mg /kg per day. We used a dosage

of 2 mg /kg per day with a maximum of 5 mg /kg per day; it
was not necessary to increase this in any case. Treatment
combined with Furosemide (I-2 mg /kg per day) was carried
ont in 5 cases; sodium intake was restricted in all cases. In
the 4 cases which involved chronic renal failure the dose was
calculated with reference to the glomerular filtration rate.

RESULTS

In all cases blood pressure became normal between I
and IO days. It may be noted that there were no secondary
effects of any gravity and treatment was never suspended.
Mild hyperpotassaemia occurred in 3 cases, reversible taste
disturbance in one case and skin rash in 2 cases.

When the patient (6) blood pressure became normal,
renal failure disappeared.

In two cases(2,4) there was a noted improvement in
the concurrent respiratory problems.

After the use of captopril there was not case of severe hypotension.

CONCLUSIONS

- Captopril when taken orally, is an effective rapidly acting hypotensive.

- It has few secondary effects.

- It simplifies the treatment of high blood pressure.

REFERENCES

American Society of Hospital Pharmacists. American Hospital
        Formulary Service. 24:08.
Friedman,A. et al. (I980). Effective use of captopril in se-
        vere childhood hypertension. J.Pediatr.97:664.
Heptinstall,R.H. et al. (1982). Informe del captopril colla-
        borarive study group. Lancet (ed. esp.) Vol. I,Nº 3.
Oberfield,S.E. et al. (I979). Use of the oral angiotensin I-
        converting enzyme inhibitor (captopril) in child-
        hood malignant hypertension. J, Pediatr. 95:64I.

DISODIUM EDETATE IN THE TREATMENT OF RESIDUAL RENAL LITHIASIS

E. Molina, A. Alfaro, C. Nagore, F. Marcotegui, E. Estaun
Servicio Farmacia, Hospital Virgen del Camino, Pamplona, Spain
A. Santiago, M. Montesino, P. García Tabar
Servicio Urología, Hospital Virgen del Camino, Pamplona, Spain

Disodium edetate is a chelating agent which forms water-soluble complexes with divalent ions such as calcium and magnesium. Thus, it seems obvious to use this substance in the treatment of residual renal lithiasis.

The aim of this study was to evaluate in a small number of patients the efficacy of a sterile solution of disodium edetate to remove residual renal calculi.

PATIENTS AND METHODS

In this study a total of 5 patients with residual caliceal lithiasis following pyelolithotomy and nephrostomy, were treated with a sterile solution of disodium edetate. Stones were chemically composed of oxalate and/or phosphate salts. All of them had a previous history of either urinary tract infections or renal lithiasis.

The following formula was utilized in the therapy: Disodium edetate (B.P.), 50 g ; Sodium hydroxide, 2.272 g ; Potassium chloride, 0.134 g ; Water for injections, to 1 litre. This solution was extemporaneously prepared in each case sterilizing it before use at 121ºC/30 minutes.

The solution was administered to the patients at a rate of 2 litres per day, by retrograde irrigation into the renal calices through an urethral catheter and drainage into the nephrostomy tube, although in some circumstances the operational procedure was carried out in the opposite direction. In order to improve its tolerance the irrigation was initiated with a 1:10 warmed dilution of the described solution, made in water for injections, increasing then gradually the concentration of disodium edetate, as patient tolerance develops.

On average the quantity of solution administered to each patient ranged between 20 and 30 litres.

RESULTS AND DISCUSSION

In 3 of the 5 patients of the study residual renal calculi disappeared at all at the end of the treatment, whereas in another one there was a significant reduction in its size. In the other patient the therapy had to be withdrawn, because he complained of a severe lumbar related pain. In this case the irrigation was carried out through the nephrostomy tube.

No problems were detected in any patient when the solution was instilled by the retrograde irrigation procedure. In contrast, a moderate lumbar discomfort was observed in 2 patients when the irrigation was firstly administered through the nephrostomy tube. These adverse effects are related to an irritating action of disodium edetate on the mucous membranes on the renal cavities.

Our experience corroborates with what other authors (Timmerman & Kallistratos 1966 ; Kallistratos 1976) have previously recommended in order to increase the tolerance of the solution. To this respect it is very important to administer the solution by the retrograde irrigation procedure and to use very high purity substances in preparing the formulation for the therapy.

CONCLUSION

In conclusion, although the experience is limited, it is pointed out that the therapy with disodium edetate constitutes an effective and safe method to remove oxalate and/or phosphate residual renal stones, when used as an adjunct to lithotomy. In preparing this type of solution Hospital Pharmacist has a good oportunity to expand Clinical Pharmacy, incorporating himself within the hospital therapeutic team.

Reference list

Kallistratos, G. (1976). Farmacoterapia de la urolitiasis y su profilaxis.
        In Litiasis renal, ed. B. Pinto, pp. 269-280. Barcelona :
        Salvat Editores S.A.
Timmerman, A. & Kallistratos, G. (1966). Modern aspects of chemical
        dissolution of human renal calculi by irrigation. J. Urol.,
        95, 469.

PHARMACY TECHNICIAN TRAINING AND PRACTICE PROGRAMS IN THE
NETHERLANDS

W.I.J. van Wieringen-van der Laan, Y.A. Hekster, T.B. Vree
and E. van der Kleijn
Department of Clinical Pharmacy, Sint Radboud Hospital,
Catholic University of Nijmegen, Geert Grooteplein Zuid no. 8
Nijmegen, the Netherlands

Until 30 years ago, the pharmacy technicians in the Netherlands
were privately educated by pharmacists and were prepared in the local
pharmacies for their state examinations. However it took a lot of time
for the pharmacist, since the number of pupils was rising. This triggered
the institution of professional schools.

Today training programs in the Netherlands are found at the secondary or
college level of education. The programs consist of a three year class
and laboratory training including a compulsory internship. Examination
leads to certification and license for the preparation and dispensing of
drugs under supervision of a licensed pharmacist. This curriculum is
standardized at the national level and also the examination is organized
centrally.

The different education training options are given below:

a. general training program

b. advanced courses

c. hospital training program

d. "Radboud" training program

GENERAL TRAINING PROGRAM FOR THE EXAMINATION

This training is divided in 2 parts, a theoretical part and
a practical part. The theoretical part consists of inorganic and organic
chemistry, some mathematics and physics, latin and especially

a. pharmacognosy

b. pharmacology

c. law

d. pharmacokinetics

Pharmacognosy includes the recognition of organic liquids, raw materials,
creamy oils, waxes, medicated gauze, liquid oils etc.

<u>Pharmacology</u> includes: Gastro intestinal systems, expiration systems, blood circulation, respiration, hormones and the nervous systems. Under <u>law</u> the following subjects are discussed: rules about narcotics, poisons, dispensing of drugs etc.

<u>Pharmacotherapeutics</u>

1. Anaesthetics
2. Analgesics
3. Anticoagulant
4. Antiepileptics
5. Antihistamines
6. Antihypertensives
7. Central nervous system
8. Cardiac
9. Chemotherapeutics
10. Diuretics
11. Hormones
12. Hypnotics etc.

In general the most frequently used drugs per pharmacotherapeutic group are mentioned, together with main effects, side effects and risks of therapy.

THE PRACTICAL EXAMINATION

The practical examination consists of the preparation of 4 prescriptions. The technicians must be able to prepare powders, mixtures, capsules, ointments, eye/eardrops, suspensions, suppositories etc. Incompatability of the substituents should be recognized and maximum doses and costs be considered.

Pharmaceutical calculations, translation and checks on medication orders in respect to age and weight of the patient, dose etc, is part of the examination.

The candidates also recognize drug-drug interactions, give some general advice on rational drug use, based upon information, given in the course. As a result of passing the examination, a national licence is obtained. Having their licence, they can follow courses such as:

<u>Post graduate courses</u>

a. pharmaceutical and chemical analysis
b. pharmacology and therapeutics
c. hospital training

The program starts with a first year basic education, containing chemistry, anatomy and physiology, microbiology, quality control and preparation and pharmacotherapy. (KNMP, 1983).

Passing a test is required for continuation for the second year. For the second year one item from the following specialisations can be chosen.

Pharmaceutical and Chemical Analysis

This part of the chemical and pharmaceutical analysis consists of the
theory of analytical chemistry, chemical calculations, instrumental and
quantitative analyses, and a practical training in drug related subjects.

Pharmacology and Therapeutics

This consists of: anatomy and physiology, pathology, medications,
pharmacotherapy and the knowledge of commodities.

Hospital training

This consists of: anatomy and physiology, pathology, pharmacotherapy,
radiopharmacy (elective), microbiology, quality control, sterility,
immunology, interactions and a practical course in the preparation of
large parenteral volumes, eyedrops, filtration techniques etc.
The knowledge obtained in this program is tested by a national examination.

SPECIAL TRAINING COURSES

Training at the Sint Radboud Hospital

        In the Sint Radboud Hospital a training program exists for
technicians for about one year. In this year the following subjects are
trained:

a. preparation for individual compounding

b. aseptic techniques as - parenteral nutrition

                         - antibiotics

                         - antineoplastic agents

c. drug distribution systems

d. ward services

e. purchase and stock control

In this hospital (950 beds), a team of 5 technicians have the responsibility for d and e.

The ward service activities consist of:

1. Maintenance of ward drug inventory: checks for expiration dates, management and control of ward stocks.

2. Maintenance of emergency sets: this set has been developed in this
   hospital, the technicians look for the expiration dates, and the re-
   placements after use.

3. <u>Dispensing of drugs into nursing medication trolley</u>: drugs are placed
   in a medication trolley per patient for a 24 hours period. On two
   wards the technician dispenses the drug. After checking the nurse dispenses the drug to the patient.

4. <u>Monitor deviances from accepted policy</u>: monitoring formulary, or non-
   formulary drug, specially by prescription.

5. <u>Provision of practical information to the nurses:</u> instruction for the
   administration of I.V. fluids or intramuscular injection. Interactions,
   trade names etc.

6. <u>Informs pharmacist of drug related problems</u>: special high doses, use
   of experimental medication, as noticed on the wards.

Once a week a general subject is chosen to be discussed with
pharmacy personnel with the intention to cover continuing education.
Recently the Journal of Drug Research has started a special Continuing
Education Program, also suitable for Pharmacy technicians. (Vree, Zelvelder, 1982).

CONCLUSION

The pharmacy technicians in the Netherlands are educated with
the intention, to be able to take responsibility, so that they are
able to work independently under the supervision of a licensed pharmacist.
This allows the technician to interact with nurses and physicians on drug
related problems in their own capacity.
These trained technicians are able to take over a large part of the work
of pharmacists. This is an essential development for clinical pharmacy
programs, especially since the number of academically trained pharmacists
in dutch hospitals is limited.

REFERENCES

KNMP (1983). Voortgezette Opleiding Apothekersassistenten, Pharmaceutisch
    Weekblad 118, 740 -743.
Vree, T.B. and Zelvelder, W.G., (1982). Schriftelijk Voortdurend Onderwijs
    Journal of Drug Research 7, 1508 - 1510.

ESTABLISHING AND OPERATING THE UNIT DOSE SYSTEM OF DISPENSING IN AHMADU
BELLO UNIVERSITY T. HOSPITAL, ZARIA, NIGERIA

Obiaga, G.O., Fanusie, E., and Jemitola, C.
AHMADU BELLO UNIVERSITY TEACHING HOSPITAL, ZARIA, NIGERIA

INTRODUCTION

In the past two or three decades, the art of dispensing drugs
in hospitals has come under constant review. (Source book on Unit Dose
Drug Distribution Systems, American Society of Hospital Pharmacists). Physicians want to see that the correct drugs are given to the patients. Phar
macists must ascertain that the dosage regimen suits each individual patient and that the drugs are given in such a way as to eliminate medication
errors. Perhaps nurses would like to perform less of pharmaceutical duties
and concentrate more on nursing duties. Hospital administrators are interested in bringing down the cost of medications for in-patients especially
where political programme for free health are the declared intentions.

The responsibility for making sure that all these objectives
are met lies to a great extent with the pharmacist. In 1963 and 1964, Barker et al. in the USA demostrated that medication errors were made in one
out of every six or seven doses administered using the traditional system
of dispensing.

The result of the search for improving the traditional system
was the Unit Dose Dispensing system (UDDS), where many of the advantages
include safety to the patient, better patient care, more efficient use of
hospital personnel and significantly reduced cost to the hospital with al-
leviation of continued drug shortages (Barker et al 1964).

There is however, a dearth of information on whether the UDDS
can been supplied in developing countries of Africa.
A pilot study evaluating the Unit Dose Dispensing System was therefore undertaken in Ahmadu Bello University Teaching Hospital, Zaria. The turnover
of patients in this hospital is about two million per year.

MATERIAL AND METHODS

A clinical Pharmacist was employed to initiate the system in
the wards to be used for the study. The objectives and intricacies of the
system were communicated and explained to hospital personnel (doctors and
nurses). The initial skepticism of the nurses who were used to the traditional system gave way to cooperation after various consultations. The system was tried in two medical female wards in the hospital. These two wards
normally hold 42 patients at a time. There are 12 wards in the hospital.

The work schedules for the pharmacist and the pharmacy technician are shown below.

(A) PHARMACIST

MON-FRI	- Daily follow-up of the wards.
7,30 AM	- Record and fill new treatment sheet orders to be delivered by 9,00 a.m.
A.M. defini-tely by noon	Check cassettes after pharmacy technician has completed fil-ling them.

9,00 A.M.   - Pharmacist goes to the ward for patients counselling and dis-
12,00 noon   cussions with physicians,
1,00 P.M.   - Fill new treatment sheet orders and place in cassettes (Phar-
(when new   macy Technicians may help here when possible)
treatment
sheet orders
arrive)
2,00 P.M.   - Pharmacist must check returned cassettes to ascertain that
               those drugs which should have been left with the patients
               have been.
2,30 P.M.   - Check for diagnoisis of patients, especially new ones.

REPLACEMENT OF WARD STOCK

MON AND THURS
ONLY 9,30 -
1,00 A.M.   - Check and replace ward stock if supplied.
FRI   - Supply enough stock for two days.

(B) PHARMACY TECHNICIAN

MON-FRI   - Daily follow-up of wards.
7,30 A.M.   - Check for new treatment sheets and inform pharmacists (20 min)
8.00 A.M.   - Fill cassettes. Put away excess drugs and organise drug cup-
12,00 noon   board in pharmacy.
1,00 P.M.   - Check for new treatment sheet (20 mins).
1,30-2,00 PM Assist pharmacist in filling new orders.
2,00-3,00 PM Deliver cassettes to wards. Returns cassettes of previous day
               to pharmacy. Put away excess drugs and organise drug cupboard.

PATIENT MEDICATION PROFILE

A patient medication profile as shown in Fig. 1 was designed
for the purposes of recording information regarding the drugs prescribed
and dispensed for each individual patient. The information obtained from
the profile include:

1. Name of patient, ward and bed number.
2. Name and strength of drug prescribed for the patient.
3. Date on which drug was started.
4. Route of administration of the drug.
5. Directions for use of the drug.
6. Cost of the drug.
7. Code number of drug.
8. Quantity of drug supplied daily.
9. Date any medication was discontinued.
10. Allergies.
11. Age and weight of patient.
12. Attending physician.
13. Diagnosis.
The profile is designed to be used for 3 weeks if the patient does not get
discharged within that time, a new profile is started. Another form, Fig.
II, was designed for use in reporting doses not taken by the patient.

AHMADU BELLO UNIVERSITY TEACHING HOSPITAL, ZARIA
PHARMACY MEDICATION PROFILE

Date	Drug	Route	Cost Code	Date	Charge	Date	Charge	Date	Charge	Remarks D/C Date
Pharm	Sig.									
Date	Drug	Route								
Pharm	Sig.									
Date	Drug	Route								
Pharm	Sig.									
Date	Drug	Route								
Pharm	Sig.									
Date	Drug	Route								
Pharm	Sig.									
Date	Drug	Route								
Pharm	Sig.									
Date	Drug	Route								
Pharm	Sig.									
			Tech/Asst Pharmacist		Total		Total		Total	
Ward	Dob Age	Attending Physician	Diagnosis			Allergies		Name		Patient's No.

PATIENT'S NAME .... WARD& BED №...............

DATE	DRUG	DOSE	NO OF DO-SES SUP-PLIED	DOSES NOT TAKEN	REMARKS

                                     PHARMACIST ....
ATTENDING PHYSICIAN .... DATE ....
ATTENDING PHYSICIAN'S COMMENTS ....
....
SIGNATURE OF ATTENDING PHYSICIAN ....
DATE..

CASSETTES.- These are receptacles in which each individual patient's medications are placed. Cardboard boxes which were cut and made into receptacles measuring 12 cm by 12 cm by 9 cm deep were initially used, but later replaced with cassettes made of perspex which were sturdier and neater.
Provision was made for labelling of the patient's name, bed number and
ward on the cassettes.

CONTAINERS FOR DISPENSING.-Plastic vials for tablets and plastic bottles
of 60 cc. and 120 cc. for liquid medicines were used since only a 24
hours supply was given. The vials and bottles were labelled using peel-off
labels.

WARD STOCK CUPBOARD.- A small lockable ward stock cupboard was provided
for keeping drugs which may be required in emergency.

        A number of drugs were kept in the cupboard as the nurses were
rather apprehensive about availability of drugs particularly at night when
the pharmacist was not there (see tables). The number and quantity of
drugs were later reduced as the patients were adequately supplied through

the Unit Dose Dispensing System. A chart for recording the drugs is placed in the cupboard (Fig. III).

FIG.III

WARD STOCK CUPBOARD

RECORD OF DRUGS USED

DATE	NAME,FORM &STRENGTH OF DRUG	QUANTITY USED	NAME OF PATIENT	PRESCRI BER	NURSE SIG.
Aug. 20, 1982	Methyldopa 25 mg Tabs	2	Sadiya	Dr.Onye Melukwe	Aladipa

TABLE 1

DRUGS KEPT IN WARD STOCK CUPBOARD

INJECTABLES	TABLETS
A. Antibiotics - Ampicillin 250 mg (5) - Cloxacillin 250mg (5) - Gentamycin 80 mg (5) - Procaine Penicillin 4 mu (5) - Crystalline Peneicil- lin 1 mu (10) - Streptomycin 1 g. (5)	A. Antibiotics - Ampicillin-Cloxacillin 500 mg (15) - Ampicillin 250 mg (20) B. Antimalarials -Chloroquine 300 mg (40) C. Analgesics - Aspirin 300 mg (40) - Paracetomol 500 mg (40)

INJECTABLES	TABLETS
B. Diuretics - Frusemide 20 mg (10) C. Antihistamines - Promethazine 20mg (10) D. Antimalarials - Chloroquine 250mg (10) E. Others - Digoxin 0,5 mg (5) -Paraldehyde I.V. (10) - Atropine 500mg (5) - Adrenaline 0,1% (5) - Aminophylline 2,5% (10)	D. Diretics - Frusemide 40mg (20) - Spironolactone 25mg (20) E. Antihypertensives - Methyldopa 25 mg (20) F. Others - Co-trimoxazole (20) - Digoxin 0,25 mg (20) - Metformin 500mg (15) - Thiacetazone/Isoniazid 75/300 mg (20)

PERSONNEL

A clinical pharmacist was put in charge of the programme. One pharmacy technician was attached the clinical pharmacist. The salary of the clinical pharmacist was N 6.800 per annum.

STATISTICAL ANALYSIS

Analysis of significance between cost of drugs using the unit dose system and the traditional method was done using the Mann-Whitney U test.

RESULTS

The cost of drugs for the patients in wards I and II was calculated on the basis of drugs supplied to each patient. Table II shows the cost of drugs using the traditional system for 6 months (June-November) and using the Unit Dose Dispensing System for 12 months (Jan-December). The difference between cost per patient based on the two systems is statistically significant ($p < .05$).

TABLE II

MONTHLY COST OF DRUGS USED FOR IN-PATIENT IN WARDS I & II

USING THE TRADITIONAL AND THE UNIT DOSE DISPENSING SYSTEM.

TABLE II

MONTHLY COST OF DRUGS USED FOR IN-PATIENT IN WARD I & II USING THE TRADITIONAL AND THE UNIT DOSE DISPENSING SYSTEM

	1981		1982	
	TRADITIONAL SYSTEM		UNIT DOSE DISPENSING SYSTEM	
Month	Amount in N	No. of Patients	Amount In N	No. of Patients
January			861.15	61
February			809.84	43
March			924.07	71
April			1,008.03	75
May			1,100.62	57
June	2,657.17	59	1,373.31	83
July	4,500.15	68	639.65	79
August	3,638.22	63	1,383.73	81
September	3,389.92	56	939.07	39
October	2,389.94	62	951.84	58
November	3,284.61	61	916.44	55
December			703.73	51
TOTAL	20,308.01	369	11,665.45	754
COST PER PATIENT	N55.035		N15.47 (Jan -Dec)	
COST PER PATIENT	N55.035 (June-Nov)		N13.14 (June-Nov)	

$p < 0.05$

DISCUSSION

This pilot study has demostrated that the Unit Dose Dispensing system is cheaper than the traditional system in Zaria in a developing country. The total cost for 6 months using the traditional system was N 20. 308.01 which was greater than for every 12 months using the Unit Dose Dispensing System. Also, per patient, per month cost showed a difference with the Unit Dose System also lower significantly ($p < 0.05$).

Another advantage of the Unit Dose Dispensing System in this study is improved patient safety and care as a result of clinically oriented pharmacists being involved in the day to day care of each patient.

Thus advise on drug side effects, dosages, and drug interaction may be offered to clinicians on the spot especially during ward rounds. With the traditional system, contact with the physicians in minimal.

A third advantage of the Unit Dose Dispensing System in this study was the better and more efficient use of hospital personnel. Nurses found the system more convenient than the traditional system as some of the pharmaceutical duties performed in the past by nurses had been taken off them.

Various Unit Dose Medication Systems are in the market, but this study has shown that locally improvised cassettes embodying the same principles can successfully be used, thus minimising total expenditure in the tropics.

The Unit Dose Dispensing System is therefore strongly recommended in hospitals in developing countries.

REFERENCES

1. Barker, K.N., Heller, W.M., Brenen, J.J. and Sheldom, C.S. "The Development of Centralised Unit Dose Dispensing System", American Journal of Hospital, Pharmacy 20: 612-623 (Dec.) 1963. (Part II), 21:66-67 (Feb.)1964. (part III), 21:230-237 (May) 1964, 21: 412-423 (Sept) 1964, 21: 609-625 (Dec) 1964.

2. American Society of Hospital Pharmacists and the American Society of Consultant Pharmacists, "Guidelines for Repackaging Oral Soilds and liquids in Single Unit and Unit Dose Packages". American Journal of Hospital Pharmacy 34: 1355. (Dec) 1977.

3. Rase, B.E., "A cost study of Single Unit Medication Packaging". American Journal of Hospital Pharmacy 25: 434-436 (Aug) 1968.

4. Shoup, L.K., "Training Technicians for Unit Dose Drug Distribution System". American Journal of Hospital Pharmacy 28:611-613 (Aug) 1968.

5. Barker, K.N., Nikeal, R.L., Pearson, R.E., Illig, N.A. and Leemorse, M. "Medication Errors in Nursing Homes and small Hospitals" American Journal of Hospital Pharmacy. Vol 39, 987-991 (Jun) 1982.

6. Stewart, G.A., Covaleski, M.A., and Taylor, S.M. "Management Control of Drug Administration Programs". American Journal of Hospital Pharmacy . Vol 38, 1681-1684 (Nov) 1981.

7. Smith, W.E. "Clinical Pharmacy in the 1980´s". American Journal of Hospital Pharmacy 40, 223-229 (Feb) 1983.

8. Obiaga, G.O. and Fanusie, C. "Establishing a Unit Dose System of Dispensing in A.B.U. Teaching Hospital, Zaria, Nigeria". Pharmacy Bulletin A.B.U. Teaching Hospital, Zaria, April 1982 No. 21 pp 1-24.

DATA PROCESSING FOR A PHARMACY SERVICE IN A GENERAL GERIATRIC HOSPITAL

M.I. GENUA
SERVICIO DE FARMACIA

A. ELOSEGUI
SERVICIO DE PROCESO DE DATOS

A. MARTINEZ
ASESOR INFORMATICO
HOSPITAL GENERAL GERIATRICO "JOSE MATIA CALVO". SAN SEBASTIAN
SPAIN

At the beginning of 1982 it was decided to computerise the
Pharmacy Service in our hospital. A commission was formed at the time, made up of the head of the Data Processing Department, a computing consultant from outside the hospital, a Management representative and the head
of the Pharmacy Service.

In the first place, the head of the Pharmacy Service informed
the rest of the team about the functioning of his service, in order to
ensure a suitable computer application.

Functions are performed within the service, which are common
to the General Hospital and others which depend on the different sections
of which it is made up, such as the distribution of medicines and
disposable material.

The sections can be differentiated according to the type of
patient, over 65 years of age who is admitted. So we have:

a)Patients who have been admitted due to an acute process.
There are 226 of these, situated in the Hospital for Short and Medium
Term Stay.

b) Patients who have been admitted due to a chronic process
(185). They are situated in the Hospital for Long and Medium Term Stay.

c) Patients who need attending in a day, as they do not
require hospitalisation, are to be found in the so called Day Hospital.

d) Patients who are at home and are attended by the Home
Assitance Team.

e) Out-patients.

The role of the pharmacist in this General Geriatric Hospital
is very diverse, however, it is as well to review our systems of drug and
disposable material distribution.

Disposable material is collected twice a week throughout the hospital, following a request made by the staff nurse in charge of the floor, and in her name.

Medicines are distributed using the unit-dose system.

a) Twice a day for the hospital for Short Term Stay because of the frequent number of changes of treatment which take place there.

b) Daily doses in the Hospital for Long Term Stay.

c) The necessary medication required by the patients of the Day Hospital during the time in which they are admitted.

d) Daily doses for those patients in the Intensive Care Unit.

e) Doses for surgery for those patients in operating theatre.

Syrups and drugs of external application are exceptions to this system of unit dose. This is because their packaging surmounts both the economic and staff possibilities of our service.

WORK OBJECTIVES

a) To know the use made of medicines and disposable material, as they are second in the list of hospital costs.

b) To make a daily update of the service's stock preventing the unnecessary accumulation of material.

c) To follow the treatment of each patient regarding the interaction of prescribed medicines, adverse reactions and duration of treatment.

d) To reduce even further, the errors resulting from the distribution of medicines.

We dispose of a computer of the type "SECOINSA" for the data processing, a piece of equipment with a central storage capacity of 128K and 78 Mbytes disc capacity. The system is also provided with 6 displays a "CONTROL DATA" line printer with a speed of 300 lines a minute and 2 satellite printers with a document feeder. The Pharmacy Service has one of the satellite printers at its disposal. At the present moment, we are trying to change this printer for one which is independent of producing 300 lines a minute.

The scheme followed for the computerisation is as follows:

I - Entries to the Pharmacy, and

II - Dispensations from the Pharmacy.

I - Entries to the Pharmacy take place in the same way as
those of medicines and disposable materials. It is necessary to emphasize
the two important points amongst the data required by the computer. They
are:

1.- The code. This is unique, and is made up of 6 digits. Five
of these refer to the therapeutic group, type of unit, medicine approved
or not by the Pharmacy and Terapeutic Commission, disposable material,
magisterial formula, etc... The sixth digit is the control one.

2.- The entry unit of the product is data which coincides
with that of dispensation from the Pharmaceutical Service. Therefore, the
unit of one clinical container of 500 tablets will be 1 tablet, that of a
box of 10 ampoules, 1 ampoule, etc...

II - Dispensations from the pharmacy may originate from the
prescriptions of a treatment, that is to say, from the distribution of
unit doses.

In this case, the computer has all the necessary up-to-date
data on the courses of treatment.

We have carried out the setting-up and bringing up-to-date of
treatments using some of the following options:

1.- New treatments (admissions).

2.- Total cancellations (discharges).

3.- Partial cancellations.

4.- Change of medicine.

5.- Change of dose and/or frequency of dose.

6.- Inclusion or consultation of order of treatment.

The computer itself takes away from the stock and attributes
to the patient each one of the medicines he is taking as part of his
treatment automatically.

When dispensations from the pharmacy are not due to a concrete
treatment, they are attributed to a patient or even to a section, service
or floor. Normally, emergency stock medicines of a particular floor and
those drugs not repacked in unit-doses are attributed to the patient that

required them and the disposable material to the section, service or floor.

The charge for medicine and/or disposable material of the intensive care unit and the operating theatre is attributed to the patient who required it.

To sum up, the application called "PHARMACY" is built up of the following options:

1) Discharge, admission or modification of file.

2) Entry to pharmacy.

3) Dispensations for treatment.

4) Dispensations without treatment to the patient.

5) Dispensations without treatment to section, service or

floor.

6) Check lists.

7) Transfer for the finalisation of an entry of correct data.

8) Listing proceeding from the preparation of unit-doses.

9) Reports.

We have already explained the first 5 options, numbers 6 and 7 are included as safety measures and numbers 8 and 9 can be regarded as the results of application, as we already obtain a list for each consignment of medicine to a floor, in which is set out in detail the medication to be taken by each of the patients during the period of time between one consignment of medicine and the next. The period will depend on which of the sections of the General Geriatric Hospital the medicine is sent to, as described in the introduction to this study.

The very fact that the medicine taken by each patient on any particular day and that the times of dosage are detailed in this way does not only mean that the preparation is applied and that the medication sent to each floor is checked, but also that the risk of error in this type of distribution is lowered considerably, as there is now no need to work out whether it is an odd or even day, if it is Tuesday or Saturday, if the medicine is to be taken at 20 hours or at 14 hours.

The option of being able to attribute dispensations to a particular patient, but not for treatment, has also made the job of preparing requests from the intensive care unit and the operating theatre a lot easier, as now, apart from knowing the expenses per patient and updating the stocks of the Pharmacy Service, we are also able to obtain a

listing, the so called accumulation listing, in which there appears a
review of everything used in conjunction with the Service.

On the other hand, updating stocks in this way daily, we are
able to ascertain when stocks of certain medicines,
disposable material or
standard magesterial formula have fallen below a level which we regard
to be a minimum. This data is obtained by a listing in which the
following information is also included: -normal supplier, the usual order
made and the average monthly consumption in the current year, whether we
are dealing with disposable material or medicines.

It is also assumed that this is of great help to the person
responsible for administration work in the Service, as time is also saved
by being able to update the stocks of material.

CONCLUSIONS

1.- The basis of the efficient computerisation of a Pharmacy
Service is to be found in the efficient organisation of the Service itself.

2.- It is possible to perfect and facilitate the
administrative work if the computerisation is carried out as described
above.

3.- At any given moment, we are able to find out the treatment
of a particular patient and the amount of medicine he has consumed during
his stay in the hospital.

4.- We are able to design a data centre storing interactions
and adverse reactions, processing them for inmediate detection, as well as
incorporating the data about patient's treatment in the computer.